Latest Advances in Clinical and Pre-Clinical Cardiovascular MRI

Volume 1

Editor

Christakis Constantinides, *Ph.D.*
Chi Biomedical Limited
Nicosia
Cyprus

CONTENTS

CHAPTERS

PART A: Clinical Advances of Cardiac MRI

PART B: Technical and Pre-Clinical Advances of Cardiac MRI

FOREWORD 1

The eBook *"Latest Advances in Cardiovascular MRI"* is an enthusiastic account of the state-of-the-art in preclinical and clinical cardiovascular MRI. The editor Christakis Constantinidis and all the individual contributors are to be congratulated for providing an excellent overview of the capabilities of this remarkable technology. Ever since the realization in the seventies that MR had extraordinary medical potential, basic scientists and clinicians alike have begun to explore its utility for *in vivo* studies of the heart and the vascular system. The cardiovascular system poses many challenges to MR imaging and spectroscopy because of the contractile motion and the flow of the blood as well as the macroscopic displacements resulting from respiratory activity. With phenomenal advances in MR hardware, pulse sequence capabilities, image reconstruction techniques and improved triggering and gating approaches, the routine acquisition of high-quality MR images of heart and blood vessels in man has become reality for quite some time. The availability of such tools for use in preclinical studies on small animals has considerably lagged behind, especially for research in mice, due to the small size of the relevant structures and the very high rates of cardiac motion and arterial blood flow. Small animal counterparts of many cardiovascular MRI techniques that had been in use for human studies for quite a while only recently became available. This process of reverse translation from the clinical to the preclinical setting is in fact of vital importance to the field as it can be expected to speed up further developments of the technology. Biomedical studies in small animals and in particular mice are crucial for gaining insights in the pathophysiological processes underlying cardiovascular diseases. For these reasons, the advancement of the field of cardiovascular MR requires a sound balance between preclinical and clinical activities and needs an active exchange of ideas on measurement concepts as well as healthcare challenges between basic biomedical and clinical researchers.

The present eBook is an excellent illustration of the remarkably broad utility of cardiovascular MRI, describing recent clinical advances and developments at the technological and preclinical level. All of the contributors are experts in their respective domains of the field. The book addresses a topic that is of great societal importance, since cardiovascular diseases continue to be main causes of death and morbidity worldwide and have an enormous impact on the costs of healthcare systems. Therefore there is a pressing need for developing more effective diagnostic procedures that can be used to guide clinical management of patients and that can provide quantitative prognostic biomarkers for steering therapy and for follow-up. MRI provides a wealth of different types of information on the cardiovascular system, ranging from plain anatomy and basic function to tissue micro-architecture and cellular metabolism and therefore is ideally suited to reshape the practice of cardiovascular patient care. The field witnesses many exciting developments to speed up the rate of MR image acquisitions, whilst maintaining high data quality. This will drastically shorten scan times and thus alleviate one of the major hurdles for advancing MRI in the clinic. The field is thereby also making big steps towards becoming more patient-friendly and more cost effective.

The eBook is highly recommended both for cardiovascular MRI experts and novices.

Klaas Nicolay, *Ph.D.* **& Gustav J. Strijkers,** *Ph.D.*
(*Professor of Biomedical NMR & Associate Professor of Biomedical NMR*)
Department of Biomedical Engineering
Eindhoven University of Technology
Eindhoven
The Netherlands
and
Centre for Imaging Research & Education
Eindhoven
The Netherlands

FOREWORD 2

Cardiac magnetic resonance imaging has witnessed tremendous advances since its introduction in the early 1990's. Although MRI has played a central role in medical imaging since the mid-1980's, cardiac MRI has only truly blossomed over the past decade. Advances in magnet hardware technology, and key developments such as segmented k-space acquisitions, advanced motion encoding techniques, ultra-rapid perfusion imaging and delayed myocardial enhancement imaging have all contributed to a revolution in how patients with ischemic and non-ischemic heart disease are diagnosed and treated.

Fundamental to this revolution has been tremendous advances, both in hardware technology and our understanding of MR physics as applied to cardiac MRI. High-field strength magnets (1.5T, 3T, and even 7T), ultra-rapid gradients, and advances in phased array coil technology with parallel imaging reconstruction algorithms that have lead to important advances in cardiac imaging strategies. Indeed, cardiac MRI is a widely accepted method as the "gold standard" for detection and characterization of many forms of cardiac disease.

Despite pessimism on the continued role of MRI in clinical care in this environment of declining reimbursement, I am highly optimistic that the safety, accuracy and increasing availability of cardiac MRI will ensure a bright future. For these reasons, this textbook is particularly timely. Dr. Constantinides has assembled a team of international recognized experts presenting a highly innovative synergistic juxtaposition of advances in clinical cardiac MRI and technical and pre-clinical advances. The two sections of this textbook are highly complementary and will be of great interest to clinicians with interests in advanced clinical applications, and to physicists and engineers interested in advanced technological advancements in cardiovascular imaging, but with a clinical context to understand the role of this important technology.

Scott Reeder, *MD. Ph.D.*
Associate Professor
Chief of MR Radiology
Cardiovascular Imaging Section
University of Wisconsin Madison
USA

PREFACE

A tremendous scientific growth has been evidenced in the field of Magnetic Resonance Imaging (MRI) over the past 70 years, ever since the inception and independent demonstration of the phenomenon in condensed matter by Felix Bloch and Edward Purcell in 1946.

Within more than a decade after the initial clinical images became available in the early 1980's, techniques such as myocardial tagging, segmented k-space, multi-slice and multi-phase cardiac imaging, introduced cardiovascular imaging to the scientific community, and opened new avenues for the study of global cardiac morphology, perfusion, flow, metabolism, and function, in health and disease. Noted advances, such as the introduction of ultrafast imaging acquisition techniques, MR microscopy, ^{1}H and ^{31}P spectroscopy, regional strain and diffusion imaging, established cardiovascular MRI as one of the prominent and advanced scientific tools available nowadays. Concurrently, clinical applications facilitated detailed studies of cardiovascular pathology, including coronary artery disease (ischemia and myocardial infarction (MI)), congenital heart disease and heart failure, both in the acute and chronic stages, under rest, and following pharmacological or exercise-induced stress. Such applications allowed assessment of critical functional, perfusion, and viability biomarkers for long-term prognosis, striving to establish MRI as the 'one-stop shop' in everyday clinical practice.

On the forefront of pre-clinical work, mouse cardiac MRI emerged as a logical consequence to the genome mapping initiatives amidst parallel developments and progress in human cardiac MRI in the late 1980's and early 1990's. With the complete characterization of the mouse and human genomes (a National Institutes of Health initiative) in 2002 and 2003 respectively, a plethora of mouse studies emerged targeting the cardiovascular system with genetic modifications, marking the onset of the molecular physiology, proteomics, and (structural and functional) genomics era.

While image-based phenotyping has been a major long-term scientific goal, aiming to high-throughput cardiac studies of pathology, to-this-date, it still remains elusive. Human and mouse cardiac pathological MRI studies have advanced mostly as parallel efforts, unsupported thus far by major National or International policies or consortia that would strategically coordinate multi-center studies under carefully-controlled and normalized protocols, as such would establish the knowledge-platform to benefit cardiovascular disease, molecular genomics, or related/emerging technological advances, with an envisaged tremendous impact for translational research to man.

Collectively, this effort summarizes extensively (with the exception of molecular imaging) the most recent clinical and basic science developments in the field of cardiac MRI, with multiple contributions from prominent researchers and scientists throughout the world. The topics are categorized in two parts; Part I concentrates on clinical advances in ischemic heart disease, heart failure, flow and quantification and cardiac and multinuclear spectroscopy. Part II focuses on pre-clinical work, including fast imaging techniques, regional functional quantification, and fiber structure characterization.

I am hopeful that the book will serve to readers as a reference guidebook for the current status and future directions of cardiac MRI.

With a great sense of responsibility I express my gratitude and dedicate this book to my parents Elpida and Demetris and to my friend Dr. Andreas Lanitis for their true love, generous encouragement, advice and support over the years.

Christakis Constantinides, *Ph.D.*
Chi Biomedical Limited
Nicosia
Cyprus
E-mail: Christakis.Constantinides@gmail.com

LIST OF CONTRIBUTORS

Andrew J. Ludman
Centre for Advanced Cardiovascular Imaging, NIHR CVBRU at Barts, London Chest Hospital, Bonner Road, London, E2 9JX, UK

Arnold D. Gomez
Department of Bioengineering, University of Utah, Utah, USA

Christakis Constantinides
Chi Biomedical Limited, 36 Parthenonos Street, Apartment 303, Strovolos 2021, Nicosia, Cyprus

Christopher J. Francois
Department of Radiology, University of Wisconsin, 600 Highland Avenue, Madison, WI 53792, USA

Christopher L. Welsh
Department of Bioengineering, University of Utah, Utah, USA

Edward Hsu
Department of Bioengineering, University of Utah, Utah, USA

Han Wen
National Heart Lung and Blood Institute, National Institutes of Health, Bethesda, MD 20892, USA

I. Jolanda M. de Vries
Radboud University Nijmegen Medical Center (RUNMC), Department of Tumor Immunology, 278, Nijmegen Center for Molecular Life Sciences (NCMLS), Nijmegen, The Netherlands

John Palios
Emory University School of Medicine, Division of Cardiology, The Emory Healthcare, 1365 Clifton Road, NE, Suite AT 503, Atlanta, Georgia 30322, USA

Jürgen E. Schneider
BHF Experimental MR Unit, Radcliffe Department of Medicine, Division of Cardiovascular Medicine, University of Oxford, Oxford, UK

L. Ceri Davies
Centre for Advanced Cardiovascular Imaging, NIHR CVBRU at Barts, London Chest Hospital, Bonner Road, London, E2 9JX, UK

Mangala Srinivas
Radboud University Nijmegen Medical Center (RUNMC), Department of Tumor Immunology, 278, Nijmegen Center for Molecular Life Sciences (NCMLS), Nijmegen, The Netherlands

Osama Abdullah
Department of Bioengineering, University of Utah, Utah, USA

Pierre Croisille
Department of Radiology, CHU Hôpital Nord, Jean-Monnet University, CREATIS Laboratory, UMR CNRS 5520 INSERM U1040, University of Lyon, 42055, Saint-Etienne, France

Stamatios Lerakis
Emory University School of Medicine, Division of Cardiology, The Emory Healthcare, 1365 Clifton Road, NE, Suite AT 503, Atlanta, Georgia 30322, USA

Steffen E. Petersen
Centre for Advanced Cardiovascular Imaging, NIHR CVBRU at Barts, London Chest Hospital, Bonner Road, London, E2 9JX, UK

Stelios Angeli
Prognosis Advanced Diagnostic Center, 2 Tefkrou Anthia Street, Larnaca 2021, Cyprus

Send Orders for Reprints to reprints@benthamscience.net

Latest Advances in Clinical and Pre-Clinical Cardiovascular MRI, 2014, *Vol. 1*, 3-40   **3**

CHAPTER 1

CMR in Heart Failure: Current and Emerging Clinical Applications

Andrew J. Ludman[1], L. Ceri Davies[2] and Steffen E. Petersen[*2]

[1]Department of Heart Failure, The Royal Brompton Hospital, London, UK; [2]Centre for Advanced Cardiovascular Imaging, National Institute for Health Research Cardiovascular Biomedical Research Unit at Barts, The London Chest Hospital, London, UK

Abstract: Heart failure is the potential result of a large number of heterogeneous diseases leaving the heart unable to provide an adequate blood supply for the body. The optimal diagnosis and management of this diverse syndrome requires the accurate synthesis of a large amount of clinical information but often the underlying diagnosis is elusive. The use of Cardiac Magnetic Resonance (CMR) is growing rapidly and it has established itself as a powerful, non-invasive, non-ionising radiation based tool. CMR is able to interrogate not only ventricular function and morphology but also characterise the tissue itself on a scale validated with histology, investigate cellular function as well as myocardial mechanics and energetics. Within this chapter we will summarise for the reader the current use of CMR in heart failure, the emerging pulse sequences and the state of the art application of CMR in specific settings within heart failure. CMR is already proven to make significant clinical impact but challenges remain in harnessing the wealth of information it can provide, proving the incremental value of each technique and in widening the availability of CMR in order to maximise its benefit. This chapter will provide an in-depth introduction to the topic, act as an update for the more advanced practitioner and provide a platform for further interest and research.

Keywords: Acquired cardiomyopathy, cardiac magnetic resonance, cardiac resynchronization, cardiac transplantation, diagnosis, dilated cardiomyopathy, fibrosis, gadolinium, heart failure, imaging, inherited cardiomyopathy, ischaemic heart disease, myocardial function, myocardial edema, myocardial characterization, perfusion, prognosis, valvular heart disease.

***Address correspondence to Steffen E. Petersen:** Centre for Advanced Cardiovascular Imaging, NIHR CVBRU at Barts, London Chest Hospital, Bonner Road, London, E2 9JX, UK; Tel: 0044-(0)207 882 6902; E-mail: s.e.petersen@qmul.ac.uk

INTRODUCTION

Heart failure is a descriptive term for the final outcome of a large number of heterogeneous conditions which damage the myocardium, manifesting as progressive failure of the heart to meet the demands of the body. As such, in order to be able to diagnose, monitor, assess treatment success and conduct research on heart failure a large amount of information is required. CMR is establishing itself as the imaging modality which can provide a breadth of information without which the contemporary management of heart failure would not be possible. The following chapter shall detail the current role of CMR in heart failure, how CMR can guide diagnosis and treatment of particular conditions and how emerging CMR techniques when applied to heart failure will further mechanistic understanding and expand therapeutic possibilities.

HEART FAILURE AND IMAGING

Heart failure is defined clinically as a syndrome of specific symptoms (breathlessness, orthopnea, paroxysmal nocturnal dyspnoea *etc.*) and signs (peripheral edema, elevated venous pressure, pulmonary crackles *etc.*) caused by an abnormality of cardiac structure and/or function [1]. The diagnosis of heart failure is not always easy and requires the synthesis of clinical, biochemical and multi-modality imaging information in order to confirm the diagnosis and then to go on and try to identify the underlying etiology. Heart failure is a significant problem worldwide; it is reported to affect approximately 900,000 individuals in the UK with an inpatient hospital mortality of 11.1% [2] and in the USA it is estimated that approximately 5.7 million individuals have heart failure with 1 in 9 death certificates mentioning heart failure [3].

Whilst the diagnosis of heart failure can often be made clinically, confirmation is almost always sought by imaging techniques and it is important to attempt to define structural and functional problems in the heart failure patient. Echocardiography is the most commonly used technique and has many positive attributes, including cost, accessibility, portability, lack of ionizing radiation, the ability to assess real time haemodynamic changes and many years of experience in its use [4]. However, echocardiography may be challenging in some patients due to body habitus and incomplete visualization may lead to inaccurate measures and tissue characterization is limited. Radio-nuclide imaging has also been used for many years to measure LV systolic function and to assess ischemia and viability. Its repeated use is limited due to high radiation doses and spatial resolution is relatively low [5]. The combined use of Computed Tomography and FDG-PET (CT-PET) is becoming very useful in some areas of heart failure (particularly sarcoidosis) but availability is still limited, radiation dose is high, a prolonged specific diet is required pre-examination and spatial resolution is not yet optimal [6]. CMR has emerged as a tool which can assess cardiac structure, function, blood flow and can characterise soft tissue (specifically myocardium) to allow insights into the underlying disease process. MRI is free from ionizing radiation and as such serial scans are less concerning. During one examination multiple imaging sequences can be performed and it is possible to use a wide range of these techniques in both animals and humans, facilitating translation of research findings and allowing exploration of physiology and mechanisms of action. CMR is unconstrained by anatomical windows and so imaging can be performed in any plane. CMR has high spatial and temporal resolution and so measurements can be made very accurately with low inter- and intra- observer variability. This has allowed CMR measures to be used as surrogate endpoints in both animal and human settings as the sample size required decreases with the reproducibility or precision of the outcome measure [7].

Practical Considerations of CMR in Heart Failure

Whilst CMR is an excellent technique for use in patients with heart failure, this particular group of patients deserves special attention in order to maximise safety as well as image quality. In the acute phase the role of CMR is limited due to the length of the examination, the requirement for the patient to lie flat and the difficulty in delivering acute treatment in the CMR environment. Once the patient is beyond the acute phase they must still be able to lie flat for approximately 45 minutes and must be able to perform multiple breath-holds. Low dose sedation and scanning the patient prone and/or feet first may allow claustrophobic patients to be successfully scanned but this can be a problem in approximately 4% of patients [8,9]. Renal dysfunction is common in heart failure and whilst the use of gadolinium contrast is safe, there is a risk of nephrogenic systemic fibrosis (NSF) in those with a glomerular filtration rate (GFR) < 30ml/min and should only be used if the benefits outweigh the risk [10]. Metallic heart valves, coronary stents and sternal wires are all safe in CMR but will cause varying amounts of artefact which must be allowed for. Other metallic implants may not be safe - generally all cardiac resynchronization devices and implantable defibrillators are not safe and preclude CMR although in some circumstances the benefit may outweigh the risk [11,12]. There are some MRI safe (conditional) permanent pacemakers now in use but one must ensure that *all* wires and the generator are MRI conditional and follow the manufacturer's programming advice pre- and post-scan [12]. www.mrisafety.com is a useful resource for further and more specific information.

Current Standard CMR Examination and Pulse Sequences in Heart Failure

Each CMR examination can be tailored to the individual, however, it is common that the protocol will be standardised depending on the clinical indication. The 'standard' protocol for heart failure is described below but other sequences can be added according to need, as described later in this section.

Structure and Function

Following initial 'scout' or 'localizer' images, axial imaging through the entire thorax is performed to evaluate gross cardiac anatomy and related extra-cardiac structures. Using oblique planes, cine image slices in 3 long axis slices (4 chamber, 2 chamber and 3 chamber) as well as multiple short axis slices along the length of the ventricles from base (level of mitral and tricuspid valves) to apex are obtained. By drawing 'regions of interest' at end-diastole and end-systole around the endocardium and epicardium in each short axis slice accurate measurement can be made of both left ventricular (LV) and right ventricular (RV) end-diastolic (EDV) and end-systolic volumes (ESV), allowing calculation of stroke volume and ejection fraction (EF) as well as myocardial volume (which can be converted to mass by multiplying by $1.05g/cm^3$ - the density of myocardium) [13].

Great Vessel Blood Flow

Flow velocity mapping imaging to assess aortic and pulmonary flow is commonly performed as a secondary check of the calculated LV/RV stroke volumes, to calculate Q_p: Q_s (looking for intra-cardiac shunts), and also to assess for any aortic or pulmonary valve disease.

Myocardial Iron

By taking advantage of the properties of iron rich myocardium within a magnetic field a rapid assessment of myocardial iron content can be made [14,15]. Increased myocardial iron content shortens the T_2* relaxation time and therefore by calculating the T_2*, myocardial iron can be quantified. This technique has been validated against histological specimens [16] and can successfully guide treatment of siderotic cardiomyopathy [17].

Myocardial Fat

Fat infiltration of RV or LV myocardium may be identified using a T_1 weighted turbo spin echo sequence. Fat saturation sequences can also be used to null the signal from fat, resulting in signal "drop out" from the ventricular wall.

Myocardial Edema

Using short tau (inversion-time) inversion recovery (STIR) imaging CMR sequences [18] it is possible to image the areas of myocardium which have increased water content. This may correlate with areas of inflammation [19] (Fig. **1**), ischemia and/or ischemia-reperfusion injury [20].

Perfusion

If ischemia is thought likely then stress and rest perfusion imaging is performed. Most commonly, adenosine (a vasodilator) is the stressor agent and 3 short axis slices of the LV are repetitively imaged in real time whilst administering gadolinium contrast to assess 'first pass perfusion'. As with other imaging modalities, other stress agents may be used in different circumstances as well as different regions imaged.

Gadolinium Contrast Enhanced Sequences

Within two minutes of administering gadolinium (early period), inversion recovery imaging allows identification of intracardiac thrombus and other non-perfused areas, such as microvascular obstruction (MVO) (Fig. **2**). Approximately

10-15 minutes following gadolinium administration (late period), inversion recovery imaging is once again performed to cover the whole LV and RV in order to identify areas of myocardial scar and/or areas of extracellular space expansion. Most commonly, the cause is myocardial infarction but the distribution and pattern of late gadolinium enhancement (LGE) may give crucial clues to other underlying pathology.

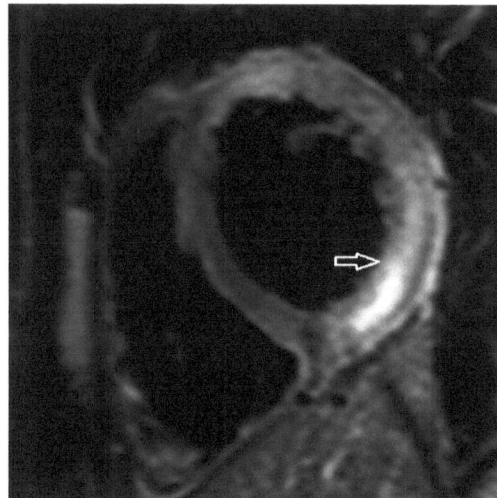

Figure 1: A short axis LV slice with a T_2 weighted sequence demonstrating an area of higher signal intensity in the inferior and inferolateral walls due to myocarditis (white arrow).

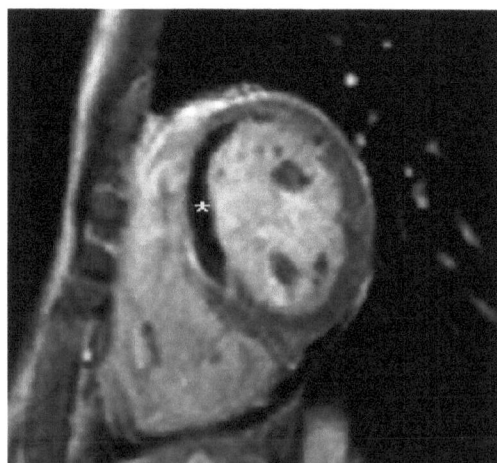

Figure 2: Early gadolinium enhanced imaging: A mid ventricular short axis slice demonstrating a dark core of microvascular obstruction (*) following an anteroseptal myocardial infarction.

EMERGING CMR SEQUENCES FOR IMAGING IN HEART FAILURE

Quantification of Regional Function

Although heart failure is often due to global myocardial dysfunction, the severity of dysfunction may vary across the myocardium or a specific disease process may preferentially affect some areas rather than others. Therefore, techniques which permit the study of regional myocardial function may allow characterization of disease type, may enhance diagnostic abilities, allow measurement of response to treatment and potentially guide targeted therapies. To this end there is increasing demand for regional quantification of function [21]. Deformation imaging by CMR allows qualitative and quantitative measures of regional myocardial function; time-to-peak contraction (assessment of dyssynchrony), regional ejection fraction (an expression of the regional contribution to the global function), torsion and myocardial strain and/or strain rate may all be quantified [21].

Strain is a measure of deformation and is defined by the change in length of an object relative to its original length and in the heart this yields radial, circumferential and longitudinal values. Depending on the technique used the measured strain may be based on a specific point in the myocardium (Lagrangian) or on a fixed point in space (Eulerian). Normal reference values are being established but as yet the numbers studied are still relatively small [22-24] and expected values in defined disease groups are being formulated [25, 26]. Strain rate is the change in strain per unit time and torsion describes the twisting, wringing, motion of the LV contraction. A number of CMR techniques offer the ability to qualitatively or quantitatively assess regional function and have varying attributes and are discussed below.

Myocardial Tissue Tagging

This is the most widely used CMR technique where by nulling the magnetization in two oblique planes a visible grid (tags) is produced through the myocardium (Fig. **3**) which can then be seen to deform during systole with cine imaging. Progressive technical advancements have improved signal and contrast to noise ratios, have increased the duration of the cardiac cycle that can be imaged (as tags fade throughout the cardiac cycle) and have reduced the time required for post-processing (notably with HARP [Harmonic Phase] analysis) [22].

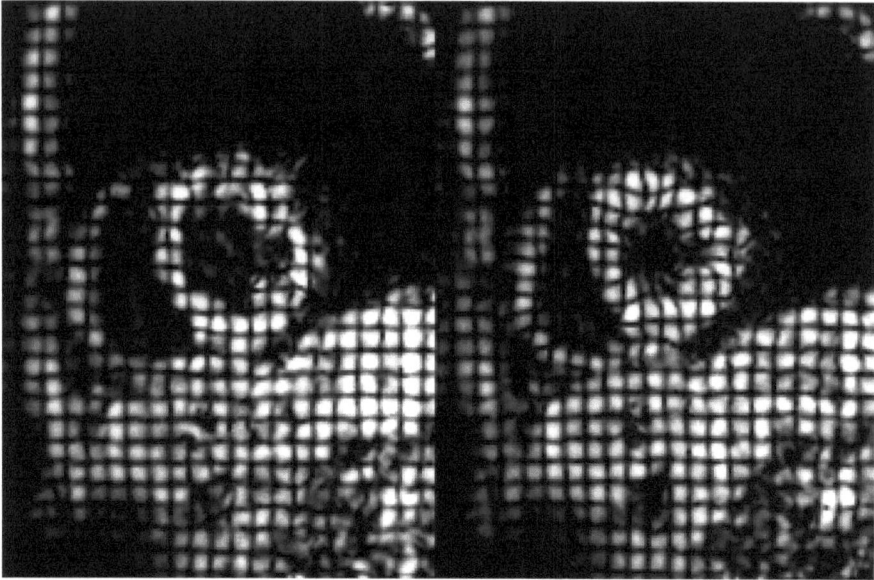

Figure 3: Diastolic (left panel) and systolic (right panel) images of myocardial tagging demonstrating myocardial deformation in a normal volunteer.

Phase Velocity Encoding

Phase velocity encoding or mapping is often used to measure flow velocity in large blood vessels but can also be used to assess regional myocardial velocity. A bipolar gradient is used to encode velocity directly into the phase of the signal. Although prone to motion artefacts and phase distortion, phase velocity encoding can measure the relative velocities of the myocardium and hence detect regional wall motion abnormalities. Peak velocity, time to peak velocity and strain rate can all be measured or calculated from the sequence [27].

Displacement Encoding with Stimulated Echoes (DENSE)

DENSE uses a stimulated echo sequence in order to encode in-plane [28] or through-plane [29] displacement directly into the phase of an image (see also chapters 3 and 7). Displacement of each pixel may be calculated at the extremes of movement or the pixels can be tracked (cine-DENSE) in order to generate strain-time curves. This technique offers rapid processing times and high precision but has not yet been widely adopted clinically due to a relatively low signal to noise ratio (SNR).

Strain Encoded Imaging (SENC)

SENC is also a technique which visually tags the myocardium, however the tags are applied in parallel, rather than perpendicular, to the imaging plane. Through-plane deformation is measured which means that longitudinal strain can be measured from the short axis views and circumferential strain from the long axis views. Radial strain cannot be measured, although SENC can be combined with other 2D-strain techniques (such as 2D-tagging or 2D DENSE [30]) in order to provide a 3D model. Strain is directly related to image pixel intensity and therefore post-processing times are short.

Feature Tracking

New post-processing techniques may allow the measurement of strain from standard steady state free precession (SSFP) cine imaging. Feature tracking offers this potential and the principle is similar to the speckle tracking echocardiography technique. The software uses the movement of myocardial features from frame-to-frame in order to calculate deformation. This technique is reasonably reproducible between studies [31], has been used in dobutamine stress studies [32] and to assess myocardial viability [32]. When compared to myocardial tagging it performs adequately for global measures of strain in the circumferential direction, but less well in the radial and longitudinal directions [33]. Therefore, it requires further development, with proven accuracy and reproducibility, prior to further clinical use.

ADVANCED TISSUE CHARACTERISATION

Diffuse Fibrosis

The focal fibrosis of a myocardial infarction is well visualised with the current LGE CMR techniques [34]. Diffuse myocardial fibrosis, however, is not visualised as it is 'nulled' along with the normal myocardium. Diffuse fibrosis of the myocardium is a slow occult process which occurs with normal aging, but is accelerated by conditions such as hypertension, diabetes, hypertrophic cardiomyopathy and aortic stenosis and may be partly responsible for the breathlessness, heart failure and arrhythmia encountered [35]. Diffuse fibrosis is universally present in end stage heart failure [36] and represents expansion of the extracellular fraction of the myocardium, and more specifically an increase in collagen deposition. There are different sub-types of diffuse fibrosis which may allow an increased diagnostic ability and if reversible, represents a target for novel therapies [35]. The ability to detect, quantify and monitor diffuse fibrosis (or its surrogate- the extracellular volume) may well become crucial for investigating and tailoring heart failure therapies [37].

T_1 Mapping and Equilibrium Contrast CMR

Currently, there are two contrast CMR techniques under investigation to identify and quantify diffuse fibrosis. Both rely on the fact that fibrosis results in an expansion of the myocardial extra-cellular volume (ECV).

T_1 mapping [38] measures the T_1 of the myocardium at baseline and then at intervals after a bolus injection of gadolinium. The T_1 of the fibrotic tissue (with an increased ECV and reduced gadolinium wash out) is shorter than that of 'normal' myocardium and by using sequences which map the T_1 signal, the percentage of ECV *versus* normal myocardium can be calculated. Histological validation has been conducted in small numbers [39,40] and this technique is promising as it is relatively easy to accomplish and is starting to provide insight into the early stages of disease in some groups (such as patients with diabetes) [41]. Unfortunately the technique is susceptible to inaccuracies at high heart rates and to variations depending on renal function and body composition. Additionally, the time that the T_1 map is obtained following gadolinium administration will affect the values obtained and may make comparisons between different research studies from different centres difficult unless exactly uniform techniques are used.

Equilibrium contrast CMR is a second technique under investigation. It requires greater acquisition time and technical expertise but aims to reduce the inaccuracies or variations in measures due to different body habitus or renal function [42]. With this technique the T_1 (of blood and myocardium) is measured before and after gadolinium but the gadolinium is given *via* a primed infusion (bolus followed by infusion) in order to equilibrate blood and myocardial levels. Once the patient's haematocrit is known, the volume of distribution of gadolinium in the blood can be calculated (1-haematocrit), which allows calculation of the volume of distribution in the myocardium. This is then expressed against the volume of myocardium to give a percentage of fibrosis. Initial validation was performed against human myocardial samples in patients undergoing surgery for aortic stenosis and the group have gone on to investigate the links with clinical outcomes [43].

Non-contrast T_1 mapping is also emerging as a method with which to attempt to quantify diffuse fibrosis. This technique may overcome some of the limitations of gadolinium based techniques. Using a shortened modified Look Locker sequence the T_1 of the myocardium is measured (a composite value of intra- and extracellular compartments is obtained) and has been found to correlate to increased wall thickness in hypertrophic cardiomyopathy (HCM) and myocardial thinning in dilated cardiomyopathy (DCM) as well as to correlate negatively with phosphocreatine/adenosine triphosphate ratios [44]. Currently non-contrast T_1 mapping is not usable on an individual patient basis but the authors postulate that at high field strengths (7T) and with further sequence optimisation, it may have a role in diagnosis and monitoring of myocardial disease.

Manganese Enhanced MRI

Manganese is one of several cations able to selectively block voltage-gated calcium channels (*via* competitive action) and has a similar structure and kinetic behaviour to calcium (Ca^{2+}) [45]. Calcium currents play a central role in the electrical and mechanical activity of cardiomyocytes. Specifically, calcium is critical for cardiomyocyte function, is involved in several pathways and may finally influence gene expression. Mn^{2+} shortens T_1 relaxation time and by this property allows the indirect assessment of calcium flux and cell viability [45]. In heart failure calcium cycling is significantly modified [46] and therefore a technique which can study this would seem to have wide application. This is so in the preclinical setting where validated indications for this method are the determination of myocardial area at risk [47] and ischemic areas [48] as well as the measurement of the effect of ischemia [49] or drugs [50] on the calcium current. Unfortunately safety concerns regarding the physiological and neurological toxic effects of manganese [51] have so far limited its application in the clinical setting and it is not currently safe for widespread use.

Myofiber Orientation (Diffusion Tensor Imaging)

The exact microstructure of the myocardium remains debated [52] but it is accepted that inherent to some diseases and due to adverse remodelling the myofiber orientation may be disturbed [53,54]. The three dimensional organisation of myocardial fibers of the mammalian ventricle is unique; being composed not only of circumferential fibers and longitudinal fibers but also of obliquely running fibres that form a helical spiral from base to apex [54]. Determination of fiber architecture may be central to the understanding of the underlying pathology and has classically been performed by *ex vivo* histological analysis [53]. Diffusion tensor resonance magnetic imaging (DT-MRI) (see also chapter 8) was initially validated in animal models [55,56] and takes advantage of the fact that MRI signal is attenuated by water diffusion in a tissue exposed to a magnetic field gradient. Water diffuses preferentially *along* the myofibers, rather than across the cell membranes, allowing the determination of the direction and inter-relation of the myofibers [56]. Technical progress has allowed the application of this method to *in vivo*, beating hearts, making it available for studies in patients [54,57,58] (Fig. **4**).

This technique allows microstructural visualization and is therefore complimentary to more macroscopic imaging techniques. Although not yet ready for routine clinical use, it is likely that with progressive technical advancement it will provide valuable insights in patients with heart failure.

Cell Tracking (Super Paramagnetic Iron Oxide Particles)

Cell therapies for cardiac regeneration in heart failure have been the subject of a huge amount of research, and in some cases promising benefits have been demonstrated in terms of systolic function and remodelling [59]. The mechanism of action however remains unclear, since long-term cell survival and engraftment after delivery in the host myocardium in large animals and humans has never been demonstrated [60]. Techniques allowing the injected cells to be tracked are pivotal in preclinical studies in order to understand their destiny and to attempt to improve survival and engraftment in the host myocardium.

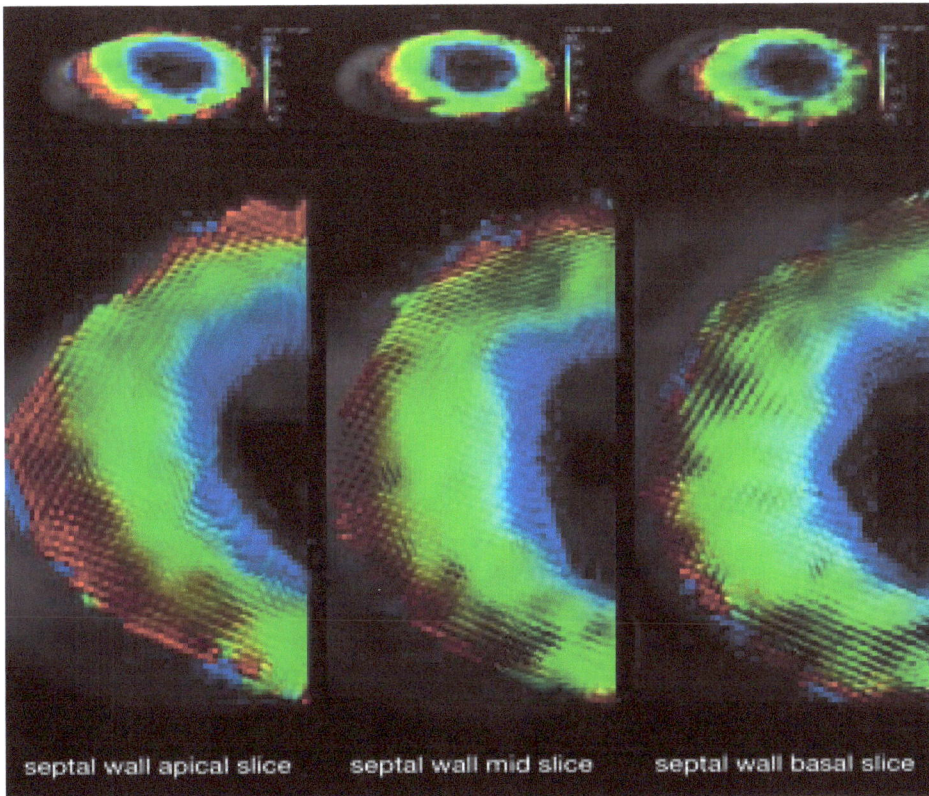

septal wall apical slice   septal wall mid slice   septal wall basal slice

Figure 4: Diffusion tensor resonance magnetic imaging has the potential to allow microstructural visualization and determination of myofiber architecture (courtesy of Dr. L.-A. McGill, The Royal Brompton Hospital CMR Department).

Superparamagnetic iron oxide particles (SPIO) have been widely used to label cells for MRI detection. The particles contain an iron oxide core surrounded by a polysaccharide polymer coat. Magnetic in-homogeneities produced by SPIO, disturb the local magnetic field and lead to decreased signal intensity on T_2-weighted and T_2^*-weighted images [60].

The major limitation of using SPIO particles for cell tracking is the absence of discrimination between living labelled stem cells and dead stem cells phagocytized by locally present macrophages. Furthermore, reports indicate that even after 40 days, no signal difference is detectable between labelled living and dead cells [61]. Currently, SPIO particles with better tissue clearance are under development.

The impact that SPIO particles have on the biological properties of the labelled cells is debated with some studies demonstrating no negative effect [62,63] and others reporting significant interference with cell migration, colony-formation and cell function [64,65,66]. In humans, intravenous solutions containing SPIO particles had been FDA-approved and intravenous administration of SPIO-labelled cells was tracked successfully by MRI [63] but safety concerns have now led to the market withdrawal of the ferumoxides and further development is awaited.

Cells labelled with "classical" MR-contrast such as gadolinium chelates are detectable as a hyperintense signal on T_1-weighted images [60]. However, the sensitivity of this method is lower than SPIO labelling and, furthermore, contrast intensity is inhomogeneous depending on the intracellular location of the contrast [67]. Safety concerns remain in terms of the possible release of free radicals [68].

Fluorine (^{19}F) contained in perfluorocarbon (PFC) is an attractive emerging MR-contrast and has a safe toxicity profile. It can be used for spectroscopy and image formation in a similar way as ^{1}H from H_2O [60]. Biological soft tissues do not contain fluorine, therefore do not contribute to any background tissue signal. A number of animal studies have been conducted on stem cell labelling and trafficking with ^{19}F-MR which, although heterogeneous in design (cell type, labelling method, delivery route *etc.*), exhibit common results in terms of the efficiency and stability of cell labelling and the specific detection of the cells throughout the body [69]. ^{19}F-MR is currently limited to preclinical research as further improvements are needed, particularly in the field of image acquisition (hardware, sequences) and in the development of approved ^{19}F contrast agents.

Myocardial Energetics (MR Spectroscopy)

Myocardial metabolism is disturbed in numerous cardiac pathologies including ischemia, hypertrophy and heart failure [70], demonstrating the fact that function and metabolism are closely linked. Creatine phosphate/ATP ratio correlates closely with clinical heart failure severity [71]. In conventional CMR, the signal arises from the position of the spins of ^{1}H nuclei contained in the water and fat molecules depending on the magnetic field. This technique provides structural and functional information but is not suitable for metabolic assessment of a particular tissue. CMR spectroscopy allows the study of several other nuclei, including ^{13}C, ^{23}Na and ^{31}P being of particular interest for cardiac metabolism [72] (see also chapter 5). In comparison to conventional CMR, MR spectroscopy offers very low sensitivity related to the low magnetic energy of the nuclear spins and the low concentration of these molecules compared to the abundance of water. To overcome this limitation, the technique of hyperpolarization has recently been developed which uses low temperatures and strong magnetic fields to increase the polarization of the spins [73].

CMR spectroscopy obviously has a role to play in the understanding of the myocardial energetics of heart failure but despite the significant technological advances achieved, it still suffers from the major limitations of poor spatial and temporal resolution, preventing its large-scale application in research or clinical practice [74]. The ability to study other molecules (such as ^{13}C-pyruvate [75]) is likely to advance this field further.

CMR APPLIED TO SPECIFIC AETIOLOGIES OF HEART FAILURE

Ischaemic Heart Disease

CMR has wide application in ischemic heart disease (IHD) (see chapter 1) and IHD is the most common cause of left ventricular systolic dysfunction and heart failure in the Western world. In patients presenting with *de novo* heart failure, often the most common initial diagnostic step is to attempt to classify the etiology as ischemic or other cause. Classically coronary angiography performs this role but recent studies demonstrate that CMR [76] (with or without CT coronary angiography (CTCA) [77]) is able to very reliably rule out coronary artery disease as the cause of the heart failure (diagnostic accuracy of 97% [76] or negative predictive value of 100% with CTCA [77]), so preventing the patient undergoing an unnecessary invasive coronary angiogram. Myocardial infarction is readily seen by LGE sequences as a region of hyperenhancement extending from the subendocardium across the myocardium to the epicardium in a coronary distribution (Fig. **5**).

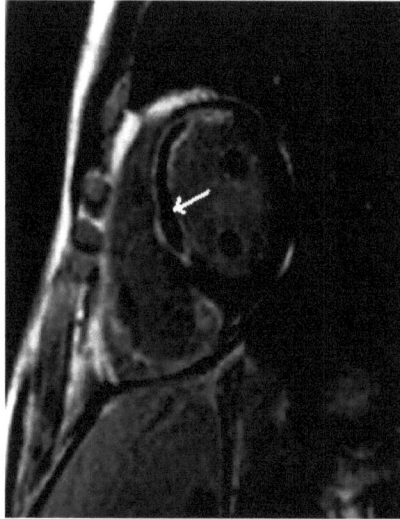

Figure 5: Late gadolinium enhanced imaging: A mid ventricular short axis slice demonstrating a transmural anteroseptal myocardial infarction with a dark core of microvascular obstruction (white arrow).

Once ischemic heart disease has been diagnosed by CMR the management can also be aided. Whether or not a myocardial segment is viable and will recover function following revascularization can be assessed by evaluating the transmurality of the LGE. In the landmark paper by Kim *et al.* [78] it was determined that, if the area of LGE with respect to the total area of myocardium in a dysfunctional segment was greater than 50% then the likelihood of recovering function following revascularization was very limited (only 10%), and if the LGE area is more than 75% then there is almost no chance that the segment will recover any function, and is thus non-viable. In myocardial segments with LGE, if there is a rim of unenhanced myocardium of 4 mm or greater, then the segment is likely to recover function with a sensitivity of 77% and a specificity of 72%. These techniques can further be enhanced by adding low dose dobutamine (LDD) to evaluate inotropic reserve in the segment. The combination of a 50% transmurality LGE cut-off with the results of the LDD-CMR produced the best prediction of segmental recovery of function at 6 months with 79-81% accuracy [79]. However, whether or not revascularization of 'viable' myocardium in patients with severe systolic dysfunction actually leads to a mortality benefit remains to be proven. The presence of myocardial viability (as assessed by SPECT and dobutamine stress echo) in a sub-study of the STICH-HF study [80] did not significantly change the outcome following coronary artery bypass graft surgery (CABG). Whether or not the enhanced spatial resolution of CMR with different cut-offs for the amount of viable (or viable and dysfunctional) myocardium and with limited viability guided revascularization can make a difference remains to be determined.

Whether there is a benefit from residual unenhanced myocardium (viable tissue) may still be in doubt, however, there is little doubt that the greater the extent of LGE (myocardial scar) the worse the outcome. In chronic ischemic cardiomyopathy (as well as non-ischemic) the extent of myocardial scar, as depicted by scoring the transmurality of late gadolinium enhancement (LGE) in the 17 segments of the LV, is strongly correlated with the progression to transplant or death [81].

Valvular Heart Disease

Due to the unrestricted imaging planes available, CMR may be a useful adjunct to echocardiography in valvular heart disease particularly when the management decision is not straight forward. Accurate assessment of ventricular volumes and function may aid decision making. The severity of aortic valvular regurgitation by CMR may predict the need for surgery [82] and aortic stenosis severity may be estimable either by direct planimetry of the valve orifice or by velocity flow mapping [83, 84]. The structure and function of the mitral valve can be precisely evaluated [85] as well as the right sided valves [86]. Early data suggest that beneficial ventricular remodeling following surgery for aortic stenosis may depend on the extent of diffuse fibrosis as measured by CMR [43].

INHERITED CARDIOMYOPATHY

Familial Dilated Cardiomyopathy

Idiopathic dilated cardiomyopathy (DCM) with a family history or genetic component to the heart failure is often a diagnosis of exclusion and CMR is very useful in identifying other etiologies. The extent of myocardial scar/fibrosis detected by LGE may confer an adverse prognosis [87,88] and the early identification of cardiac involvement in the dystrophinopathies may allow early institution of heart failure treatment [89]. The LGE distribution is most commonly mid-myocardial in patients with DCM. In patients with lamin A/C mutations (an inherited condition resulting in mutations of the nuclear lamin proteins) myocardial fibrosis can be accurately identified and is directly correlated with diastolic dysfunction [90].

Hypertrophic Cardiomyopathy

Hypertrophic cardiomyopathy (HCM) (Fig. **6**) is an autosomal dominant inherited disease characterized by ventricular muscle hypertrophy and myocardial fibre disarray. Due to the unlimited imaging planes available and excellent spatial resolution characterization of left ventricular hypertrophy (LVH) is often easier with CMR than with echocardiography- particularly in apical HCM [91]. The extent of myocardial scar/fibrosis is linked to risk of progression to heart failure and sudden cardiac death [92,93] and the presence of increased T_2 signal may indicate added risk [94].

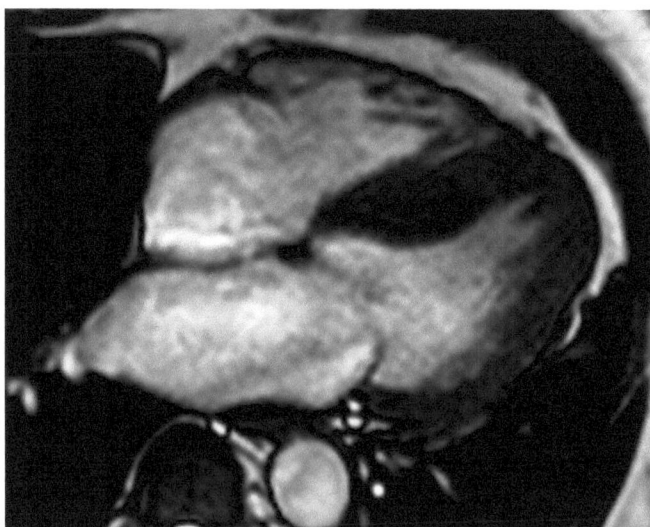

Figure 6: Four chamber image demonstrating significant septal hypertrophy due to Hypertrophic Cardiomyopathy. CMR allows views in any plane and precise quantification of myocardial dimensions.

Arrhythmogenic Right Ventricular Cardiomyopathy

Arrhythmogenic Right Ventricular Cardiomyopathy (ARVC) is challenging to diagnose and is based on a number of clinical and investigational factors [95]. Histologically, ARVC is characterized by fibro-fatty replacement of myocardium in the RV (and sometimes the LV), which can be detected by CMR although is not currently a diagnostic criteria. Evaluation of RV volumes, function and the identification of RV regional wall motion abnormalities is often easier than through limited echo windows [96] and the modified Task Force assigns a major criterion to the following CMR findings: regional RV akinesia or dyskinesia or dyssynchronous RV contraction and either, a ratio of RV end-diastolic volume to body surface area (BSA) of 110 mL/m^2 (male) or 100 mL/m^2 (female), or a RV ejection fraction of less than or equal to ≤40% [95] (Fig. **7**).

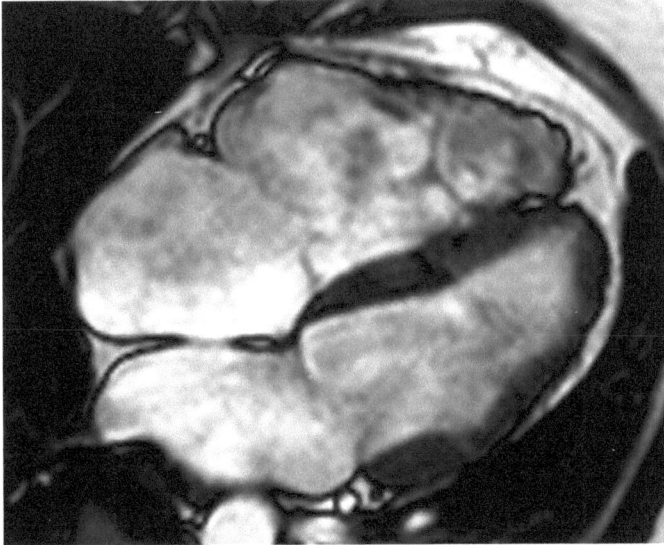

Figure 7: Four chamber systolic view from a patient with Arrhythmogenic Right Ventricular Cardiomyopathy (ARVC). Note the dilated right ventricle with aneurysmal akinetic areas of the free wall. CMR gives excellent visualisation of the RV which is sometimes difficult by echocardiography.

Left Ventricular Non-Compaction

This cardiomyopathy remains poorly understood [97], is often over-diagnosed by echocardiography [98] and CMR may provide morphological diagnosis with greater sensitivity and specificity [99]. The extent of LGE is correlated with disease severity and lower LV ejection fraction [100].

Anderson Fabry Disease

An X-linked deficiency in the enzyme alpha-galactosidase A leads to multi-system deposition of glycosphingolipid and in the heart results in concentric hypertrophy, arrhythmia and can progress to heart failure. Focal myocardial collagen scarring characteristically occurs in the inferolateral segments of the left ventricle [101] and treatment with enzyme replacement gives symptomatic and morphological improvement [102].

ACQUIRED CARDIOMYOPATHY

Myocarditis

Myocarditis is an inflammatory process which may be precipitated by a number of different causes but is often difficult to diagnose and sometimes to differentiate from acute coronary syndromes [103]. Myocarditis may rapidly lead to heart failure and as such an early diagnosis is important. Some believe that CMR with its multiple different imaging sequences is now key in the diagnosis [104], and certainly when faced with a patient with chest pain, troponin elevation and normal coronary arteries, CMR allows one to narrow the differential [105]. Specifically, beyond quantification of ventricular function, the most useful sequences are T_2 weighted images evaluating for edema/inflammation (see Fig. **1**), T_1 weighted images in the early phase following gadolinium administration evaluating for hyperaemia and late gadolinium enhanced images evaluating for necrosis/fibrosis [106]. In acute myocarditis CMR has a diagnostic accuracy of 79% when compared to clinical data and endomyocardial biopsy, however, in chronic myocarditis the accuracy falls to 52% and so cannot yet be reliably used alone [107]. When found, the LGE is commonly subepicardial, patchy and does not correspond to a coronary artery territory (Fig. **8**). Lack of LGE on CMR in patients with biopsy positive viral myocarditis predicts a good outcome, with no sudden cardiac death reported in a subgroup of 77 patients from one series at a median follow-up of 4.7 years [108].

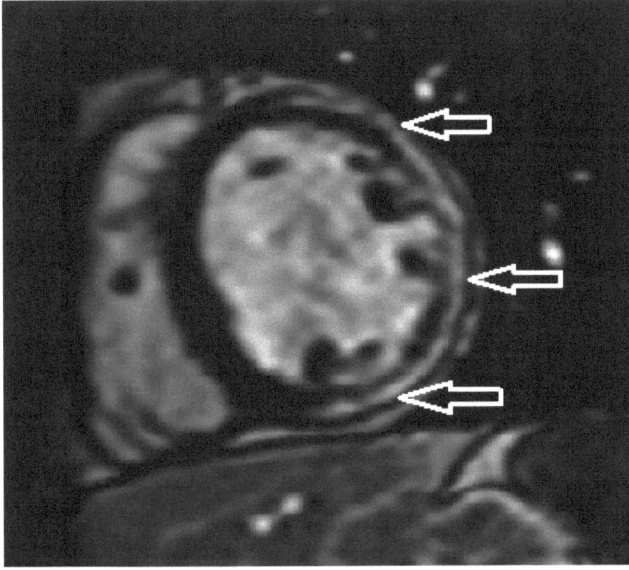

Figure 8: Mid ventricular short axis slice demonstrating extensive mid wall and epicardial late gadolinium enhancement in the anterior, lateral and inferior walls following myocarditis (white arrows).

Siderotic Cardiomyopathy

As discussed earlier, CMR T_2* sequences are able to reliably quantify myocardial iron [16]. In patients with thalassaemia, myocardial iron overload puts them at significant risk of mortality from heart failure [109] and the use of T_2* techniques allows chelation therapy to be tailored [110], which has a significant effect on mortality [111].

Sarcoidosis

A multisystem, non-caseating, granulomatous disease which is a great mimic of other diseases and may lead to death either through arrhythmia or progressive heart failure. The diagnostic role of CMR may be summarized as two fold; firstly to detect the presence of cardiac involvement in those with established extra-cardiac disease and secondly to make the diagnosis of cardiac sarcoid in those patients presenting '*de novo*' with chest pain, arrhythmia or heart failure (Fig. **9**). The Japanese criteria for the diagnosis of cardiac sarcoid have long been the comparable gold standard, but it is now recognized that they lack sensitivity and that CMR [112] or PET-CT [113] should be used as the non-invasive imaging techniques of choice in conjunction with other clinical features. Early data suggest that CMR may also give prognostic information in sarcoid, with a lack of LGE conferring an excellent event free survival at a mean of 2.7 years follow up [114]. The pattern of LGE in sarcoid may mimic other conditions but commonly is mid myocardial or epicardial and most frequently in the basal septal or inferior/inferolateral segments and classically involves the papillary muscles [115]. The use of T_2 weighted sequences to assess disease activity with the potential to guide immunosuppressive therapy is a tantalizing prospect but is not yet attainable and is likely to be limited by the requirement for implantable defibrillators in a large number of patients.

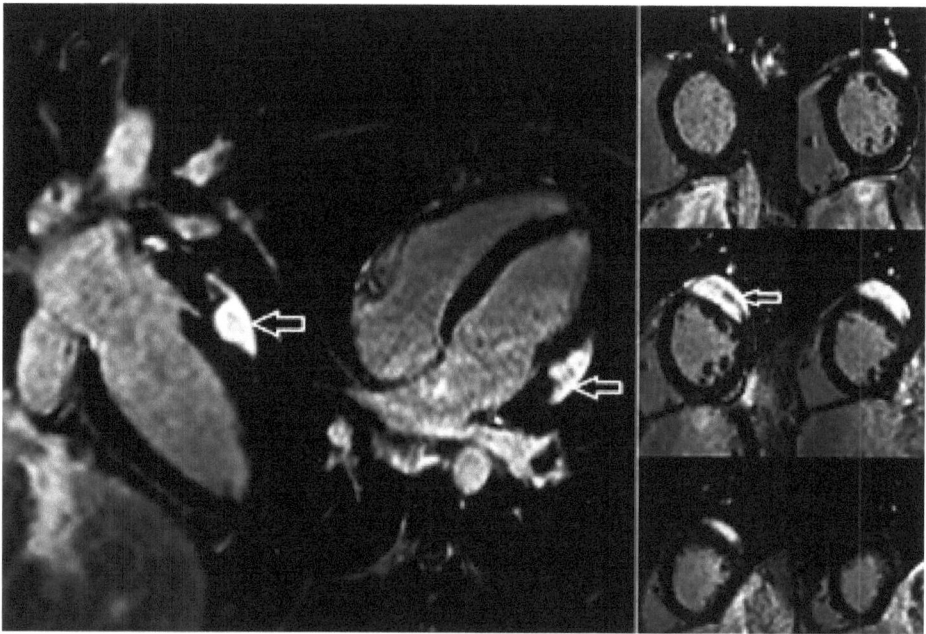

Figure 9: Two-chamber, four-chamber and short axis late gadolinium enhanced images of a patient following an acute presentation with cardiac sarcoidosis. The basal anterior wall is thickened with a brightly enhancing area extending from mid myocardium to epicardium with associated thickening and inflammation of the pericardium (white arrows).

Amyloidosis

Cardiac deposition of amyloid fibrils may occur in primary (AL) amyloid, inherited amyloid or senile systemic amyloid and is associated with a progressive restrictive cardiomyopathy which has a poor prognosis [116]. Gadolinium kinetics alter with avid uptake to the myocardium giving a characteristically dark blood pool and 'difficulty' nulling the myocardial signal (Fig. **10**). Early on in the disease process LGE may be patchy, and later, there is commonly circumferential sub-endocardial LGE which is due to the high degree of protein deposition in this area [117]. CMR is extremely useful in the non-invasive assessment of potential cardiac amyloid with a 90% negative predictive value and 88% positive predictive value [118]. A CMR study which is positive for cardiac amyloid confers an adverse prognosis with only 14% survival at 2 years in one series [119]. CMR may offer the potential to quantify the burden of disease through measurement of the ventricular extra-cellular volume which may add further insights, and perhaps allow more detailed prognostic assessment and tailored therapy [120,121].

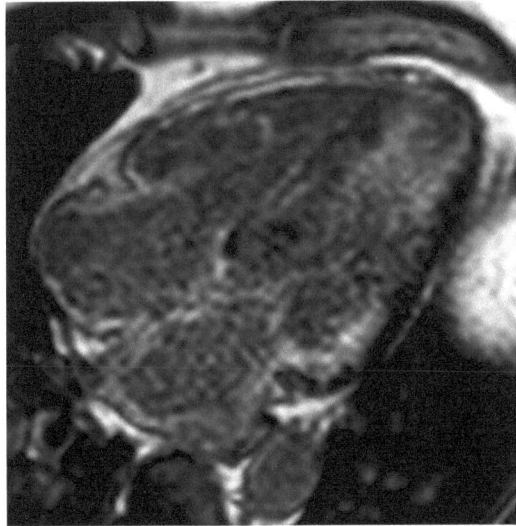

Figure 10: Four-chamber late gadolinium enhanced image demonstrating cardiac amyloidosis. The blood pool is unusually bright and it has been difficult to 'null' the myocardium. In addition there is predominantly subendocardial LGE of the lateral LV wall from base to apex.

Chemotherapy Induced Systolic Dysfunction

The role of CMR in chemotherapy induced cardiomyopathy is currently mainly related to accurate assessment, serial study and in excluding other causes. Interestingly, in anthracycline related cardiomyopathy, myocardial LGE is rare and there is an inverse relationship between cumulative dose and myocardial mass [122].

Peripartum Cardiomyopathy

Peripartum cardiomyopathy (PPCM) is an idiopathic cardiomyopathy presenting towards the end of pregnancy or in the months following delivery with no other apparent cause [123]. When used, CMR provides a more accurate assessment of LV function and excludes other causes. Unless essential, the administration of gadolinium should be avoided until after delivery but breastfeeding does not need to be interrupted after its use [124].

Eosinophilia and Cardiac Disease

Hyper-eosinophilic syndromes, which includes Churg-Strauss syndrome amongst others, may cause a progressive heart failure which can be difficult to diagnose. The eosinophil is strongly attracted to the heart and causes endocardial fibrosis which is readily seen on CMR with a characteristic circumferential endocardial pattern including the papillary muscles [125]. CMR has excellent accuracy for identification of disease but whether it can accurately differentiate fibrosis *versus* inflammation in order to guide treatment, remains to be determined [126].

Chagas Cardiomyopathy

A source of considerable mortality and morbidity in Latin America and, due to migratory movements, an increasing problem in non-endemic areas - Chagas disease is caused by infection from Trypanosoma Cruzi - it may cause progressive heart failure and ventricular arrhythmias [127]. The use of LGE imaging allows detection of cardiac involvement and may do so before symptoms develop. The pattern of LGE is not specific and may mimic that of myocardial infarction or other infiltrative cardiomyopathies (such as Fabry's disease), however there does appear to be a predilection to LGE in the infero-lateral and apical segments [128].

Thiamine Deficiency and Cardiomyopathy

Wet beriberi caused by deficiency of vitamin B1 (Thiamine) may cause severe cardiomyopathy and cardiogenic shock in combination with other largely neurological manifestations. Although rare, it may be underdiagnosed and so should be considered in patients with dietary deficiency, malabsorption or in unknown etiologies of heart failure. A diffuse increase in T_2 signal suggestive of myocardial inflammation has been reported but requires further verification in larger numbers of patients [129].

Takotsubo Cardiomyopathy

Stress induced or Takotsubo cardiomyopathy is being increasingly recognised as a largely reversible ventricular dysfunction in varying patterns, but most commonly affecting the LV apex with hyperdynamic basal function (Fig. **11**). There is often a discrete cut off between normal and abnormal myocardium that does not correspond to a coronary artery territory. LGE is only found in a small percentage of patients, whereas increased T_2 signal suggesting myocardial inflammation is found in approximately 80% of patients and corresponds with the regional wall motion abnormality [130]. Demonstration of normalization of LV systolic function after 1-2 months confirms the diagnosis.

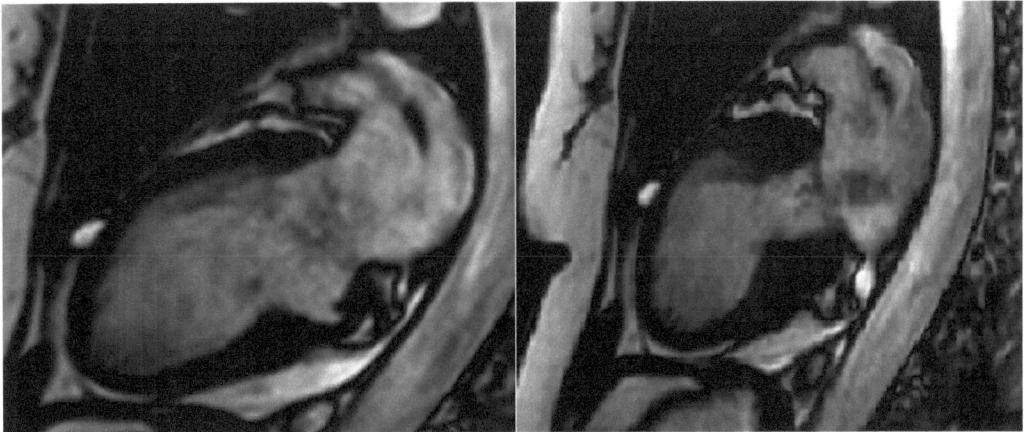

Figure 11: Diastolic (left panel) and systolic (right panel) phases of a two-chamber LV view demonstrating extensive apical akinesia with hyperdynamic basal function typical of Takotsubo cardiomyopathy.

CMR AND CARDIAC RESYNCHRONISATION THERAPY

The use of echocardiographic measures of dyssynchrony to guide the use of cardiac resynchronization therapy (CRT) has, so far, largely been disappointing [131]. Approximately 70% of suitable patients will respond to CRT but the reasons for non-response are numerous; it may be however, that in specific patient groups, imaging techniques can explain the reason for non-response or, with the correct parameters, be able to improve the response rate. Whilst advanced echocardiography is extremely important in this area, CMR with its added tissue characterization capability may also play a significant role.

A number of CMR techniques can be used to measure dyssynchrony and a number of dyssynchrony ratios produced, as yet no single index or measure has shown superiority in enough patient numbers to recommend its routine application [132]. CMR derived dyssynchrony measures may directly relate to outcome, with the more dyssynchrony equating to worse outcome and potentially those with the most severe intraventricular dyssynchrony not actually benefiting from CRT [133]. However, the burden and position of LV scar also appears to play an important role in response; the addition of LGE scar imaging to a tissue tagging measure of dyssynchrony allowed a 95% accurate prediction of CRT response defined as improvement in functional class [134]. Using CMR to define the location of LV scar and then positioning the LV lead away from regions with scar (particularly from the usual target of the inferolateral LV segments [135]) improves clinical outcome at a median follow-up period of 666 days; in fact LV pacing in areas with CMR identified scar was associated with the worse outcomes in this cohort of 559 patients [136]. CMR is superior to SPECT in accurately identifying significant inferolateral LV scar which may predict poor CRT response [137]. Poor RV function (EF<30%) as measured by CMR is also a predictor of low response rate (likelihood of response 18%) [138].

More recently investigators have used CMR images (venous anatomy [139], coronary artery anatomy [140], myocardial scar and dyssynchrony) fused with fluoroscopy in order to plan and then perform CRT procedures [141]. Shetty *et al.* [141] demonstrated feasibility in a cohort of 20 patients and improved the acute response rate by 10% (as measured by improved LV dp/dt) and in those where the ideal myocardial segment identified by CMR was successfully paced, 92% responded by echo criteria (reduction in end-systolic volume of >15%). However, the added time required for CMR interpretation and image fusion was at least 2.5 hours per patient, and so this technique is not yet ready for routine clinical use, but it does suggest that CMR will play an important role in maximising CRT response in the future.

CMR FOLLOWING CARDIAC TRANSPLANTATION

In the period following cardiac transplantation there is relatively intense surveillance in order to monitor cardiac function and to detect organ rejection. CMR is more accurate than echocardiography and more reproducible in measuring LV volumes and ejection fraction in this group [142]. The ability to non-invasively detect transplant rejection, preventing the need for repeated myocardial biopsies would have the potential to avoid significant morbidity. A number of different CMR sequences have been studied [143] and the most promising is the measurement of myocardial T_2 signal intensity [144] or T_2 relaxation time [145]. Increasing T_2 weighted signal intensity and/or relaxation time appears to correlate with inflammation suggesting graft rejection. Validation in larger numbers is needed, but if confirmed, it may be possible to reduce the number of myocardial biopsies required in transplant recipients. Alongside this, the discovery of LGE in transplant recipients is an adverse sign, correlating with increased hospitalization and death at 1 year [146].

CONCLUSION

CMR has become a powerful tool for use in heart failure. Established and emerging CMR techniques now enable multi-parametric *in vivo* characterization of the heart, from changes in global LV structure and function, to changes in tissue composition, mechanics, perfusion, as well as exploration of calcium channel function and gene expression. In addition, novel techniques for cell tracking and molecular imaging can be used in both clinical and preclinical research. Many of the techniques described in this chapter can be combined in a single imaging study, providing a comprehensive assessment of the heart as a function of disease progression or treatment, thereby allowing unprecedented insight into the patho-physiology of the diverse diseases that result in heart failure. Major challenges for the future include harnessing the huge volume of information that CMR is capable of providing in order to guide our clinical decision making, showing consistent incremental benefit through its use, and by making CMR more accessible, allowing its benefit to reach as many people as possible. This chapter has summarized the current and emerging CMR techniques as applied to the syndrome of heart failure, has related their use to the different clinical areas and provided the reader with a springboard for further interest and research - there is likely to be continued rapid growth in the use of CMR in heart failure in the future.

CONFLICT OF INTEREST

The author(s) confirm that this chapter content has no conflict of interest.

ACKNOWLEDGEMENTS

The authors would like to thank Dr. Filip Zemrak, Dr. Redha Boubertakh and Dr. Laura-Ann Mcgill for valuable assistance with images.

REFERENCES

[1]   McMurray JJV, Adamopoulos S, Anker SD, Auricchio A, Böhm M, Dickstein K, *et al*. ESC guidelines for the diagnosis and treatment of acute and chronic heart failure 2012: The Task Force for the Diagnosis and Treatment of Acute and Chronic Heart Failure 2012 of the European Society of Cardiology. Developed in collaboration with the Heart Failure Association (HFA) of the ESC. Eur J Heart Fail 2012; 14: 803-69.

[2]   British Society of Heart Failure. National Heart Failure Audit (April 2011-March2012) 2012.

[3]   Roger VL, Go AS, Lloyd-Jones DM, Benjamin EJ, Berry JD, Borden WB, *et al*. Heart Disease and Stroke Statistics—2012 Update A Report From the American Heart Association. Circulation 2012; 125: e2-e220.

[4]   Slaughter RE, Mottram PM. What should be the principle imaging test in heart failure--CMR or echocardiography? JACC Cardiovasc Imaging 2010; 3: 776-82.

[5]   Notghi A, Low CS. Myocardial perfusion scintigraphy: past, present and future. Br J Radiol 2011; 84 Spec No 3: S229-236.

[6]   Gewirtz H. Cardiac PET: A Versatile, Quantitative Measurement Tool for Heart Failure Management. JACC: Cardiovascular Imaging 2011; 4: 292-302.

[7]   Karamitsos TD, Francis JM, Myerson S, Selvanayagam JB, Neubauer S. The role of cardiovascular magnetic resonance imaging in heart failure. J Am Coll Cardiol 2009; 54: 1407-24.

[8]   Francis JM, Pennell DJ. Treatment of claustrophobia for cardiovascular magnetic resonance: use and effectiveness of mild sedation. J Cardiovasc Magn Reson 2000; 2: 139-41.

[9]   Von Knobelsdorff-Brenkenhoff F, Bublak A, El-Mahmoud S, Wassmuth R, Opitz C, Schulz-Menger J. Single-centre survey of the application of cardiovascular magnetic

resonance in clinical routine. Eur Heart J Cardiovasc Imaging 2012; doi: 10.1093/ehjci/jes125.

[10]   Chopra T, Kandukurti K, Shah S, Ahmed R, Panesar M. Understanding Nephrogenic Systemic Fibrosis. International Journal of Nephrology 2012; 2012: 1-14.

[11]   Naehle CP, Kreuz J, Strach K, Schwab JO, Pingel S, Luechinger R, *et al.* Safety, feasibility, and diagnostic value of cardiac magnetic resonance imaging in patients with cardiac pacemakers and implantable cardioverters/defibrillators at 1.5 T. Am Heart J 2011; 161: 1096-105.

[12]   Beinart R, Nazarian S. MRI-Conditional Cardiac Implantable Electronic Devices: What's New and What Can We Expect in the Future? Curr Treat Options Cardiovasc Med 2012; 14: 558-64.

[13]   Teo KSL, Carbone A, Piantadosi C, Chew DP, Hammett CJK, Brown MA, *et al.* Cardiac MRI assessment of left and right ventricular parameters in healthy Australian normal volunteers. Heart Lung and Circulation 2008; 17: 313-7.

[14]   Anderson LJ, Wonke B, Prescott E, Holden S, Walker JM, Pennell DJ. Comparison of effects of oral deferiprone and subcutaneous desferrioxamine on myocardial iron concentrations and ventricular function in beta-thalassaemia. Lancet 2002; 360: 516-20.

[15]   Westwood M, Anderson LJ, Firmin DN, Gatehouse PD, Charrier CC, Wonke B, *et al.* A single breath-hold multiecho T2* cardiovascular magnetic resonance technique for diagnosis of myocardial iron overload. J Magn Reson Imaging 2003; 18: 33-9.

[16]   Carpenter J-P, He T, Kirk P, Roughton M, Anderson LJ, De Noronha SV, *et al.* On T2* magnetic resonance and cardiac iron. Circulation 2011; 123: 1519-28.

[17]   Chouliaras G, Berdoukas V, Ladis V, Kattamis A, Chatziliami A, Fragodimitri C, *et al.* Impact of magnetic resonance imaging on cardiac mortality in thalassemia major. J Magn Reson Imaging 2011; 34: 56-9.

[18]   Simonetti OP, Finn JP, White RD, Laub G, Henry DA. Black blood'' T2-weighted inversion-recovery MR imaging of the heart. Radiology 1996; 199: 49-57.

[19]   Abdel-Aty H, Boye P, Zagrosek A, Wassmuth R, Kumar A, Messroghli D, *et al.* Diagnostic performance of cardiovascular magnetic resonance in patients with suspected acute myocarditis - Comparison of different approaches. Journal of the American College of Cardiology 2005; 45: 1815-22.

[20]   Phrommintikul A, Abdel-Aty H, Schulz-Menger J, Friedrich MG, Taylor AJ. Acute oedema in the evaluation of microvascular reperfusion and myocardial salvage in reperfused myocardial infarction with cardiac magnetic resonance imaging. Eur J Radiol 2009.

[21]   Petersen JW, Forder JR, Thomas JD, Moyé LA, Lawson M, Loghin C, *et al.* Quantification of myocardial segmental function in acute and chronic ischemic heart disease and implications for cardiovascular cell therapy trials: a review from the NHLBI-Cardiovascular Cell Therapy Research Network. JACC Cardiovasc Imaging 2011; 4: 671-9.

[22]   Shehata ML, Cheng S, Osman NF, Bluemke DA, Lima JAC. Myocardial tissue tagging with cardiovascular magnetic resonance. J Cardiovasc Magn Reson 2009; 11: 55.

[23]   Kuijer JPA, Marcus JT, Götte MJW, Van Rossum AC, Heethaar RM. Three-dimensional myocardial strains at end-systole and during diastole in the left ventricle of normal humans. J Cardiovasc Magn Reson 2002; 4: 341-51.

[24]   Moore CC, Lugo-Olivieri CH, McVeigh ER, Zerhouni EA. Three-dimensional systolic strain patterns in the normal human left ventricle: characterization with tagged MR imaging. Radiology 2000; 214: 453-66.

[25]   Hollingsworth KG, Blamire AM, Keavney BD, Macgowan GA. Left ventricular torsion, energetics, and diastolic function in normal human aging. Am J Physiol Heart Circ Physiol 2012; 302: H885-892.

[26]   Ahmed MI, Desai RV, Gaddam KK, Venkatesh BA, Agarwal S, Inusah S, *et al.* Relation of torsion and myocardial strains to LV ejection fraction in hypertension. JACC Cardiovasc Imaging 2012; 5: 273-81.

[27]   Simpson RM, Keegan J, Firmin DN. MR assessment of regional myocardial mechanics. Journal of Magnetic Resonance Imaging: JMRI 2012; 10.1002/jmri.23756.

[28]   Aletras AH, Ding S, Balaban RS, Wen H. DENSE: displacement encoding with stimulated echoes in cardiac functional MRI. J Magn Reson 1999; 137: 247-52.

[29]   Spottiswoode BS, Zhong X, Lorenz CH, Mayosi BM, Meintjes EM, Epstein FH. 3D myocardial tissue tracking with slice followed cine DENSE MRI. J Magn Reson Imaging 2008; 27: 1019-27.

[30]   Hess AT, Zhong X, Spottiswoode BS, Epstein FH, Meintjes EM. Myocardial 3D strain calculation by combining cine displacement encoding with stimulated echoes (DENSE) and cine strain encoding (SENC) imaging. Magn Reson Med 2009; 62: 77-84.

[31]   Morton G, Schuster A, Jogiya R, Kutty S, Beerbaum P, Nagel E. Inter-study reproducibility of cardiovascular magnetic resonance myocardial feature tracking. J Cardiovasc Magn Reson 2012; 14: 43.

[32]   Schuster A, Kutty S, Padiyath A, Parish V, Gribben P, Danford DA, *et al.* Cardiovascular magnetic resonance myocardial feature tracking detects quantitative wall motion during dobutamine stress. J Cardiovasc Magn Reson 2011; 13: 58.

[33]   Augustine D, Lewandowski AJ, Lazdam M, Rai A, Francis J, Myerson S, *et al.* Global and regional left ventricular myocardial deformation measures by magnetic resonance feature tracking in healthy volunteers: comparison with tagging and relevance of gender. J Cardiovasc Magn Reson 2013; 15: 8.

[34]   Klein C, Schmal TR, Nekolla SG, Schnackenburg B, Fleck E, Nagel E. Mechanism of late gadolinium enhancement in patients with acute myocardial infarction. Journal of Cardiovascular Magnetic Resonance 2007; 9: 653-8.

[35]   Mewton N, Liu CY, Croisille P, Bluemke D, Lima JAC. Assessment of myocardial fibrosis with cardiovascular magnetic resonance. J Am Coll Cardiol 2011; 57: 891-903.

[36]   Schaper J, Speiser B. The extracellular matrix in the failing human heart. Basic Res Cardiol 1992; 87 Suppl 1: 303-9.

[37]   Ugander M, Oki AJ, Hsu L-Y, Kellman P, Greiser A, Aletras AH, *et al.* Extracellular volume imaging by magnetic resonance imaging provides insights into overt and sub-clinical myocardial pathology. Eur Heart J 2012; 33: 1268-78.

[38]   Messroghli DR, Radjenovic A, Kozerke S, Higgins DM, Sivananthan MU, Ridgway JP. Modified Look-Locker inversion recovery (MOLLI) for high-resolution T1 mapping of the heart. Magn Reson Med 2004; 52: 141-6.

[39]   Iles L, Pfluger H, Phrommintikul A, Cherayath J, Aksit P, Gupta SN, *et al.* Evaluation of diffuse myocardial fibrosis in heart failure with cardiac magnetic resonance contrast-enhanced T1 mapping. J Am Coll Cardiol 2008; 52: 1574-80.

[40]   Sibley CT, Noureldin RA, Gai N, Nacif MS, Liu S, Turkbey EB, *et al*. T1 Mapping in Cardiomyopathy at Cardiac MR: Comparison with Endomyocardial Biopsy. Radiology 2012; 265: 724-32.

[41]   Ng ACT, Auger D, Delgado V, Van Elderen SGC, Bertini M, Siebelink H-M, *et al*. Association between diffuse myocardial fibrosis by cardiac magnetic resonance contrast-enhanced T₁ mapping and subclinical myocardial dysfunction in diabetic patients: a pilot study. Circ Cardiovasc Imaging 2012; 5: 51-9.

[42]   Flett AS, Hayward MP, Ashworth MT, Hansen MS, Taylor AM, Elliott PM, *et al*. Equilibrium contrast cardiovascular magnetic resonance for the measurement of diffuse myocardial fibrosis: preliminary validation in humans. Circulation 2010; 122: 138-44.

[43]   Flett AS, Sado DM, Quarta G, Mirabel M, Pellerin D, Herrey AS, *et al*. Diffuse myocardial fibrosis in severe aortic stenosis: an equilibrium contrast cardiovascular magnetic resonance study. Eur Heart J Cardiovasc Imaging 2012; 10.1093/ehjci/jes102.

[44]   Dass S, Suttie JJ, Piechnik SK, Ferreira VM, Holloway CJ, Banerjee R, *et al*. Myocardial tissue characterization using magnetic resonance noncontrast T1 mapping in hypertrophic and dilated cardiomyopathy. Circ Cardiovasc Imaging 2012; 5: 726-33.

[45]   Geelen T, Paulis LEM, Coolen BF, Nicolay K, Strijkers GJ. Contrast-enhanced MRI of murine myocardial infarction - Part I. NMR in Biomedicine 2012; 25: 953-68.

[46]   Bers DM. Altered cardiac myocyte Ca regulation in heart failure. Physiology (Bethesda) 2006; 21: 380-7.

[47]   Natanzon A, Aletras AH, Hsu L-Y, Arai AE. Determining canine myocardial area at risk with manganese-enhanced MR imaging. Radiology 2005; 236: 859-66.

[48]   Hu TC-C, Christian TF, Aletras AH, Taylor JL, Koretsky AP, Arai AE. Manganese enhanced magnetic resonance imaging of normal and ischemic canine heart. Magn Reson Med 2005; 54: 196-200.

[49]   Waghorn B, Edwards T, Yang Y, Chuang K-H, Yanasak N, Hu TC-C. Monitoring dynamic alterations in calcium homeostasis by T (1)-weighted and T (1)-mapping cardiac manganese-enhanced MRI in a murine myocardial infarction model. NMR Biomed 2008; 21: 1102-11.

[50]   Waghorn B, Yang Y, Baba A, Matsuda T, Schumacher A, Yanasak N, *et al*. Assessing manganese efflux using SEA0400 and cardiac T1-mapping manganese-enhanced MRI in a murine model. NMR Biomed 2009; 22: 874-81.

[51]   Zheng W, Kim H, Zhao Q. Comparative toxicokinetics of manganese chloride and methylcyclopentadienyl manganese tricarbonyl (MMT) in Sprague-Dawley rats. Toxicol Sci 2000; 54: 295-301.

[52]   Gilbert SH, Benson AP, Li P, Holden AV. Regional localisation of left ventricular sheet structure: integration with current models of cardiac fibre, sheet and band structure. Eur J Cardiothorac Surg 2007; 32: 231-49.

[53]   St John Sutton MG, Lie JT, Anderson KR, O'Brien PC, Frye RL. Histopathological specificity of hypertrophic obstructive cardiomyopathy. Myocardial fibre disarray and myocardial fibrosis. Br Heart J 1980; 44: 433-43.

[54]   Wu M-T, Tseng W-YI, Su M-YM, Liu C-P, Chiou K-R, Wedeen VJ, *et al*. Diffusion tensor magnetic resonance imaging mapping the fiber architecture remodeling in human myocardium after infarction: correlation with viability and wall motion. Circulation 2006; 114: 1036-45.

[55]   Hsu EW, Muzikant AL, Matulevicius SA, Penland RC, Henriquez CS. Magnetic resonance myocardial fiber-orientation mapping with direct histological correlation. Am J Physiol 1998; 274: H1627-1634.

[56]   Scollan DF, Holmes A, Winslow R, Forder J. Histological validation of myocardial microstructure obtained from diffusion tensor magnetic resonance imaging. Am J Physiol 1998; 275: H2308-2318.

[57]   Edelman RR, Gaa J, Wedeen VJ, Loh E, Hare JM, Prasad P, *et al. In vivo* measurement of water diffusion in the human heart. Magn Reson Med 1994; 32: 423-8.

[58]   McGill L-A, Ismail TF, Nielles-Vallespin S, Ferreira P, Scott AD, Roughton M, *et al.* Reproducibility of *in vivo* diffusion tensor cardiovascular magnetic resonance in hypertrophic cardiomyopathy. Journal of Cardiovascular Magnetic Resonance 2012; 14: 86.

[59]   Chong JJH. Cell therapy for left ventricular dysfunction: an overview for cardiac clinicians. Heart Lung Circ 2012; 21: 532-42.

[60]   Ruggiero A, Thorek DLJ, Guenoun J, Krestin GP, Bernsen MR. Cell tracking in cardiac repair: what to image and how to image. Eur Radiol 2012; 22: 189-204.

[61]   Winter EM, Hogers B, Van der Graaf LM, Gittenberger-de Groot AC, Poelmann RE, Van der Weerd L. Cell tracking using iron oxide fails to distinguish dead from living transplanted cells in the infarcted heart. Magn Reson Med 2010; 63: 817-21.

[62]   Hsiao J-K, Chu H-H, Wang Y-H, Lai C-W, Chou P-T, Hsieh S-T, *et al.* Macrophage physiological function after superparamagnetic iron oxide labeling. NMR Biomed 2008; 21: 820-9.

[63]   Richards JMJ, Shaw CA, Lang NN, Williams MC, Semple SIK, MacGillivray TJ, *et al. In vivo* mononuclear cell tracking using superparamagnetic particles of iron oxide: feasibility and safety in humans. Circ Cardiovasc Imaging 2012; 5: 509-17.

[64]   Schäfer R, Kehlbach R, Müller M, Bantleon R, Kluba T, Ayturan M, *et al.* Labeling of human mesenchymal stromal cells with superparamagnetic iron oxide leads to a decrease in migration capacity and colony formation ability. Cytotherapy 2009; 11: 68-78.

[65]   Yang J-X, Tang W-L, Wang X-X. Superparamagnetic iron oxide nanoparticles may affect endothelial progenitor cell migration ability and adhesion capacity. Cytotherapy 2010; 12: 251-9.

[66]   Kostura L, Kraitchman DL, Mackay AM, Pittenger MF, Bulte JWM. Feridex labeling of mesenchymal stem cells inhibits chondrogenesis but not adipogenesis or osteogenesis. NMR Biomed 2004; 17: 513-7.

[67]   Aime S, Castelli DD, Crich SG, Gianolio E, Terreno E. Pushing the sensitivity envelope of lanthanide-based magnetic resonance imaging (MRI) contrast agents for molecular imaging applications. Acc Chem Res 2009; 42: 822-31.

[68]   Brekke C, Morgan SC, Lowe AS, Meade TJ, Price J, Williams SCR, *et al.* The *in vitro* effects of a bimodal contrast agent on cellular functions and relaxometry. NMR Biomed 2007; 20: 77-89.

[69]   Chen J, Lanza GM, Wickline SA. Quantitative magnetic resonance fluorine imaging: today and tomorrow. Wiley Interdiscip Rev Nanomed Nanobiotechnol 2010; 2: 431-40.

[70]   Balschi JA. *In vivo* clinical measures of intermediary metabolism are inadequate: can a new magnetic resonance spectroscopy technology do better? Circ Cardiovasc Imaging 2012; 5: 171-4.

[71] Neubauer S, Krahe T, Schindler R, Horn M, Hillenbrand H, Entzeroth C, *et al*. 31P magnetic resonance spectroscopy in dilated cardiomyopathy and coronary artery disease. Altered cardiac high-energy phosphate metabolism in heart failure. Circulation 1992; 86: 1810-8.

[72] Myerson S, Francis JM, Neubauer S. Cardiovascular Magnetic Resonance. Oxford University Press; 2010.

[73] Ardenkjaer-Larsen JH, Fridlund B, Gram A, Hansson G, Hansson L, Lerche MH, *et al*. Increase in signal-to-noise ratio of > 10,000 times in liquid-state NMR. Proc Natl Acad Sci USA 2003; 100: 10158-63.

[74] Holloway C, Clarke K. Is MR spectroscopy of the heart ready for humans? Heart Lung Circ 2010; 19: 154-60.

[75] Schroeder MA, Clarke K, Neubauer S, Tyler DJ. Hyperpolarized magnetic resonance: a novel technique for the *in vivo* assessment of cardiovascular disease. Circulation 2011; 124: 1580-94.

[76] Assomull RG, Shakespeare C, Kalra PR, Lloyd G, Gulati A, Strange J, *et al*. Role of cardiovascular magnetic resonance as a gatekeeper to invasive coronary angiography in patients presenting with heart failure of unknown etiology. Circulation 2011; 124: 1351-60.

[77] Hamilton-Craig C, Strugnell WE, Raffel OC, Porto I, Walters DL, Slaughter RE. CT angiography with cardiac MRI: non-invasive functional and anatomical assessment for the etiology in newly diagnosed heart failure. Int J Cardiovasc Imaging 2012; 28: 1111-22.

[78] Kim RJ, Wu E, Rafael A, Chen EL, Parker MA, Simonetti O, *et al*. The use of contrast-enhanced magnetic resonance imaging to identify reversible myocardial dysfunction. N Engl J Med 2000; 343: 1445-53.

[79] Glaveckaite S, Valeviciene N, Palionis D, Skorniakov V, Celutkiene J, Tamosiunas A, *et al*. Value of scar imaging and inotropic reserve combination for the prediction of segmental and global left ventricular functional recovery after revascularisation. J Cardiovasc Magn Reson 2011; 13: 35.

[80] Bonow RO, Maurer G, Lee KL, Holly TA, Binkley PF, Desvigne-Nickens P, *et al*. Myocardial viability and survival in ischemic left ventricular dysfunction. N Engl J Med 2011; 364: 1617-25.

[81] Cheong BYC, Muthupillai R, Wilson JM, Sung A, Huber S, Amin S, *et al*. Prognostic significance of delayed-enhancement magnetic resonance imaging: survival of 857 patients with and without left ventricular dysfunction. Circulation 2009; 120: 2069-76.

[82] Myerson SG, D' Arcy J, Mohiaddin R, Greenwood JP, Karamitsos TD, Francis JM, *et al*. Aortic regurgitation quantification using cardiovascular magnetic resonance: association with clinical outcome. Circulation 2012; 126: 1452-60.

[83] Kilner PJ, Manzara CC, Mohiaddin RH, Pennell DJ, Sutton MG, Firmin DN, *et al*. Magnetic resonance jet velocity mapping in mitral and aortic valve stenosis. Circulation 1993; 87: 1239-48.

[84] Caruthers SD, Lin SJ, Brown P, Watkins MP, Williams TA, Lehr KA, *et al*. Practical value of cardiac magnetic resonance imaging for clinical quantification of aortic valve stenosis: comparison with echocardiography. Circulation 2003; 108: 2236-43.

[85] Gabriel RS, Kerr AJ, Raffel OC, Stewart RA, Cowan BR, Occleshaw CJ. Mapping of mitral regurgitant defects by cardiovascular magnetic resonance in moderate or severe mitral regurgitation secondary to mitral valve prolapse. J Cardiovasc Magn Reson 2008; 10: 16.

[86]   Myerson SG. Heart valve disease: investigation by cardiovascular magnetic resonance. J Cardiovasc Magn Reson 2012; 14: 7.

[87]   Assomull RG, Prasad SK, Lyne J, Smith G, Burman ED, Khan M, *et al.* Cardiovascular magnetic resonance, fibrosis, and prognosis in dilated cardiomyopathy. J Am Coll Cardiol 2006; 48: 1977-85.

[88]   Lehrke S, Lossnitzer D, Schöb M, Steen H, Merten C, Kemmling H, *et al.* Use of cardiovascular magnetic resonance for risk stratification in chronic heart failure: prognostic value of late gadolinium enhancement in patients with non-ischaemic dilated cardiomyopathy. Heart 2011; 97: 727-32.

[89]   Yilmaz A, Gdynia H-J, Baccouche H, Mahrholdt H, Meinhardt G, Basso C, *et al.* Cardiac involvement in patients with Becker muscular dystrophy: new diagnostic and pathophysiological insights by a CMR approach. J Cardiovasc Magn Reson 2008; 10: 50.

[90]   Raman SV, Sparks EA, Baker PM, McCarthy B, Wooley CF. Mid-myocardial fibrosis by cardiac magnetic resonance in patients with lamin A/C cardiomyopathy: possible substrate for diastolic dysfunction. J Cardiovasc Magn Reson 2007; 9: 907-13.

[91]   Moon JCC, Fisher NG, McKenna WJ, Pennell DJ. Detection of apical hypertrophic cardiomyopathy by cardiovascular magnetic resonance in patients with non-diagnostic echocardiography. Heart 2004; 90: 645-9.

[92]   Moon JCC, McKenna WJ, McCrohon JA, Elliott PM, Smith GC, Pennell DJ. Toward clinical risk assessment in hypertrophic cardiomyopathy with gadolinium cardiovascular magnetic resonance. J Am Coll Cardiol 2003; 41: 1561-7.

[93]   Bruder O, Wagner A, Jensen CJ, Schneider S, Ong P, Kispert E-M, *et al.* Myocardial scar visualized by cardiovascular magnetic resonance imaging predicts major adverse events in patients with hypertrophic cardiomyopathy. J Am Coll Cardiol 2010; 56: 875-87.

[94]   Hen Y, Iguchi N, Machida H, Takada K, Utanohara Y, Sumiyoshi T. High signal intensity on T2-weighted cardiac magnetic resonance imaging correlates with the ventricular tachyarrhythmia in hypertrophic cardiomyopathy. Heart Vessels 2012; doi: 10.1007/s00380-012-0300-3.

[95]   Marcus FI, McKenna WJ, Sherrill D, Basso C, Bauce B, Bluemke DA, *et al.* Diagnosis of arrhythmogenic right ventricular cardiomyopathy/dysplasia: proposed modification of the Task Force Criteria. Eur Heart J 2010; 31: 806-14.

[96]   Fairbairn TA, Motwani M, Greenwood JP, Plein S. CMR for the Diagnosis of Right Heart Disease. JACC: Cardiovascular Imaging 2012; 5: 227-9.

[97]   Val-Bernal JF, Garijo MF, Rodriguez-Villar D, Val D. Non-compaction of the ventricular myocardium: a cardiomyopathy in search of a pathoanatomical definition. Histol Histopathol 2010; 25: 495-503.

[98]   Habib G, Charron P, Eicher J-C, Giorgi R, Donal E, Laperche T, *et al.* Isolated left ventricular non-compaction in adults: clinical and echocardiographic features in 105 patients. Results from a French registry. Eur J Heart Fail 2011; 13: 177-85.

[99]   Petersen SE, Selvanayagam JB, Wiesmann F, Robson MD, Francis JM, Anderson RH, *et al.* Left ventricular non-compaction: insights from cardiovascular magnetic resonance imaging. J Am Coll Cardiol 2005; 46: 101-5.

[100]   Nucifora G, Aquaro GD, Pingitore A, Masci PG, Lombardi M. Myocardial fibrosis in isolated left ventricular non-compaction and its relation to disease severity. Eur J Heart Fail 2011; 13: 170-6.

[101] Moon JC, Sheppard M, Reed E, Lee P, Elliott PM, Pennell DJ. The histological basis of late gadolinium enhancement cardiovascular magnetic resonance in a patient with Anderson-Fabry disease. J Cardiovasc Magn Reson 2006; 8: 479-82.

[102] Imbriaco M, Pisani A, Spinelli L, Cuocolo A, Messalli G, Capuano E, *et al.* Effects of enzyme-replacement therapy in patients with Anderson-Fabry disease: a prospective long-term cardiac magnetic resonance imaging study. Heart 2009; 95: 1103-7.

[103] Pellaton C, Monney P, Ludman AJ, Schwitter J, Eeckhout E, Hugli O, *et al.* Clinical features of myocardial infarction and myocarditis in young adults: a retrospective study. BMJ Open 2012; 2.

[104] Friedrich MG, Sechtem U, Schulz-Menger J, Holmvang G, Alakija P, Cooper LT, *et al.* Cardiovascular Magnetic Resonance in Myocarditis: A JACC White Paper. J Am Coll Cardiol 2009; 53: 1475-87.

[105] Monney PA, Sekhri N, Burchell T, Knight C, Davies C, Deaner A, *et al.* Acute myocarditis presenting as acute coronary syndrome: role of early cardiac magnetic resonance in its diagnosis. Heart 2011; 97: 1312-8.

[106] Guglin M, Nallamshetty L. Myocarditis: Diagnosis and Treatment. Myocarditis: diagnosis and treatment. Curr Treat Options Cardiovasc Med 2012; 14(6): 637-51

[107] Lurz P, Eitel I, Adam J, Steiner J, Grothoff M, Desch S, *et al.* Diagnostic performance of CMR imaging compared with EMB in patients with suspected myocarditis. JACC Cardiovasc Imaging 2012; 5: 513-24.

[108] Grün S, Schumm J, Greulich S, Wagner A, Schneider S, Bruder O, *et al.* Long-term follow-up of biopsy-proven viral myocarditis: predictors of mortality and incomplete recovery. J Am Coll Cardiol 2012; 59: 1604-15.

[109] Kirk P, Roughton M, Porter JB, Walker JM, Tanner MA, Patel J, *et al.* Cardiac T2* magnetic resonance for prediction of cardiac complications in thalassemia major. Circulation 2009; 120: 1961-8.

[110] Anderson LJ, Westwood MA, Holden S, Davis B, Prescott E, Wonke B, *et al.* Myocardial iron clearance during reversal of siderotic cardiomyopathy with intravenous desferrioxamine: a prospective study using T2* cardiovascular magnetic resonance. Br J Haematol 2004; 127: 348-55.

[111] Modell B, Khan M, Darlison M, Westwood MA, Ingram D, Pennell DJ. Improved survival of thalassaemia major in the UK and relation to T2* cardiovascular magnetic resonance. J Cardiovasc Magn Reson 2008; 10: 42.

[112] Smedema J-P, Snoep G, Van Kroonenburgh MPG, Van Geuns R-J, Dassen WRM, Gorgels APM, *et al.* Evaluation of the accuracy of gadolinium-enhanced cardiovascular magnetic resonance in the diagnosis of cardiac sarcoidosis. J Am Coll Cardiol 2005; 45: 1683-90.

[113] Langah R, Spicer K, Gebregziabher M, Gordon L. Effectiveness of prolonged fasting 18f-FDG PET-CT in the detection of cardiac sarcoidosis. J Nucl Cardiol 2009; 16: 801-10.

[114] Ashwath, M, Kim, HW, Parker, M, Kim, RJ. Prognostic value of delayed enhancement cardiovascular magnetic resonance in patients with sarcoidosis. Journal of Cardiovascular Magnetic Resonance 2012; 14(Suppl 1): O13.doi: 10.1186/1532-429X-14-S1-O13.

[115] Patel AR, Klein MR, Chandra S, Spencer KT, DeCara JM, Lang RM, *et al.* Myocardial damage in patients with sarcoidosis and preserved left ventricular systolic function: an observational study. Eur J Heart Fail 2011; 13: 1231-7.

[116] Sharma N, Howlett J. Current state of cardiac amyloidosis. Current Opinion in Cardiology 2013; 28: 242-8.

[117] Leone O, Longhi S, Quarta CC, Ragazzini T, De Giorgi LB, Pasquale F, *et al.* New pathological insights into cardiac amyloidosis: implications for non-invasive diagnosis. Amyloid 2012; 19: 99-105.

[118] Austin BA, Tang WHW, Rodriguez ER, Tan C, Flamm SD, Taylor DO, *et al.* Delayed hyper-enhancement magnetic resonance imaging provides incremental diagnostic and prognostic utility in suspected cardiac amyloidosis. JACC Cardiovasc Imaging 2009; 2: 1369-77.

[119] Mekinian A, Lions C, Leleu X, Duhamel A, Lamblin N, Coiteux V, *et al.* Prognosis assessment of cardiac involvement in systemic AL amyloidosis by magnetic resonance imaging. Am J Med 2010; 123: 864-8.

[120] Mongeon F-P, Jerosch-Herold M, Coelho-Filho OR, Blankstein R, Falk RH, Kwong RY. Quantification of Extracellular Matrix Expansion by CMR in Infiltrative Heart Disease. J Am Coll Cardiol Img 2012; 5: 897-907.

[121] Banypersad SM, Sado DM, Flett AS, Gibbs SDJ, Pinney JH, Maestrini V, *et al.* Quantification of myocardial extracellular volume fraction in systemic Al amyloidosis: an equilibrium contrast cardiovascular magnetic resonance study. Circ Cardiovasc Imaging 2013; 6: 34-9.

[122] Neilan TG, Coelho-Filho OR, Pena-Herrera D, Shah RV, Jerosch-Herold M, Francis SA, *et al.* Left ventricular mass in patients with a cardiomyopathy after treatment with anthracyclines. Am J Cardiol 2012; 110: 1679-86.

[123] Sliwa K, Hilfiker-Kleiner D, Petrie MC, Mebazaa A, Pieske B, Buchmann E, *et al.* Current state of knowledge on aetiology, diagnosis, management, and therapy of peripartum cardiomyopathy: a position statement from the Heart Failure Association of the European Society of Cardiology Working Group on peripartum cardiomyopathy. Eur J Heart Fail 2010; 12: 767-78.

[124] Webb JAW, Thomsen HS, Morcos SK. The use of iodinated and gadolinium contrast media during pregnancy and lactation. Eur Radiol 2005; 15: 1234-40.

[125] Looi JL, Ruygrok P, Royle G, Raos Z, Hood C, Kerr AJ. Acute eosinophilic endomyocarditis: early diagnosis and localisation of the lesion by cardiac magnetic resonance imaging. Int J Cardiovasc Imaging 2010; 26 Suppl 1: 151-4.

[126] Moosig F, Richardt G, Gross WL. A fatal attraction: eosinophils and the heart. Rheumatology (Oxford) 2013.

[127] Machado FS, Jelicks LA, Kirchhoff LV, Shirani J, Nagajyothi F, Mukherjee S, *et al.* Chagas heart disease: report on recent developments. Cardiol Rev 2012; 20: 53-65.

[128] Regueiro A, García-Álvarez A, Sitges M, Ortiz-Pérez JT, De Caralt MT, Pinazo MJ, *et al.* Myocardial involvement in Chagas disease: Insights from cardiac magnetic resonance. Int J Cardiol 2011.

[129] Essa E, Velez MR, Smith S, Giri S, Raman SV, Gumina RJ. Cardiovascular magnetic resonance in wet beriberi. J Cardiovasc Magn Reson 2011; 13: 41.

[130] Eitel I, Von Knobelsdorff-Brenkenhoff F, Bernhardt P, Carbone I, Muellerleile K, Aldrovandi A, *et al.* Clinical characteristics and cardiovascular magnetic resonance findings in stress (takotsubo) cardiomyopathy. JAMA 2011; 306: 277-86.

[131] Chung ES, Leon AR, Tavazzi L, Sun J-P, Nihoyannopoulos P, Merlino J, *et al.* Results of the Predictors of Response to CRT (PROSPECT) trial. Circulation 2008; 117: 2608-16.

[132] Leyva F, Foley PWX. Current and future role of cardiovascular magnetic resonance in cardiac resynchronization therapy. Heart Fail Rev 2011; 16: 251-62.

[133]   Chalil S, Stegemann B, Muhyaldeen S, Khadjooi K, Smith REA, Jordan PJ, *et al.* Intraventricular dyssynchrony predicts mortality and morbidity after cardiac resynchronization therapy: a study using cardiovascular magnetic resonance tissue synchronization imaging. J Am Coll Cardiol 2007; 50: 243-52.

[134]   Bilchick KC, Dimaano V, Wu KC, Helm RH, Weiss RG, Lima JA, *et al.* Cardiac magnetic resonance assessment of dyssynchrony and myocardial scar predicts function class improvement following cardiac resynchronization therapy. JACC Cardiovasc Imaging 2008; 1: 561-8.

[135]   Chalil S, Stegemann B, Muhyaldeen SA, Khadjooi K, Foley PW, Smith REA, *et al.* Effect of posterolateral left ventricular scar on mortality and morbidity following cardiac resynchronization therapy. Pacing Clin Electrophysiol 2007; 30: 1201-9.

[136]   Leyva F, Foley PWX, Chalil S, Ratib K, Smith REA, Prinzen F, *et al.* Cardiac resynchronization therapy guided by late gadolinium-enhancement cardiovascular magnetic resonance. J Cardiovasc Magn Reson 2011; 13: 29.

[137]   Yokokawa M, Tada H, Toyama T, Koyama K, Naito S, Oshima S, *et al.* Magnetic resonance imaging is superior to cardiac scintigraphy to identify nonresponders to cardiac resynchronization therapy. Pacing Clin Electrophysiol 2009; 32 Suppl 1: S57-62.

[138]   Alpendurada F, Guha K, Sharma R, Ismail TF, Clifford A, Banya W, *et al.* Right ventricular dysfunction is a predictor of non-response and clinical outcome following cardiac resynchronization therapy. J Cardiovasc Magn Reson 2011; 13: 68.

[139]   Duckett SG, Chiribiri A, Ginks MR, Sinclair S, Knowles BR, Botnar R, *et al.* Cardiac MRI to investigate myocardial scar and coronary venous anatomy using a slow infusion of dimeglumine gadobenate in patients undergoing assessment for cardiac resynchronization therapy. J Magn Reson Imaging 2011; 33: 87-95.

[140]   White JA, Fine N, Gula LJ, Yee R, Al-Admawi M, Zhang Q, *et al.* Fused whole-heart coronary and myocardial scar imaging using 3-T CMR. Implications for planning of cardiac resynchronization therapy and coronary revascularization. JACC Cardiovasc Imaging 2010; 3: 921-30.

[141]   Shetty AK, Duckett SG, Ginks MR, Ma Y, Sohal M, Bostock J, *et al.* Cardiac magnetic resonance-derived anatomy, scar, and dyssynchrony fused with fluoroscopy to guide LV lead placement in cardiac resynchronization therapy: a comparison with acute haemodynamic measures and echocardiographic reverse remodelling. Eur Heart J Cardiovasc Imaging 2012; doi: 10.1093/ehjci/jes270.

[142]   Bellenger NG, Marcus NJ, Rajappan K, Yacoub M, Banner NR, Pennell DJ. Comparison of techniques for the measurement of left ventricular function following cardiac transplantation. J Cardiovasc Magn Reson 2002; 4: 255-63.

[143]   Butler CR, Thompson R, Haykowsky M, Toma M, Paterson I. Cardiovascular magnetic resonance in the diagnosis of acute heart transplant rejection: a review. J Cardiovasc Magn Reson 2009; 11: 7.

[144]   Taylor AJ, Vaddadi G, Pfluger H, Butler M, Bergin P, Leet A, *et al.* Diagnostic performance of multisequential cardiac magnetic resonance imaging in acute cardiac allograft rejection. Eur J Heart Fail 2010; 12: 45-51.

[145]   Usman AA, Taimen K, Wasielewski M, McDonald J, Shah S, Giri S, *et al.* Cardiac magnetic resonance T2 mapping in the monitoring and follow-up of acute cardiac transplant rejection: a pilot study. Circ Cardiovasc Imaging 2012; 5: 782-90.

[146]   Butler CR, Kumar A, Toma M, Thompson R, Chow K, Isaac D, *et al*. Late Gadolinium Enhancement in Cardiac Transplant Patients Is Associated With Adverse Ventricular Functional Parameters and Clinical Outcomes. Can J Cardiol 2013; doi: 10.1016/j.cjca.2012.10.021.

Send Orders for Reprints to reprints@benthamscience.net

Latest Advances in Clinical and Pre-Clinical Cardiovascular MRI, 2014, Vol. 1, 41-63   **41**

CHAPTER 2

CMR Applications in Ischemic Heart Disease

Stamatios Lerakis[*] and John Palios

Emory University Hospital, Cardiology Division, and Emory University, School of Medicine, Atlanta, Georgia, USA

Abstract: Ischemic heart disease is the most frequent cause of cardiovascular morbidity and mortality. Early detection and accurate evaluation are essential to guide optimal patient treatment and assess the individual's prognosis. Cardiovascular Magnetic Resonance (CMR) has proven accuracy and is an established technique for the assessment of myocardial function both at rest and during stress. CMR is widely used for structural heart disease and its use in ischemic cardiomyopathy evaluation is growing. It allows stress perfusion analysis with high spatial and temporal resolution and applies to differentiate tissue, such as distinguishing between reversibly and irreversibly injured myocardium. Evaluation of ischemic heart disease with CMR includes imaging of coronary arteries, assessment of ventricular morphology and function, myocardial perfusion and viability. Late Gadolinium Enhancement (LGE) CMR techniques can clearly differentiate necrotic to viable areas of the myocardium leading to proper patients' revascularization management. CMR is considered to be a safe imaging modality with limited restrictions mainly to patients with implantable defibrillators and pacemakers. It is noninvasive and radiation-free and the burden of the high cost appears to diminish as it becomes more popular. CMR is considered to be a safe imaging modality with limited restrictions mainly to patients with implantable defibrillators and pacemakers. It is noninvasive and radiation-free and the burden of the high cost appears to diminish as it becomes more popular. CMR is an established imaging modality for both functional and structural ischemic heart disease.

Keywords: Cardiac imaging, coronary disease, gadolinium enhancement, ischemic cardiomyopathy, magnetic resonance, molecular imaging, myocardial viability, myocardial ischemia, perfusion imaging, stress imaging.

INTRODUCTION

Increased morbidity and mortality is described in patients suffering from ischemic cardiomyopathy [1]. Despite general medical progress, there is concern that the

*Address correspondence to Stamatios Lerakis: Division of Cardiology, Department of Medicine, Emory University School of Medicine, 1365 Clifton Rd NE, Suite AT-503, Atlanta GA 30322, USA; Tel: 404-778-5414; Fax: 404-778-3540; E-mail: sleraki@emory.edu

predominance of cardiovascular mortality will even increase in the future considering the growing prevalence of the cardiovascular disease risk factors such as hypertension, metabolic syndrome, obesity, diabetes and hypercholesterolemia. Cardiovascular magnetic resonance imaging (CMR) has a proven diagnostic accuracy and it is increasingly applied for the assessment of cardiovascular structure and function [2]. Applications of CMR imaging in ischemic cardiomyopathy include heart failure investigation, anomalous coronary artery identification, atherosclerotic coronary artery disease early detection and ischemic heart disease evaluation as well as myocardial tissue characterization [3].

CMR provides cine imaging of the heart, mostly based on steady-state free-precession acquisitions, with high blood-tissue contrast to allow for accurate cardiac chamber quantification and wall motion analysis both at rest and at stress. It enables myocardial perfusion studies to detect myocardial ischemia and gives insights into the morphology of the myocardial tissue. The latter characteristic enables CMR imaging to noninvasively differentiate various causes of myocardial injury like ischemia or inflammation, various stages of myocardial injury, like acute *versus* chronic and various severity grades of myocardial cell damage like reversible *versus* irreversible (scar). CMR appears to be the prominent part of multimodality imaging for patients with ischemic heart disease [4] and its use in managing patients with ischemic cardiomyopathy has been widely expanding during the last few years [5], successfully taking over other imaging techniques used for the investigation of ischemic heart disease such as dobutamine stress echocardiography (DSE), single photon emission computed tomography (SPECT), positron emission tomography (PET) and multidetector computed tomography (MDCT). Myocardial perfusion imaging techniques, stress CMR, late gadolinium enhancement (LGE) CMR have already been established in clinical practice for ischemic cardiomyopathy assessment [6], while the use of CMR spectroscopy, speckle tracking/strain CMR and molecular CMR in patients with ischemic heart disease is under investigation.

CMR IN CORONARY ARTERY DISEASE

CMR has already been widely used for cardiac structure abnormalities assessment [7]. Anomalous coronary artery identification is a common application for CMR since arterial tree visualization can be rapidly achieved with this test without radiation exposure [8]. Although unusual (less than 1%) of the general population and usually benign, congenital coronary anomalies in which the anomalous segment courses between the aorta and the main pulmonary artery are a well-recognized cause of myocardial ischemia especially among young adults. Congenital coronary abnormalities may also be a cause of sudden cardiac death. Catheter-based X-ray angiography has traditionally been the diagnostic imaging test to identify these anomalies, but the extended use of radiation and iodinated contrast agents and the minimal risk of vascular complications during the procedure is a concern, especially in young patients. On the other hand, CMR does not require ionizing radiation or iodinated contrast agents. Both two-dimensional breath-hold and targeted three-dimensional or whole-heart free-breathing navigator coronary CMR methods have been used with similar excellent results. The use of coronary CMR for suspected anomalous coronary disease is also very helpful when an intramural course is suspected or present (myocardial bridge). In addition to coronary artery anomalies, CMR is highly advantageous for identifying aneurysms or vascular fistulas without the use of contrast materials and without exposing patients to ionizingradiation.

In general, non invasive assessment of coronary arteries by coronary magnetic resonance angiography (CMRA) has become a promising non-invasive diagnostic method for both congenital coronary abnormalities and for CAD [9]. The small size of coronary arteries, their complex course, and the constant motion with cardiac contraction and respiration are the most common reasons for a CMRA to be described as technically difficult. In comparison with the native coronary arteries, reverse saphenous vein and internal mammary artery grafts are relatively easy to image due to their minimal motion during the cardiac and respiratory cycles and the larger lumen of reverse saphenous vein grafts. However, limitations of coronary CMR bypass graft assessment include difficulties related to local signal loss or artifact due to various metallic objects implanted such as hemostatic clips, ostial stainless steel graft markers, sternal wires, co-existent prosthetic valves and supporting struts or rings and graft stents. Using modern free-breathing, electrocardiogram (ECG) navigator-gated three dimensional segmented methods, good results have been shown, especially for the proximal coronary segments and in subjects with high image quality scans. The physiological relevance of a coronary stenosis can be established by the coronary flow reserve which is calculated by the ratio of hyperemic to baseline coronary flow. CMR can evaluate coronary flow reserve by assessment of myocardial perfusion with first-pass contrast enhanced imaging [10] or by determining coronary artery blood flow *via* fast velocity encoded cine MRI before and after pharmacologically induced hyperemia (usually using adenosine or dipyridamole).

Myocardial perfusion and myocardial perfusion reserve can be used as indirect measures of coronary flow. CMR first-pass perfusion has been reported to have high diagnostic accuracy for detection of coronary artery disease. A meta-analysis of all CMR perfusion studies demonstrated a sensitivity of 91% and specificity of 81% for the diagnosis of CAD [11]. The combination of CMR stress perfusion, function, and LGE allows the use of CMR as a primary form of testing for identifying patients with ischemic heart disease in cases of existing resting ECG abnormalities or inability to exercise and thereby define patients with CAD who might be candidates for revascularization.

THE ROLE OF CMR IN ACUTE CHEST PAIN PRESENTATION

Acute chest pain is one of the most common reasons for presentation to the emergency room. Stress testing is a valuable risk-stratifying technique reserved for the subset of patients who have intermediate clinical probability of obstructive CAD. Management of intermediate-risk patients with possible acute coronary syndrome with stress CMR may reduce coronary artery revascularization, hospital readmissions, and recurrent cardiac testing [6]. Given the risks of radiation inherent to nuclear and computed tomography imaging, both adenosine stress cardiovascular magnetic resonance (AS-CMR) imaging and dobutamine stress echocardiography (DSE) are attractive alternative stress modalities. Identification of patients who could safely be discharged is of great significance because on one hand, the non necessary admission of these patients would pose a great burden of cost, while on the other, missing a diagnosis of chest pain of cardiac origin is associated with increased risk for adverse cardiac events in follow-up [12].

Patients presenting with low-risk acute chest pain to emergency department, both normal AS-CMR and normal DSE have excellent negative prognostic values. Accordingly, both of these tests appear to be attractive options void of ionizing radiation suitable for use in selected intermediate risk patients requiring further stratification [13]. AS-CMR appears to be preferable to DSE for patients without contraindications at well equipped advanced cardiovascular imaging centers due to improved prognostic performance and diagnostic quality. Additionally, suspicion for alternative causes of acute chest pain readily diagnosed with AS-CMR further favors the use of this modality over DSE. Furthermore, AS-CMR should be considered in patients with poor echocardiographic acoustic windows or a contraindication to intravenous dobutamine administration. Approximately 5% of patients with an acute coronary syndrome are discharged from the emergency room with an erroneous diagnosis of non-cardiac chest pain. CMR, which can detect smaller myocardial infarctions can be prognostically important with no radiation. Together with its ability to detect ventricular thrombus, edema and inflammation, CMR is a promising test for the acute pain management and furthermore, allows monitoring of revascularization procedures′ success.

AS-CMR is an imaging modality with increasing application due to its high sensitivity and negative predictive value [14]. It is also considered a safe and well tolerated procedure with only minimal risk to the patient. It has specific advantages over other imaging modalities in addition to the avoidance of radiation, iodinated contrast, and dobutamine administration with its risks. Furthermore, gold standard quantification of ejection fraction as well as assessment of valvular function is inherent to the exam. In the case of acute chest presentation AS-CMR images (Fig. **1**) can be read immediately and clinical decisions made quickly, as there is no post-processing required.

CMR imaging during acute chest pain presentation can also apply for the diagnosis of cardiomyopathies mimicking acute coronary syndromes such as apical ballooning syndrome know also as Takotsubo cardiomyopathy (Fig. **2**). Transient catecholaminergic myocardial stunning appears to be the underlying mechanism of this syndrome. Takotsubo cardiomyopathy, known as well as stress cardiomyopathy or broken heart syndrome, is typically characterized by the

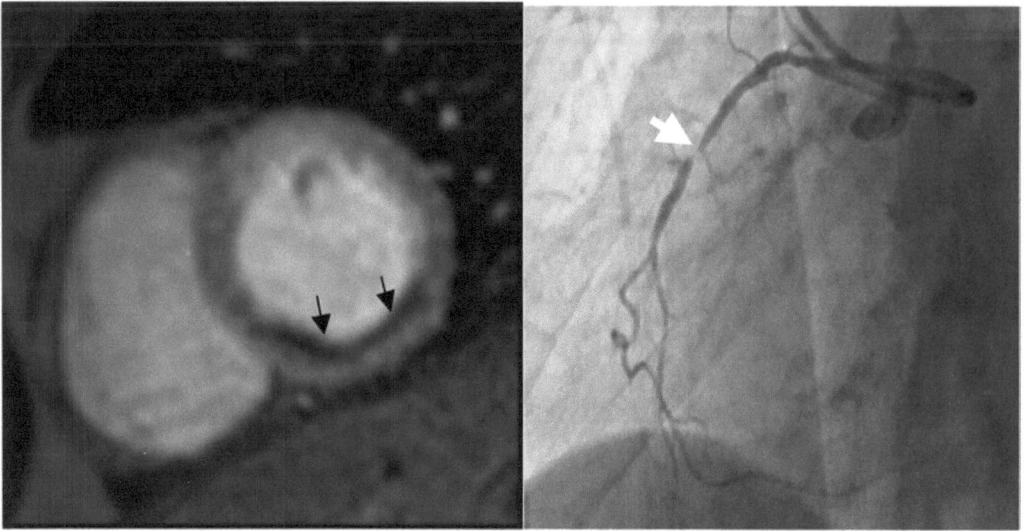

Figure 1: CMR perfusion imaging for CAD assessment in acute chest pain presentation. Adenosine stress test images showing that the basal inferior wall of the left ventricle has an ischemic lesion (black arrows indicating darker areas at the endocardium). In the coronary angiography, critical stenosis of the mid-right coronary artery was present (white arrow).

following: 1) acute onset of ischemic-like chest pain 2) transient apical regional wall-motion abnormality, 3) minor elevation of cardiac biomarkers, 4) dynamic electrocardiographic changes, and 5) the absence of epicardial coronary artery disease as confirmed with coronary angiography.

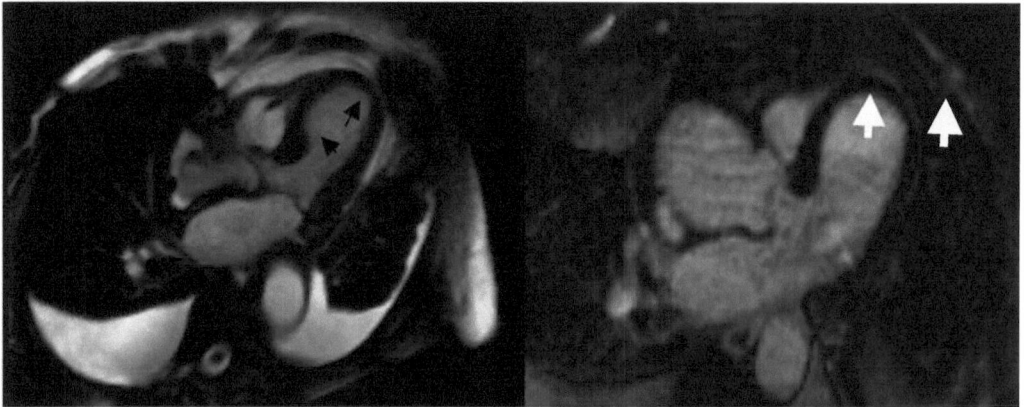

Figure 2: CMR imaging in acute chest pain presentation. Cine images of Takotsubo cardiomyopathy (black arrows indicating apical ballooning) and LGE images showing no signs of ischemic heart disease (white arrow).

CMR is also useful in acute chest pain presentation due to its ability to recognize acute aortic syndromes. It is used for defining the location and extent of aortic aneurysms, erosions, ulcers, dissections; evaluating post-surgical processes involving the aorta and surrounding structures, and the aortic size, the blood flow and the cardiac cycle-dependent changes in aortic area [15].

Acute myocarditis may also be a common case for acute chest pain presentation especially for younger patients visiting the emergencies. It is usually combined with low fever and elevated inflammatory and myocardial necrosis blood markers. CMR is considered one of the most important diagnostic tools in the workup of patients with acute myocarditis (Fig. **3**). It can detect inflammation and especially myocardial edema offering a high diagnostic accuracy to reveal acute myocarditis [16]. Reflecting irreversible injury, a typical pattern of regional, typically subepicardial fibrosis can be visualized. With combined analysis of T_1 and T_2 weighted scans, heightened diagnostic accuracy for identifying active myocarditis can be achieved.

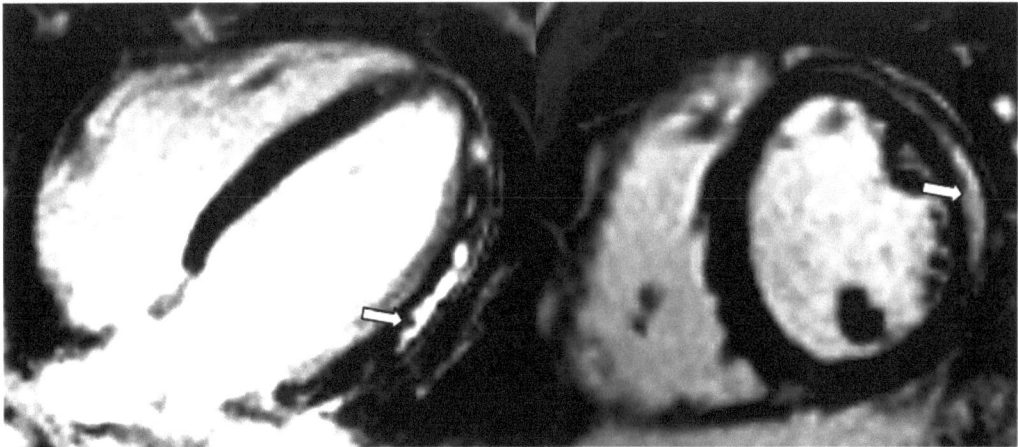

Figure 3: CMR T_2-weighted delayed gadolinium enhancement images showing sub epicardial lesions of high signal intensity at the lateral and apical wall of the left ventricle indicative of edematous tissue with inflammation consistent with the diagnosis of acute myocarditis (white arrows indicating bright areas).

CMR can also be used as a noninvasive imaging modality to diagnose patients with suspected pericardial disease. Acute pericarditis is often the diagnosis for patients presenting with chest pain, low fever and possibly previous respiratory infection. CMR can provide a comprehensive structural and functional assessment of the pericardium as well as evaluate the physiological consequences of pericardial effusion [17].

Patients suffering from acute pulmonary embolism may also present with acute chest pain. CMR imaging can be used to assess the major pulmonary arteries both for acute and chronic thromboembolic disease. There are few studies regarding the utility of data for pulmonary contrast enhanced magnetic resonance angiography (CE-MRA) for the diagnosis of severe acute pulmonary embolism [18]. Data from small single center studies are promising, with the sensitivity for pulmonary CE-MRA to detect pulmonary emboli ranging from 77% to 100% and the specificity ranging from 95% to 100% [19]. Real-time CE-MR pulmonary perfusion methods can be added to raise the sensitivity for pulmonary embolism detection. Techniques used for this purpose have a lower spatial resolution, which may preclude direct visualization of emboli; however, these methods display segmental and sub-segmental perfusion defects analogous to nuclear medicine techniques, which can be used to indirectly predict the presence of emboli.

CMR IN ISCHEMIC CARDIOMYOPATHY

There is an emerging role of CMR in the detection and management of patients with ischemic cardiomyopathy. CMR can detect many of the physiologic consequences of ischemia through the assessment of myocardial abnormalities of perfusion, diastolic and systolic performance, and metabolism. CMR provides high spatial and temporal resolution images of myocardial perfusion, myocardial function, and identification of infarcts using LGE techniques [20].

Myocardial Perfusion Imaging

Myocardial perfusion imaging (MPI) is based on the coronary flow reserve. Coronary flow reserve refers to the capacity of the coronary circulation to increase blood flow through the coronary tree, when the perfusion bed is maximally dilated. In a clinical CMR examination, coronary vasodilatation can be achieved with the use of a variety of pharmacological agents, typically adenosine [21-23].The determination of the coronary flow reserve entails a measurement of resting coronary flow and a second measurement during maximal vasodilatation. The coronary flow reserve can be measured with CMR imaging by means of direct visualization of the myocardial perfusion lumen of the proximal coronary artery and with quantification of blood flow velocity in the vessel lumen by using the phase-contrast technique. Perfusion imaging with CMR is performed by acquiring a series of ECG-gated T_1weighted images during the first pass of the contrast media, most commonly gadolinium, during one breath-hold.

Signal intensity of evoked MRI signals correlates with contrast concentration. Following peripheral injection, gadolinium is detected against the background of nulled (dark) myocardium with rapid enhancement during vasodilatation stress. This is done during simultaneous infusion of a vasodilator drug such as adenosine or dipyridamol, which causes myocardial hyperemia. The hyperemic flow is compromised in myocardial segments that are supplied by a coronary artery with significant stenosis because of the drop of coronary perfusion pressure downstream of the coronary stenosis. Microcirculatory dysfunction can also lead to an impaired perfusion reserve despite the absence of any significant stenosis of the epicardial coronary arteries. Segments with a perfusion defect in relation to the hyperemic myocardium will, therefore, be identifiable by a lower signal intensity on the CMR images. Image analysis can be performed either visually or quantitatively by calculating the rate of myocardial signal change (upslope) during the contrast medium first pass. Studies demonstrated that even for patients after surgical revascularization, stress perfusion CMR presents good diagnostic accuracy for the detection and localization of significant stenosis (above 50%), although the sensitivity is reduced compared to patients without coronary bypass.

MPI can successfully replace the traditional nuclear imaging techniques used in the ischemic cardiomyopathy assessment such as SPECT and PET despite the fact that it not currently used as a routine test due to its relative complexity and high cost. MPI has been used to assess biventricular function, regional myocardial wall function (wall thickening and strain imaging), edema and infarction imaging. Stress myocardial perfusion CMR is considered to be the primary form of testing for identifying patients with ischemic heart disease when there are resting electrocardiographic abnormalities or they present with inability to exercise, identifying patients with large-vessel CAD and patients who are appropriate candidates for interventional procedures [24]. MPI is ideally suited to resolve imaging challenges posed by particular patient populations such as women with breast attenuation artifacts, patients suffering from obesity, smaller-sized hearts, and limited exercise tolerance.

Overall, perfusion CMR is regarded as a safe imaging method. By using a T_1weighted sequence to visualize first passage of a gadolinium based contrast agent in transit through the heart, CMR perfusion imaging appears to be an established technique to evaluate myocardial ischemia especially when is supplemented by LGE imaging, which delineates even small or subendocardiac infarcted myocardium with high accuracy.

Stress CMR Imaging of Ventricular Function

Dobutamine is commonly used to evaluate stress CMR with a qualitative evaluation of regional wall motion abnormalities similar to the protocols used during dobutamine stress echocardiography. Wall motion imaging during high-dose dobutamine stress CMR (DSCMR) as well as perfusion imaging during vasodilator stress are highly accurate for assessing ischemia and are appropriate tests for patients with stable angina [25]. They are particularly helpful in combination with LGE to determine whether there are areas with ischemia on the borders of scarred myocardium. Finding ischemic areas in the myocardium with LGE-CMR is of great significance for the further therapeutic management of the patients with ischemic cardiomyopathy and may help the clinical decision for revascularization.

Studies have shown DSCMR to have a high accuracy for detecting ischemia, related in part to excellent visualization of the LV endocardium. CMR tagging may further improve the accuracy of DSCMR for detecting ischemia [26]. In addition, in patients with resting LV wall motion abnormalities, low-dose DSCMR is useful for identifying contractile reserve indicative of potential for recovering systolic thickening after coronary arterial revascularization. Quantitative assessment of strain at peak stress is mildly more accurate for ischemia detection than visual analysis alone. This may be of specific importance in patients with ischemic cardiomyopathy because LV remodeling results to complex wall motion abnormalities at rest. In addition to being more accurate, quantitative analysis of strain and strain rate wall motion could also apply for the detection of ischemia below peak stress, potentially reducing the need for high-dose dobutamine stress and the patient's risks deriving from the high dosage of inotropic agents.

Advanced first-pass perfusion CMR imaging during adenosine-induced coronary vasodilatation may detect ischemia in thinned and remodeled segments. Prognostic data are now available using both vasodilator and DSCMR methods. Three-year event-free survival has been reported at 99.2% for patients with normal stress perfusion CMR or DSCMR and 83.5% for those with abnormal stress perfusion or DSCMR [27].

Detecting hibernating myocardium which reflects an incomplete adaptation to reduced myocardial blood supply can alter patients' prognosis through revascularization. Various tests are available for identifying hibernating myocardium. SPECT imaging is sensitive for detecting cellular integrity and is widely available to detect hibernating myocardium. Dobutamine stress echocardiography (DSE) is also widely available since it is relatively simple, safe and low cost imaging modality. However, the sensitivity of this technique appears to be inferior compared to LGE-CMR or PET. In patients with severely depressed LV ejection fraction, PET imaging may be useful for assessment of hibernating myocardium because it has high sensitivity and superior resolution to SPECT. Contrast-enhanced CMR in combination with low-dose dobutamine stimulation seems to be the most accurate of all the imaging modalities for the detection of hibernating myocardium [28].

In summary, CMR appears to be an established imaging method to assess biventricular structural and functional status and myocardial viability at the same time [29]. The abnormalities observed during stress CMR serve as independent predictors of adverse cardiac events. Its safety and efficacy have been assessed extensively. CMR exhibits major complications in less than 0.1% of subjects, findings that are similar to those observed with dobutamine stress echocardiography.

CMR in Assessment of Myocardial Infarction

LGE CMR can be used for identifying the extent and location of myocardial necrosis in individuals suffering from ischemic cardiomyopathy. First attempts to visualize myocardial infarction (MI) by contrast enhanced CMR date back to the 1980s. In the mid and late 1990s, techniques using contrast-enhanced CMR for infarction detection were significantly improved, leading to image acquisitions specifically designed to achieve maximum contrast between infarcted and non-infarcted myocardium. The technique involves T_1 weighted inversion-recovery imaging after intravenous administration of gadolinium contrast.

During LGE CMR imaging, normal myocardium appears black or nulled, whereas necrotic myocardium appears bright (Fig. **3**). The mechanism of LGE relies upon two assumptions: (a) The tissue volume of normal myocardium is predominately intracellular, because myocytes are densely packed; (b) Gadolinium is an extracellular agent that cannot cross intact sarcolemmal membranes. Therefore, the gadolinium distribution volume is small and tissue concentration is low in normal myocardium, whereas cell membrane rupture in acute necrosis allows gadolinium to diffuse into myocytes leading to increased gadolinium concentration, shortened T_1 relaxation, and thus hyperenhancement, resulting to the bright image appearance.

LGE imaging detects the presence of MI lesions with higher accuracy than any other non-invasive diagnostic modality [30-32]. Studies have confirmed a low observer dependency for MI detection by LGE. Even microcirculation infarctions, such as may occur during percutaneous coronary angioplasty, are detectable by CMR. LGE detects right ventricular involvement in MI more often than measurements based on standard echocardiography, which is important as right ventricular dysfunction following MI is associated with a worse prognosis [33, 34].

Myocardial edema which is characterized by increased myocardial water content is a feature of many forms of acute myocardial injury that are associated with inflammation, such as ischemia or myocarditis. T_2-weighted CMR imaging is sensitive to regional or global increases in myocardial water. Free water appears to be the most significant contributor to the T_2 signal intensity in myocardial tissue and therefore myocardial segments with myocardial edema appear bright. Similar to LGE, the pattern of distribution of bright zones on T$_2$-weighted images may help to indicate the etiology of myocardial injury. In general, tissue alterations caused by ischemia lead to increased signal intensity in segments corresponding to the supplying coronary artery territories. Furthermore, the combination of T$_2$weighted imaging with LGE imaging has been proven to be helpful in differentiating acute from chronic MI. While chronic MI is represented by LGE alone, acute MI is characterized by high signal intensity in both T$_2$weighted images and LGE images in the infarcted region (Fig. **4**). The hyper-enhanced area in T$_2$-weigthed images can also be used as a measure of area at risk in the acute phase after myocardial infarction.

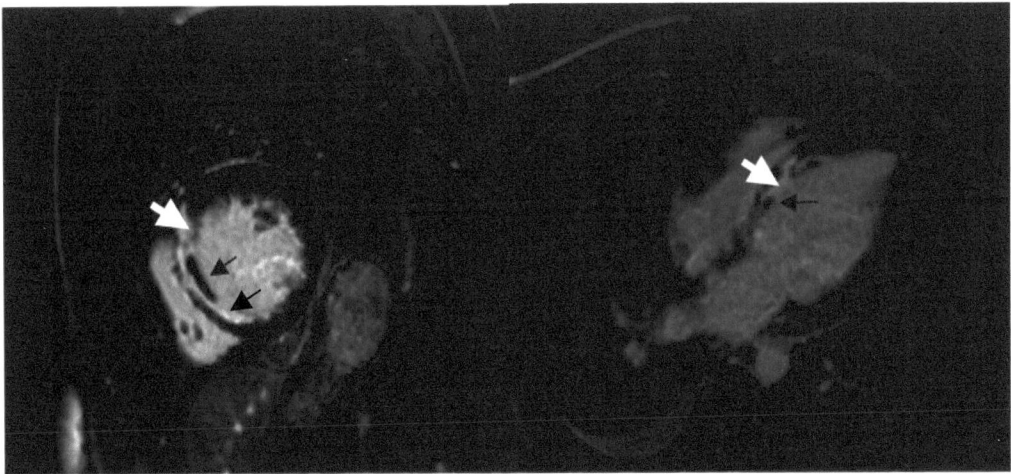

Figure 4: LGE-CMR imaging of a patient with scar tissue due to myocardial infraction (white arrows indicating brighter areas at the endocardium of the septum) and micro vascular obstruction (black arrows indicating darker areas).

CMR Spectroscopy

Spectroscopy provides the CMR basis for the assessment of myocardial metabolism without the need for gadolinium. Hydrogen spectroscopy may be useful for assessing myocardial cellular triglyceride levels. Phosphorus spectroscopy has been used to measure myocardial energetics. In an early clinical application CMR spectroscopy showed independent prognostic information on cardiovascular mortality [35]. Myocardial CMR spectroscopy is a sensitive method of identifying ischemia and ischemic damage in a number of diseases. It has been demonstrated that the resting phosphocreatine (PCr) to ATP ratio was decreased in patients with myocardial infarction. The resting PCr to ATP ratio correlates with the clinical severity of myocardial dysfunction and is increased after pharmacologic treatment. A significant decrease in the PCr to ATP ratio during isometric handgrip exercise is seen in patients with significant coronary stenosis. This ratio does not seem to change significantly during exercise in either normal subjects or patients with non-ischemic heart disease.

There is evidence of altered myocardial metabolism on stress testing combined with CMR spectroscopy in patients with coronary angiographies negative for the presence of significant CAD suggesting the presence of ischemia. These findings suggest that microvascular coronary artery disease is a likely mechanism for myocardial ischemia in the absence of angiographically significant stenosis. Microvascular coronary artery obstruction is claimed to be the underlying factor for the 'no-reflow' phenomenon. This phenomenon is believed to be the result of coronary microvascular obstruction but may as well have complex, multifactorial pathogenesis including: distal embolization, ischemia-reperfusion myocardial tissue injury, and individual coronary microcirculation predisposition to injury. It is of great significance to early detect the 'no reflow' phenomenon because it is related to severe myocardial damage and is independently associated with lack of functional recovery, adverse ventricular remodeling and worse patient outcome.

CMR spectroscopy is a non-invasive and non-traumatic method to identify a metabolic abnormality in the subgroup of patients presenting with chest-pain syndromes and have coronary arteries negative for the presence of significant CAD. In this case CMR spectroscopy test may facilitate the development of further management of these patients. Overall CMR spectroscopy seems to be a promising method for the myocardial characterization in patients with ischemic cardiomyopathy but further evaluation is needed to establish this method in clinical practice.

Comparing CMR with Other Cardiac Imaging Modalities

Studies comparing CMR with PET and SPECT protocols for assessment of reversible myocardial dysfunction in patients with chronic ischemic heart disease undergoing revascularization indicated a higher sensitivity and a comparable specificity for CMR [29, 32, 36]. CMR appear to be superior to a PET/SPECT combined protocol for identification of segments unlikely to recover function after revascularization. For assessment of global functional improvement, CMR studies show a good correlation of the overall patient-related viability score and improvement of ejection fraction after revascularization. As compared to SPECT, a technique frequently used to make clinical decisions concerning revascularization in patients with chronic ischemic heart disease, there seems to be superior accuracy of CMR for the prediction of improvement in regional and global LV function in the setting of chronic myocardial ischemia.

CMR and MDCT infusion protocols have an excellent sensitivity and very good specificity for the detection of functionally significant CAD [37, 38]. CMR appears to be superior and safer for diagnosis and evaluation of ischemic cardiomyopathy compared to MDCT. Low-dose MDCT perfusion protocols are ready for routine use in clinical practice, without a significant increase of radiation exposure, using standard 64 MDCT scanners: the entire MDCT protocol is completed with an effective radiation exposure that represents less than one half of the exposure usually reported for SPECT. On the other hand, no radiation exposure is present on CMR perfusion protocols and the excellent accuracy of the method in symptomatic intermediate risk patients is already well established [39, 40]. Stress and rest perfusion are simultaneously visualized with LGE images resulting in very good accuracy for ischemia detection. Overall, CMR has several advantages over MDCT for the detection of myocardial ischemia: it does not expose patients to ionizing radiation and provides dynamic real-time imaging of myocardial perfusion over the first-passage of contrast. MDCT perfusion is limited to the "one-shot" opportunity to visualize differences of x-ray attenuation between the ischemic and remote myocardium. A potential advantage of MDCT protocol over CMR protocol is the ability to acquire high-resolution isotropic three dimensional whole heart datasets that allow for simultaneous coronary anatomy and myocardial perfusion analysis. This may be of particular interest for decision and management of revascularization.

Echocardiographic assessments of myocardial thickening and endocardiac excursion during dobutamine infusion provide a highly specific marker for myocardial viability, but with relatively less sensitivity. The additional modalities of myocardial contrast agent echocardiography and tissue Doppler imaging have been proposed to provide further, quantitative measures of myocardial viability assessment. Speckle tracking advanced echocardiography techniques using strain and strain rate measurements may help for the left and the right ventricle systolic and diastolic dysfunction assessment. CMR though appears to be a better choice for the assessment of myocardial viability as it can assess cardiac function, volumes, myocardial scar, and perfusion with high-spatial resolution. CMR methods may provide overall greater diagnostic certainty in the majority of patients. Data from everyday clinical practice though support the continuing role of dobutamine echocardiographic techniques as reliable, widespread, economic, easy to use methods for those patients in sinus rhythm and with excellent acoustic windows.

Safety of CMR in Ischemic Cardiomyopathy Imaging

CMR is generally considered an established imaging modality for patients with ischemic cardiomyopathy, but there are a few important safety concerns [41]. The first would be the general safety considerations for usual implanted devices in patients with ischemic cardiomyopathy such as implantable cardioverter defibrillators (ICD) or cardiac pacemakers [42]. Pacemakers and ICDs contain metal components with ferromagnetic properties, as well as complex electrical systems with one or more leads implanted into the myocardium. Potential complications of CMR under these circumstances include damage or movement of the device, inhibition of the pacing output, activation of the tachyarrhythmia therapy of the device, cardiac stimulation, and heating of the electrode tips. These factors may lead to clinical deterioration of these patients due to changes in pacing/defibrillation thresholds, pacemaker ICD dysfunction or damage. Consequently, CMR examination of patients with a pacemaker or ICD is discouraged and should only be considered at highly experienced centers in cases in which there is a strong clinical indication and where the benefits clearly outweigh the risks [43].

The second concern would be in critically ill ischemic patients who need hemodynamic support devices such as ventricular assist devices and intra-aortic balloon pumps. Formal CMR testing of these devices has not been conducted. However, it is believed that these hemodynamic support devices represent absolute contraindications to CMR examination.

A third concern would be the use of contrast agents in critically ill ischemic patients especially to those with impaired renal function. Gadolinium contrast agents are used for imaging the heart with LGE and perfusion imaging techniques. Mild-to-moderate reactions to Gadolinium contrast agents have been reported to occur in approximately one in five thousands patients [44]. Most common reactions include hives, flushing, shortness of breath. Severe anaphylactic reactions occur in one in three hundred thousands patients. Nephrogenic systemic fibrosis (NSF) is a rare but important complication of administration associated with acute renal failure or severe renal failure due to advanced chronic kidney disease. Because of the risk of NSF, screening for reduced renal function prior to a CMR test should be considered in all patients with ischemic cardiomyopathy.

CMR Future Perspectives

Over the next years novel CMR technology will not rely on the use of an exogenous contrast agent and will be sufficiently fast and cost effective for routine clinical use. It will provide quantitative read outs of myocardial tissue status and multi-parametric information on structural and functional heart disease [45]. Molecular CMR will enable imaging of various processes involved in atherosclerotic cardiovascular disease such as apoptosis, necrosis, macrophage infiltration, enzyme activity, angiogenesis and development of fibrosis [46]. It is expected that molecular CMR technology eventually will find its way in clinical practice. Diffusion tensor imaging (DTI) of myocardial fiber architecture is rapidly emerging as a technique to characterize the myocardial fiber structure, offering diagnostic utility in the differential diagnosis of adverse left ventricle remodeling [47]. Furthermore while investigating complex arrhythmias, functional CMR techniques may be used to determine local electrical tissue properties and assess the presence of abnormal electrical activation and conductivity. Hybrid imaging protocols will be developed to assess anatomical and functional information at the same time [48]. CMR will be combined with other imaging modalities for a full structural and functional assessment of ischemic heart disease. Novel data acquisition and reconstruction strategies such as retrospective imaging, compressed sensing techniques for image reconstruction, parallel imaging using multiple receiver coils and accelerated real-time cardiac cine MRI pulse sequences using a combination of compressed sensing and parallel imaging (k-t SPARSE-SENSE) are already under development, and will increase CMR efficacy in the future. Ultra high field CMR used at 7 Tesla is a challenge and first tests have already been performed successfully [49]. Further steps are based on further technical developments both on software and hardware. Feature tracking (FT) CMR [50, 51] and strain encoded (SENC) CMR [52, 53] allow real time visualization of cardiac regional function and allow rapid imaging data analysis. Developments still need to be made to resolve all the technical issues of the novel CMR techniques. Another challenge would be to reduce the time consumed and the high cost of the CMR test in order to enable researchers and physicians to widely apply these techniques in everyday clinical practice.

CONCLUSION

CMR has become an important diagnostic element during the clinical work-up of patients with known or suspected ischemic heart disease. Hence, ischemic heart disease has become the most frequent indication to perform a CMR study. The American College of Cardiology Foundation (ACCF), American College of Radiology (ACR), Society of Cardiovascular Computed Tomography (SCCT), Society for Cardiovascular Magnetic Resonance (SCMR), American Society of Nuclear Radiology (ASNC), North American Society for Cardiac Imaging (NASCI), Society for Cardiovascular Angiography and Interventions (SCAI) and Society of Interventional Radiology (SIR) 2006 Appropriateness Criteria for Cardiac CT and Cardiac MRI indicates that the use of CMR stress testing is appropriate in individuals with intermediate pretest probability of CAD, those with an uninterpretable ECG, or those who are unable to exercise. CMR is also appropriate to determine viability prior to revascularization and establish the likelihood of recovery of systolic function with revascularization. Furthermore, CMR is appropriate to assess myocardial viability when determinations from other forms of noninvasive testing exhibit indeterminate results. Finally, CMR stress testing is appropriate for identifying cardiac risk in patients with prior coronary angiography or coronary artery stenosis of unclear significance.

Overall, CMR provides information about cardiac dimensions, function, and myocardial perfusion with high robustness and accuracy. It gives unique insights into myocardial tissue alterations during acute and chronic ischemic heart disease. This non-invasive and radiation-free combined approach of functional and morphologic cardiac assessment with CMR provides unique characteristics and strengths compared with other imaging modalities since it allows the early detection of ischemic heart disease, diagnostic differentiation of non ischemic disorders, patient risk stratification and guidance of therapy.

AUTHORS STATEMENT

Informed consent was sought and secured from patients for publishing images for this chapter.

CONFLICT OF INTEREST

This is to certify that the authors do not have any conflict of interest.

ACKNOWLEDGEMENT

None declared.

REFERENCES

[1]   Cannon CP, Brindis RG, Chaitman BR, Cohen DJ, Cross JT Jr, Drozda JP Jr, Fesmire FM, Fintel DJ, Fonarow GC, Fox KA, Gray DT, Harrington RA, Hicks KA, Hollander JE, Krumholz H, Labarthe DR, Long JB, Mascette AM, Meyer C, Peterson ED, Radford MJ, Roe MT, Richmann JB, Selker HP, Shahian DM, Shaw RE, Sprenger S, Swor R, Underberg JA, Van de Werf F, Weiner BH, Weintraub WS; American College of Cardiology Foundation/American Heart Association Task Force on Clinical Data Standards; American College of Emergency Physicians; Emergency Nurses Association; National Association of Emergency Medical Technicians; National Association of EMS Physicians; Preventive Cardiovascular Nurses Association; Society for Cardiovascular Angiography and Interventions; Society of Cardiovascular Patient Care; Society of Thoracic Surgeons. 2013 ACCF/AHA key data elements and definitions for measuring the clinical management and outcomes of patients with acute coronary syndromes and coronary artery disease: a report of the American College of Cardiology Foundation/American Heart

Association Task Force on Clinical Data Standards (Writing Committee to Develop Acute Coronary Syndromes and Coronary Artery Disease Clinical Data Standards). Circulation 2013; 127: 1052-89.

[2]   Hendel RC, Patel MR, Kramer CM, Poon M, Hendel RC, Carr JC, Gerstad NA, Gillam LD, Hodgson JM, Kim RJ, Kramer CM, Lesser JR, Martin ET, Messer JV, Redberg RF, Rubin GD, Rumsfeld JS, Taylor AJ, Weigold WG, Woodard PK, Brindis RG, Hendel RC, Douglas PS, Peterson ED, Wolk MJ, Allen JM, Patel MR; ACCF/ACR/SCCT/SCMR/ASNC/NASCI/SCAI/SIR 2006 appropriateness criteria for cardiac computed tomography and cardiac magnetic resonance imaging: a report of the American College of Cardiology Foundation Quality Strategic Directions Committee Appropriateness Criteria Working Group, American College of Radiology, Society of Cardiovascular Computed Tomography, Society for Cardiovascular Magnetic Resonance, American Society of Nuclear Cardiology, North American Society for Cardiac Imaging, Society for Cardiovascular Angiography and Interventions, and Society of Interventional Radiology. J Am CollCardiol 2006; 48: 1475-97.

[3]   Hundley WG, Bluemke DA, Finn JP, Flamm SD, Fogel MA, Friedrich MG, Ho VB, Jerosch-Herold M, Kramer CM, Manning WJ, Patel M, Pohost GM, Stillman AE, White RD, Woodard PKl. ACCF/ACR/AHA/NASCI/SCMR 2010 expert consensus document on cardiovascular magnetic resonance: a report of the American College of Cardiology Foundation Task Force on Expert Consensus Documents. J Am CollCardiol 2010; 55: 2614-62.

[4]   Von Knobelsdorff-Brenkenhoff F, Schulz-Menger J. Cardiovascular Magnetic Resonance Imaging in Ischemic Heart Disease. J MagnReson Imaging 2012; 36: 20-38.

[5]   Schuster A, Morton G, Chiribiri A, Perera D, Vanoverschelde JL, Nagel E. Imaging in the management of ischemic cardiomyopathy: special focus on magnetic resonance. J Am Coll Cardiol 2012; 59: 359-70.

[6]   Miller CD, Case LD, Little WC, Mahler SA, Burke GL, Harper EN, Lefebvre C, Hiestand B, Hoekstra JW, Hamilton CA, Hundley WG. Stress CMR reduces revascularization, hospital readmission, and recurrent cardiac testing in intermediate-risk patients with acute chest pain. JACC Cardiovasc Imaging 2013; 7: 785-94.

[7]   Constantine G, Shan K, Flamm SD, Sivananthan MU. Role of MRI in clinical cardiology. Lancet 2004; 363: 2162-71.

[8]   Jahnke C, Paetsch I, Nehrke K, Schnackenburg B, Gebker R, Fleck E, Nagel E.. Rapid and complete coronary arterial tree visualization with magnetic resonance imaging: feasibility and diagnostic performance. Eur Heart J 2005; 26: 2313-9.

[9]   Kim WY, Danias PG, Stuber M, Flamm SD, Plein S, Nagel E, Langerak SE, Weber OM, Pedersen EM, Schmidt M, Botnar RM, Manning WJ. Coronary magnetic resonance angiography for the detection of coronary stenoses. N Engl J Med 2001; 345: 1863-9.

[10]   Lockie T, Ishida M, Perera D, Chiribiri A, De Silva K, Kozerke S, Marber M, Nagel E, Rezavi R, Redwood S, Plein S. High-resolution magnetic resonance myocardial perfusion imaging at 3.0-Tesla to detect hemodynamically significant coronary stenoses as determined by fractional flow reserve. J Am Coll Cardiol 2011; 57: 70-5.

[11]   Nandalur KR, Dwamena BA, Choudhri AF, Nandalur MR, Carlos RC. Diagnostic performance of stress cardiac magnetic resonance imaging in the detection of coronary artery disease: a meta-analysis. J Am Coll Cardiol 2007; 50: 1343-53.

[12]   Lerakis S, Janik M, McLean DS, Anadiotis AV, Zaragoza-Macias E, Veledar E, Oshinski J, Stillman AE. Adenosine stress magnetic resonance imaging in women with low risk chest pain: the Emory University experience. Am J Med Sci 2010; 339: 216-20.

[13]   Hartlage G, Janik M, Anadiotis A, Veledar E, Oshinski J, Kremastinos D, Stillman A, Lerakis S. Prognostic value of adenosine stress cardiovascular magnetic resonance and dobutamine stress echocardiography in patients with low-risk chest pain. Int J Cardiovasc Imaging 2012; 28: 803-12.

[14]   Lerakis S, McLean D, Anadiotis A, Janik M, Oshinski J, Alexopoulos N, Zaragoza-Macias E, Veledar E, Stillman A. Prognostic value of adenosine stress cardiovascular magnetic resonance in patients with low-risk chest pain. J Cardiovasc Magn Reson 2009; 21: 37.

[15]   Macura KJ, Szarf G, Fishman EK, Bluemke DA. Role of computed tomography and magnetic resonance imaging in assessment of acute aortic syndromes. Semin Ultrasound CT MR. 2003; 24:232-54.

[16]   Liu PP, Yan AT. Cardiovascular magnetic resonance for the diagnosis of acute myocarditis: prospects for detecting myocardial inflammation. J Am Coll Cardiol 2005; 45:1823-5.

[17]   Kojima S, Yamada N, Goto Y. Diagnosis of constrictive pericarditis by tagged cine magnetic resonance imaging. N Engl J Med 1999; 341:373- 4.

[18]   Oudkerk M, van Beek EJ, Wielopolski P, van Ooijen PM, Brouwers-Kuyper EM, Bongaerts AH, Berghout A. Comparison of contrast-enhanced magnetic resonance angiography and conventional pulmonary angiography for the diagnosis of pulmonary embolism: a prospective study. Lancet 2002; 359: 1643-7.

[19]   Kluge A, Luboldt W, Bachmann G. Acute pulmonary embolism to the subsegmental level: diagnostic accuracy of three MRI techniques compared with 16-MDCT. AJR Am J Roentgenol 2006; 187: 7-14.

[20]   Florian A, Jurcut R, Ginghina C, Bogaert J. Cardiac Magnetic Resonance Imaging in Ischemic Heart Disease: A Clinical Review. J Med Life 2011; 4: 330-345.

[21]   Cury RC, Cattani CA, Gabure LA, Racy DJ, de Gois JM, Siebert U, Lima SS, Brady TJ. Diagnostic performance of stress perfusion and delayed-enhancement MR imaging in patients with coronary artery disease. Radiology 2006; 240: 39-45.

[22]   Giang TH, Nanz D, Coulden R, Friedrich M, Graves M, Al-Saadi N, Lüscher TF, von Schulthess GK, Schwitter J. Detection of coronary artery disease by magnetic resonance myocardial perfusion imaging with various contrast medium doses: first European multi-centre experience. Eur Heart J 2004; 25: 1657- 65.

[23]   Klem I, Heitner JF, Shah DJ, Sketch MH Jr, Behar V, Weinsaft J, Cawley P, Parker M, Elliott M, Judd RM, Kim RJ. Improved detection of coronary artery disease by stress perfusion cardiovascular magnetic resonance with the use of delayed enhancement infarction imaging. J Am Coll Cardiol 2006; 47: 1630-8.

[24]   Nandalur KR, Dwamena BA, Choudhri AF, Nandalur MR, Carlos RC. Diagnostic performance of stress cardiac magnetic resonance imaging in the detection of coronary artery disease: a meta-analysis. J Am Coll Cardiol 2007; 50: 1343-53.

[25]   Wahl A, Paetsch I, Gollesch A, Roethemeyer S, Foell D, Gebker R, Langreck H, Klein C, Fleck E, Nagel E. Safety and feasibility of high-dose dobutamine-atropine stress cardiovascular magnetic resonance for diagnosis of myocardial ischaemia: experience in 1000 consecutive cases. Eur Heart J 2004; 25: 1230-6.

[26] Kuijpers D, Ho KY, van Dijkman PR, Vliegenthart R, Oudkerk M. Dobutamine cardiovascular magnetic resonance for the detection of myocardial ischemia with the use of myocardial tagging. Circulation 2003; 107: 1592-7.

[27] Jahnke C, Nagel E, Gebker R, Kokocinski T, Kelle S, Manka R, Fleck E, Paetsch I. Prognostic value of cardiac magnetic resonance stress tests: adenosine stress perfusion and dobutamine stress wall motion imaging. Circulation 2007; 115: 1769-76.

[28] Selvanayagam JB, Jerosch-Herold M, Porto I. Resting myocardial blood flow is impaired in hibernating myocardium. A magnetic resonance study of quantitative perfusion assessment. Circulation 2005; 112: 3289-3296.

[29] Regenfus M, Schlundt C, von Erffa J, Schmidt M, Reulbach U, Kuwert T, Daniel W, Schmid M. Head-to-head comparison of contrast-enhanced cardiovascular magnetic resonance and 201-Thallium single photon emission computed tomography for prediction of reversible left ventricular dysfunction in chronic ischaemic heart disease. Int J Cardiovasc Imaging 2012; 28: 1427-1434.

[30] Tomlinson D, Becher H, Selvanayagam J. Assessment of Myocardial Viability: Comparison of Echocardiography *versus* Cardiac Magnetic Resonance Imaging in the Current Era. Heart, Lung and Circulation 2008; 17: 173-185.

[31] Fieno DS, Kim RJ, Chen EL, Lomasney JW, Klocke FJ, Judd RM. Contrast-enhanced magnetic resonance imaging of myocardium at risk: distinction between reversible and irreversible injury throughout infarct healing. J Am Coll Cardiol 2000; 36: 1985-91.

[32] Ibrahim T, Bülow HP, Hackl T, Hörnke M, Nekolla SG, Breuer M, Schömig A, Schwaiger M. Diagnostic value of contrast enhanced magnetic resonance imaging and single-photon emission computed tomography for detection of myocardial necrosis early after acute myocardial infarction. J Am Coll Cardiol 2007; 49: 208 -16.

[33] Kumar A, Abdel-Aty H, Kriedemann I, Schulz-Menger J, Gross CM, Dietz R, Friedrich MG. Contrast-enhanced cardiovascular magnetic resonance imaging of right ventricular infarction. J Am Coll Cardiol 2006; 48: 1969-76.

[34] Choi KM, Kim RJ, Gubernikoff G, Vargas JD, Parker M, Judd RM. Transmural extent of acute myocardial infarction predicts long-term improvement in contractile function. Circulation 2001; 104: 1101-7.

[35] Buchthal SD, den Hollander JA, Merz CN, Rogers WJ, Pepine CJ, Reichek N, Sharaf BL, Reis S, Kelsey SF, Pohost GM. Abnormal myocardial phosphorus-31 nuclear magnetic resonance spectroscopy in women with chest pain but normal coronary angiograms. N Engl J Med 2000; 342: 829-35.

[36] Carlson M, Ubachs JFA, Hedström E. Myocardium at risk after acute infarction in humans on cardiac magnetic resonance. Quantitative assessment during follow-up and validation with single-photon emission computed tomography. J Am Coll Cardiol Img 2009; 2: 569-576.

[37] Bettencourt N, Chiribiri A, Schuster A, Ferreira N, Sampaio F, Gustavo P, Santos L, Bruno M, Rodrigues A, Braga P, Azevedo L, Teixeira M, Leite-Moreira A, Silva-Cardoso J, Nagel E, Gama V. Direct Comparison of Cardiac Magnetic Resonance and Multidetector Computed Tomography Stress-Rest Perfusion Imaging for Detection of Coronary Artery Disease. J Am Coll Cardiol 2013; 61: 1099-107.

[38] Morton G, Plein S, Nagel E. Noninvasive coronary angiography using computed tomography *versus* magnetic resonance imaging. Ann Intern Med 2010; 152: 827-828.

[39]   Cheong BYC, Muthupillai R, Wilson JM, Sung A. Prognostic significance of delayed enhancement magnetic resonance imaging. Survival of 857 patients with and without left ventricular dysfunction. Circulation 2009; 120: 2069-2076.

[40]   Romero J, Xue X, Gonzalez W, Garcia MJ. CMR imaging assessing viability in patients with chronic ventricular dysfunction due to coronary artery disease: a meta-analysis of prospective trials. J Am Coll Cardiol Imaging 2012; 5: 494-508.

[41]   Kanal E, Barkovich AJ, Bell C, Borgstede JP, Bradley WG Jr, Froelich JW, Gilk T, Gimbel JR, Gosbee J, Kuhni-Kaminski E, Lester JW Jr, Nyenhuis J, Parag Y, Schaefer DJ, Sebek-Scoumis EA, Weinreb J, Zaremba LA, Wilcox P, Lucey L, Sass N; ACR Blue Ribbon Panel on MR Safety. ACR guidance document for safe MR practices: 2007. Am J Roentgenol 2007; 188: 1447-74.

[42]   Prasad SK, Pennell DJ. Safety of cardiovascular magnetic resonance in patients with cardiovascular implants and devices. Heart 2004; 90: 1241-4.

[43]   Gimbel JR, Kanal E. Can patients with implantable pacemakers safely undergo magnetic resonance imaging? J Am Coll Cardiol 2004; 43: 1325-7.

[44]   Perazella MA. Current status of gadolinium toxicity in patients with kidney disease.Clin J Am Soc Nephrol 2009; 4: 461-9.

[45]   Paterson I, Mielniczuk LM, O'Meara E, So A, White JA. Imaging heart failure: current and future applications. Can J Cardiol 2013; 29: 317-28.

[46]   Won S, Davies-Venn C, Liu S, Bluemke DA. Noninvasive imaging of myocardial extracellular matrix for assessment of fibrosis.Curr Opin Cardiol 2013; 28: 282-9.

[47]   Ellims AH, Iles LM, Ling LH, Hare JL, Kaye DM, Taylor AJ. Diffuse myocardial fibrosis in hypertrophic cardiomyopathy can be identified by cardiovascular magnetic resonance, and is associated with left ventricular diastolic dysfunction. J Cardiovasc Magn Reson 2012; 14: 76.

[48]   Rischpler C, Nekolla SG, Dregely I, Schwaiger M. Hybrid PET/MR imaging of the heart: potential, initial experiences, and future prospects. J Nucl Med 2013; 53: 402-15.

[49]   von Knobelsdorff-Brenkenhoff F, Tkachenko V, Winter L, Rieger J, Thalhammer C, Hezel F, Graessl A, Dieringer MA, Niendorf T, Schulz-Menger J. Assessment of the right ventricle with cardiovascular magnetic resonance at 7 Tesla. J Cardiovasc Magn Reson 2013; 15: 23.

[50]   Augustine D, Lewandowski AJ, Lazdam M, Rai A, Francis J, Myerson S, Noble A, Becher H, Neubauer S, Petersen SE, Leeson P. Global and regional left ventricular myocardial deformation measures by magnetic resonance feature tracking in healthy volunteers: comparison with tagging and relevance of gender. J Cardiovasc Magn Reson 2013; 15: 8.

[51]   Morton G, Schuster A, Jogiya R, Kutty S, Beerbaum P, Nagel E. Inter-study reproducibility of cardiovascular magnetic resonance myocardial feature tracking. J Cardiovasc Magn Reson 2012; 14: 43.

[52]   Altiok E, Neizel M, Tiemann S, Krass V, Becker M, Zwicker C, Koos R, Kelm M, Kraemer N, Schoth F, Marx N, Hoffmann R. Layer-specific analysis of myocardial deformation for assessment of infarct transmurality: comparison of strain-encoded cardiovascular magnetic resonance with 2D speckle tracking echocardiography. Eur Heart J Cardiovasc Imaging 2013; 14: 570-8.

[53]   Heiberg E, Pahlm-Webb U, Agarwal S, Bergvall E, Fransson H, Steding-Ehrenborg K, Carlsson M, Arheden H. Longitudinal strain from velocity encoded cardiovascular magnetic resonance: a validation study. J Cardiovasc Magn Reson 2013; 15: 15.

Send Orders for Reprints to reprints@benthamscience.net

CHAPTER 3

Applications of Displacement-Encoded MRI in Cardiovascular Disease

Han Wen[*,1] and Pierre Croisille[2]

[1]*National Heart, Lung and Blood Institute, National Institutes of Health, Bethesda, Maryland, USA;* [2]*Department of Radiology, CHU Hôpital Nord, Jean-Monnet University, CREATIS Laboratory, UMR CNRS 5520 INSERM U1040, University of Lyon, 42055, Saint-Etienne, France*

Abstract: Displacement-encoded MRI is a class of imaging sequences and protocols that are based on the idea of displacement-encoding with stimulated echo (DENSE). Due to its ability to encode the displacement information over an extended period of time into the phase value of individual pixels in the image, it is a suitable method for track tissue motion at high resolution, which is valuable imaging tool in the assessment of cardiovascular diseases. This chapter describes the application of displacement-encoded MRI in the assessment of ischemic heart disease through strain mapping, and in the assessment of carotid artery lesions through wall strain measurements in compliance to arterial pressure fluctuations.

Keywords: Human, swine model, heart, myocardium, cardiovascular disease, carotid artery, atherosclerotic plaque, strain, compliance, circumferential, radial, phase, DENSE.

INTRODUCTION

Among clinical imaging modalities for assessing soft tissue motion, MRI is often the preferred standard due to its flexible view planes and quantitative accuracy. Since the first demonstration of myocardial tissue motion tracking using a displacement-encoded stimulated-echo (DENSE) pulse sequence [1], the method has been continually improved over time. Prior to DENSE, there were two major MRI techniques for quantitative imaging of tissue motion: tagged [2,3] and cine phase-contrast (PC) velocity imaging [4-6]. Tagged imaging is well-suited for tracking the movement of tissue over time [7,8], but its resolution is somewhat

---

*****Address correspondence to Han Wen:** National Heart Lung and Blood Institute, National Institutes of Health, Bethesda, MD 20892, USA; Tel: (301)496-2694 ; E-mail: han.wen@nih.gov

limited since displacement vectors can only be measured at the intersects of tag lines. Cine PC can measure velocity at the resolution of the anatomical images, but lacks the inherent tissue tracking capability of tagged imaging [9].

The technique of DENSE [1,10-12] is able to combine the advantages of the above methods. It provides directly the 3D displacement vector of each image pixel. This is realized by encoding tissue position into the phase of the MRI signal, and preserving that phase in the longitudinal magnetization such that it remains coherent for as long as the T_1 relaxation time. This then allows the direct measurement of tissue displacement over long periods of time. DENSE imaging has been validated against tagged imaging in phantom and human studies [13,14]. In the context of cardiac imaging, displacement-encoded MRI provides a quantitatively accurate means for evaluating myocardial contractile function [14, 15]. The high spatial resolution also found applications in non-invasive assessment of the stiffness of the carotid artery wall based on the circumferential strain in the wall in response to the pulsatile arterial pressure [16].

Two additional properties of DENSE images that are relevant to clinical applications are the dark blood pool signal and T_1 weighting of the image intensity. The dark appearance of flowing blood in the ventricular cavities and in vessel lumens is the result of phase-scrambling by the rapid flow. The advantage of the dark-blood contrast is that it reduces ringing and blood-flow related artifacts, and it reduces measurement errors at the tissue/blood boundary. The second characteristic is the positive T_1 weighting of the image intensity - shorter T_1 leads to lower intensity. In the presence of a T_1 contrast agent such as the common Gadolinium compounds, the higher the contrast concentration the lower the signal level. This positive contrast is the opposite of standard saturation or inversion recovery perfusion sequences. It has the advantage of very low blood pool intensity and associated artifacts.

The following are a few representative examples of how displacement-encoded MRI is used in clinical research studies.

SENSITIVITY AND SPECIFICITY IN THE DETECTION OF ABNORMAL WALL MOTION IN PATIENTS USING DISPLACEMENT-ENCODED MRI WITH ADAPTIVE IMAGE PROCESSING

Since DENSE is a quantitative technique, image processing is a key step from raw data to diagnostic indices. Two components in the post-processing of displacement-encoded images are phase-unwrapping and noise suppression. Myocardial motion is sufficient to induce phase-shifts that are greater than $360°$ and requires phase-unwrapping. In patient scans standard phase-unwrapping techniques can cause substantial errors [17]. An adaptive phase-unwrapping (APU) algorithm was therefore developed to reduce the rate of failure. APU incorporates the dynamic location of the myocardial wall as guidance for the unwrapping procedure and thereby keep the errors out of the areas of the wall.

This idea also proved to be effective in reducing the noise level in the myocardial strain images. Strain measures the amount of tissue deformation in the myocardial wall during systolic contraction and diastolic relaxation. It is calculated from the displacement-encoded phase data, and random noise in the phase data eventually leads to noise in strain. Noise suppression by spatial filtering is applicable to both cine and single-phase DENSE data, but conventional fixed-kernel filters are susceptible to partial volume effects at the endo- and epicardial borders of the myocardial wall, and tend to smooth out strain gradients across the wall. An adaptive spatial filter is the solution to these issues. As illustrated in Fig. (**1**), spatial filtering reduces the noise of an image pixel by assigning to it the averaged value of several pixels in its neighborhood. The shape of this neighborhood is the filter kernel. It is a fixed shape in conventional filters, but can be made to adapt to local anatomical features [18]. For example, the filter kernels can be thin arcs of one pixel thick and several pixels long. They are automatically aligned with the ventricular contours for all pixels. These kernels avoid the smoothing and partial volume effects across the wall.

In a study that included 16 patients (male-female ratio 11:5, age range of 26 - 74 years, 5 heart failure, 9 acute myocardial infarction, and 2 diabetic) and 12 volunteers (male-female ratio 6:6, age range of 29-53 years), adaptive phase-

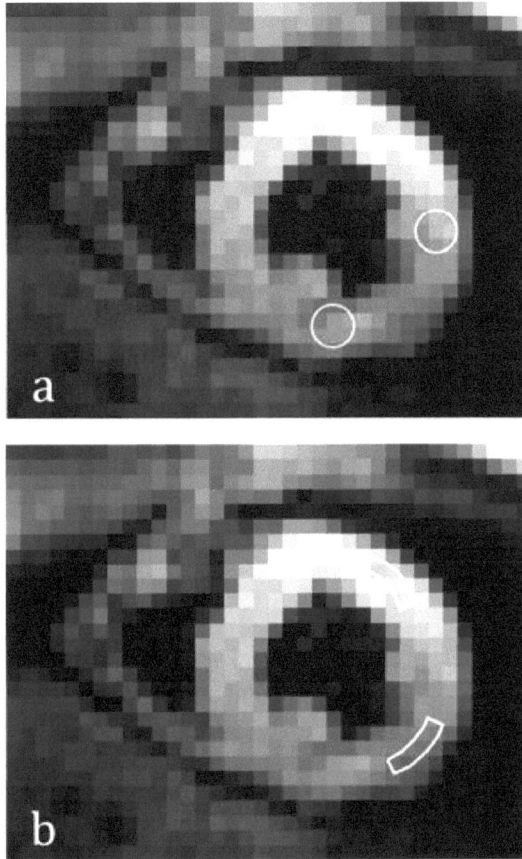

Figure 1: (**a**) Conventional filter kernels are location independent. (**b**) Adaptive filter kernels follow the wall contour.

unwrapping lowered the error rate from 5.05% to 0.089% when compared with conventional phase-unwrapping (P = 0.00031). The adaptive filter also significantly reduced the strain noise level (Fig. **2**).

The end result is that adaptive image processing significantly (P = 0.034) improves the sensitivity in detecting abnormal wall motion in the patient group according to Receiver-Operating Curve (ROC) analysis (Fig. **3**). The mean and 95% confidence interval of the sensitivity with and without the adaptive techniques were (82.5 ± 4.6)% and (87.7 ± 4.0)%, respectively. This study shows that detection based on a systolic circumferential strain (Ecc) threshold achieves 87.7% sensitivity and specificity in reference to echocardiography as the gold standard. This strain threshold was found to be -0.122 [15].

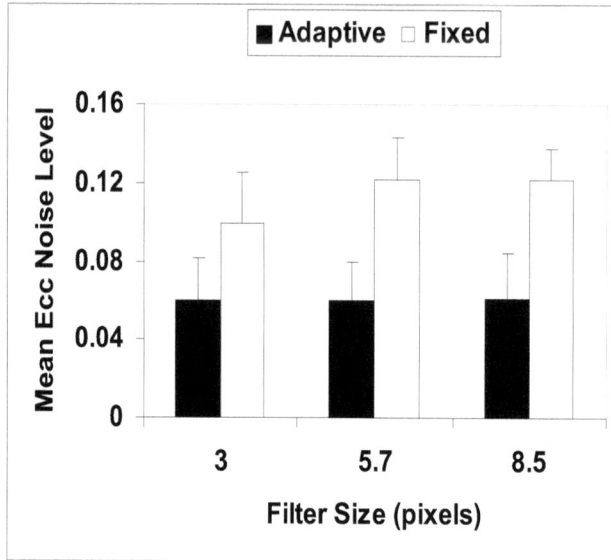

Figure 2: Circumferential strain (Ecc) strain noise is significantly lower with adaptive than with conventional filters (P < 0.02).

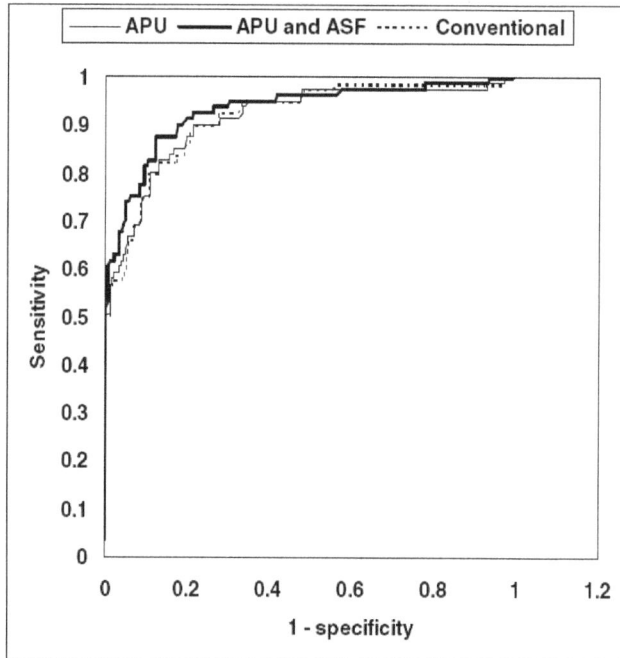

Figure 3: ROC analysis of strain-threshold-based detection of abnormal wall motion *vs* 2D echocardiography reading. APU - adaptive phase-unwrapping. ASF - adaptive filter.

SYSTOLIC MYOCARDIAL DYSFUNCTION IN PATIENTS WITH TYPE 2 DIABETES MELLITUS

Cardiovascular disease is and remains the leading cause of morbidity and mortality in diabetic patients, largely due to an accelerated atherosclerosis that involves macro- and microvasculature, with a prevalence growing rapidly, and an estimated number of diabetic patients increasing from 135 million in 1995 to 300 million in 2025 [19]. In addition, a true diabetic cardiomyopathy has also been identified and is defined as ventricular dysfunction that occurs independently of coronary artery disease and hypertension, which becomes more apparent in presence of hypertension or myocardial ischemia [20]. Diabetic cardiomyopathy is largely unrecognized but plays an important role in the increase cardiovascular morbidity and mortality associated with diabetic patients [21].

At a preclinical stage of type 2 diabetes mellitus (DM), echocardiographic studies have shown subclinical systolic myocardial dysfunction in patients without patent cardiomyopathy, suggestive of early signs of diabetic cardiomyopathy [22-25]. Whereas a reduced longitudinal myocardial strain has been demonstrated in this population, circumferential and radial abnormalities remain controversial, particularly due to technical limitations commonly associated with ultrasound techniques [26].

To evaluate how cine-DENSE can help in identifying sub-clinical myocardial systolic dysfunction and its patterns in a diabetic population, we studied 37 (50.7±5 y.o.) type 2 DM patients without overt heart disease and 23 (48.6±9 y.o.) age-matched controls. 2D cine-DENSE sequences were acquired at 3 short-axis and 2 long-axis locations [27].

While the left ventricular ejection fraction was normal and similar between the patients and controls, the DM patients showed a decrease in circumferential (Ecc) (-14.4±1.6% *vs* -17.0±1.6%, P<.0001) (Fig. **4**), radial (Err) (36.2±10.9% *vs* 44.4±9.9%, P=.006) and longitudinal (Ell) strain (-12.9±2.1% *vs* -15.5±1.6%, P<.0001) compared to controls. Finally, DM was independently associated with Ecc (P<.0001), Err (P=.05) and Ell (P=.01) after adjustment for age, sex, hypertension, body mass index and left ventricular mass [27].

In this setting, we showed that cine-DENSE is both feasible and reproducible in clinical practice. The intraobserver and interobserver variability were low, but there were higher intraobserver and interobserver limits of agreement of strain values in the radial direction compared with Ecc and Ell, confirming that Err is more susceptible to noise than Ecc [28]. Off course, further research is needed to assess whether the detection of subclinical myocardial dysfunction is of prognostic value, especially in patients with diabetes mellitus, as well as whether such detection may be useful in preventing the development of overt heart disease.

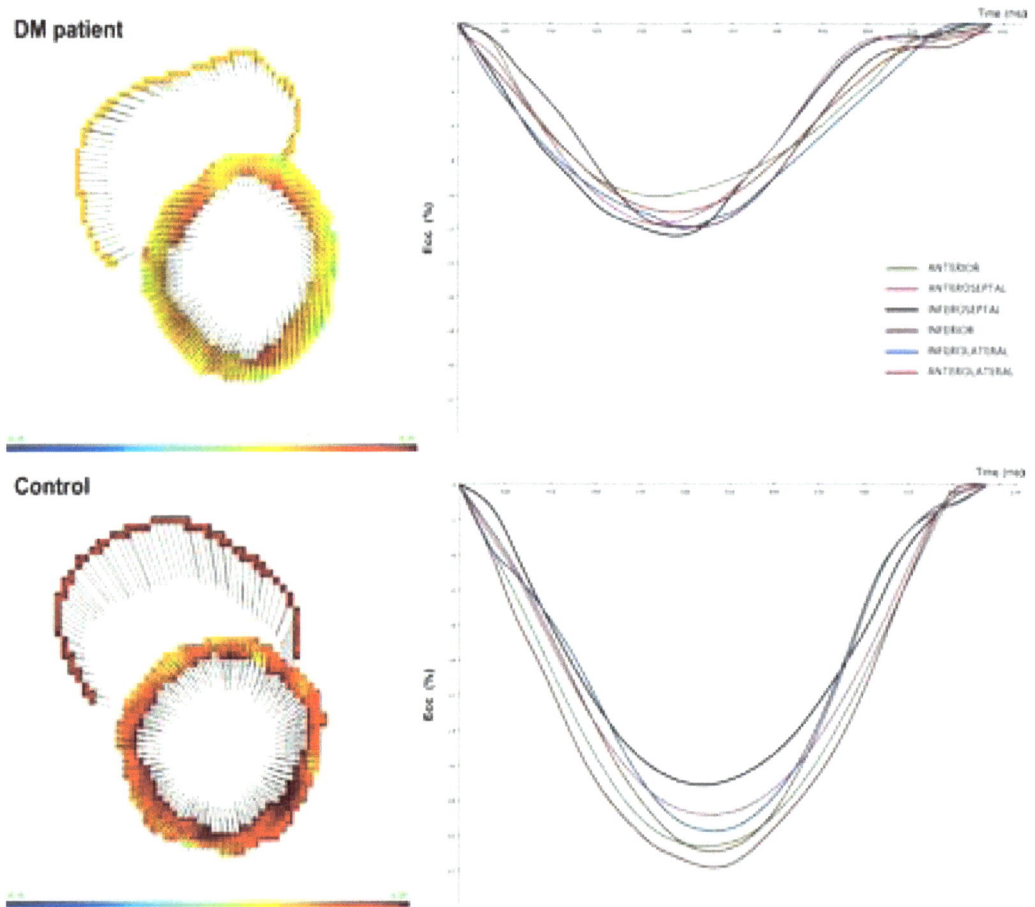

Figure 4: Example of circumferential systolic strain (Ecc) maps (left) and strain curves over time (right) in a 50 year-old male patient with type 2 diabetes mellitus (DM) (top), and a 50 year-old male control (bottom) (data are from short axis views at the mid-ventricular level).

DENSE BASED SIMULTANEOUS STRAIN AND POSITIVE-CONTRAST PERFUSION IMAGING

Because DENSE images are T_1 weighted, an early test in a pig acute myocardial infarction (AMI) protocol showed that when these images were acquired repeatedly with a single-shot pulse sequence during gadolinium (Gd) contrast agent infusion, the area of shortened T_1 from the contrast agent became dark, while the area that lacked blood flow had persistent signal intensity (Fig. **5**).

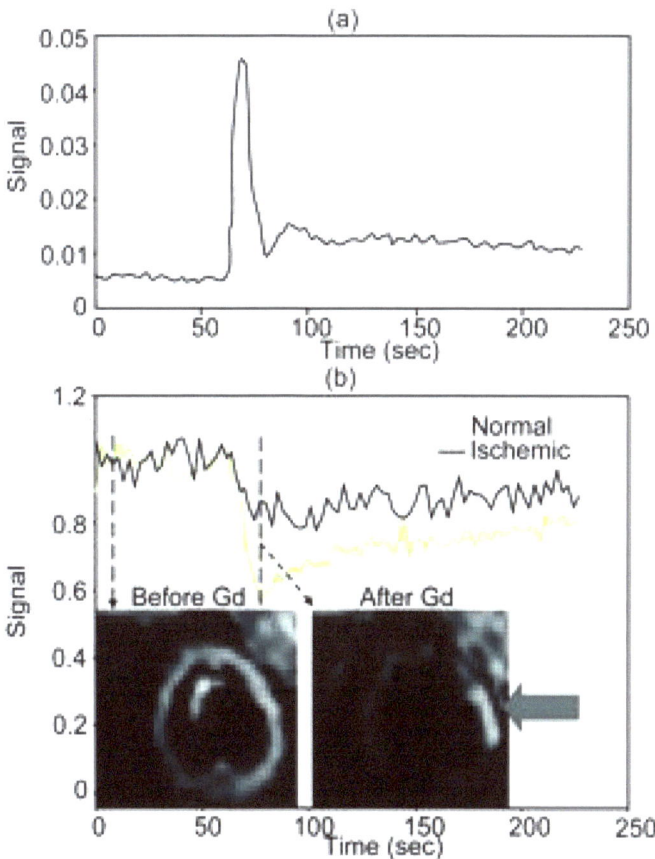

Figure 5: DENSE imaging during gadolinium contrast agent infusion and washout. Signal time-intensity curves in a swine study are shown. (**a**) Intensity of the LV blood pool in the saturation-recovery image provides the arterial input function for quantifying perfusion in the myocardium. (**b**) Intensity of the myocardium in a DENSE slice after Gd infusion. Arrow points to the ischemic segment. Due to the positive T_1 contrast of the image, normally perfused tissue became dark upon contrast arrival, while ischemic tissue retained its brightness. Ventricular cavities are dark due to rapid blood flow and high contrast concentration.

Based on this observation, we hypothesized that it would be feasible to optimize the pulse sequence for simultaneous perfusion and strain imaging, where the phase of the signal encodes tissue motion as usual, and the signal time-intensity curve allows the measurement of tissue perfusion [29].

Two key components of this approach are the arterial input function (AIF), and elastic registration of the images during free-breathing. To obtain the first, the DENSE pulse sequence was modified to acquire a saturation-recovery AIF image during the time gap between displacement-encoding and multi-slice image acquisition [30, 31]. The AIF slice was placed at or above the mitral valve plane. Signal in the descending aorta in the AIF slice provided a quantitative measure of the arterial contrast concentration. Images were acquired during free breathing with ECG gating. Thus, the position and shape of the heart varied from frame to frame, which required elastic registration before quantitative analysis could be performed on the image intensity.

The application of displacement-encoded MRI for simultaneous strain and perfusion imaging was carried out in a swine AMI study followed by a patient study [32]. The purpose of the animal study was to verify the perfusion values with gold-standard microsphere measurements. The animal study included 10 Yorkshire farm pigs. Permanent occlusion of the left anterior descending artery distal to the first diagonal branch was effected either by ligation following left side thoracotomy (n = 7) or with a balloon occluder in a fluoroscope-guided percutaneous procedure (n = 3). Fluorescent microspheres were injected into the left atrium immediately after the MR scan. Simultaneous arterial blood samples were taken from the femoral artery for calibration of the microsphere counts. The animal was then sacrificed and the heart was embedded in agarose gel for fluorescence imaging and microsphere counting.

The patient study subsequently tested the performance of the imaging protocol in a realistic setting, and evaluated how perfusion, strain, contrast washout rate and tissue viability are inter-correlated in a small patient group. Under an IRB approved protocol, 13 Acute Myocardial Infarction (AMI) patients (11 men, 2 women, age 39-82) were recruited on the criteria that they had angiographic evidence of one- or two-vessel coronary artery disease; had undergone percutaneous revascularization and deemed stable for MRI scans at least two days after the procedure. The data from one patient (a 52-year-old man) were excluded due to the failure of ECG triggering.

All MR scans were performed on clinical 1.5T scanners The single-shot DENSE sequence acquired 3 to 4 short-axis slices in every other heart beat and was repeated for 3 (encoding directions) × 30(repetitions) = 90 times over a period of 3.5 to 4 minutes. During this time a bolus of Gd-DOPA (Dotarem, Guerbet, France) or Gd-DTPA (Magnevist, Bayer HealthCare Pharmaceuticals Inc. Wayne, NJ) was given intravenously at the dose of 0.1 mmol/kg and an infusion rate of 2.0 ml/sec in the pigs and 4.0 ml/sec in patients. Other imaging parameters were matrix size of 128 × 40 with inner-volume excitation equivalent to 128 × 96 and 3/4 phase-encode FOV, resolution of 2.5 mm in pigs and 3.5 mm in patients, and slice thickness of 6-8 mm. After elastic image registration, pixel-wise perfusion and short term washout rate maps were obtained with Marquardt-Levenberg fitting using the Fermi transfer function model [33]. The 30 repetitions of strain maps were averaged into a single systolic strain map for each slice.

In the pig study, segmental MRI perfusion values were validated against microsphere values (Fig. **6**). Microsphere data showed that the perfusion levels obtained with the DENSE images were accurate.

A complete set of results from a patient is shown in Fig. (**7**). Statistically a strong correlation was found between regional absolute perfusion and contrast washout rate in the patient group (R^2 = 0.796). The slope, or ratio, between the two values is the capillary extraction fraction. This indicates that the extraction fraction was constant over the range of conditions in the patient group. This has been also found previously in canine AMI models [34].

The correlation between regional strain and perfusion was weaker in the patients (R^2 = 0.374). The Ecc strain measurements were generally less noisy than the radial strain [15]. The weaker strain-perfusion correlation was most likely due to the resting condition under which the scans were performed as compared with stress tests. In the literature this has been the consensus in both animal and human studies [35,36].

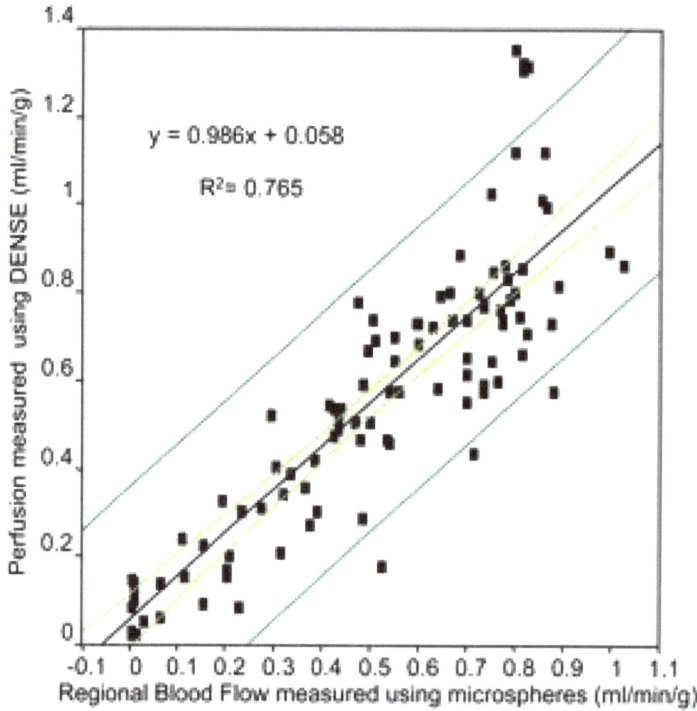

Figure 6: Validation of DENSE perfusion against microsphere values.

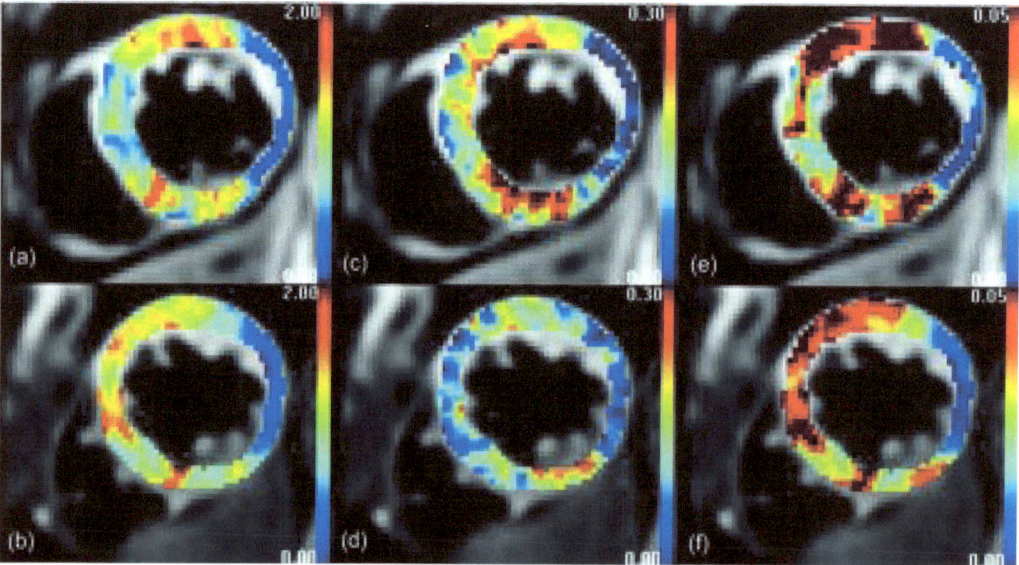

Figure 7: The perfusion, circumferental strain and short-term washout rate in the basal and mid-level short axis slices of a patient. All were derived from the same DENSE images.

In the patient group, tissue viability was assessed with separate inversion-recovery T_1 weighted scans at 4 and 10 minutes after contrast infusion. The myocardial segments were classified into three groups of delayed hyper-enhanced (DHE) with no-reflow, DHE with reflow, or non-DHE. The histograms of normalized perfusion values relative to remote normal myocardium for the three groups are shown in Fig. (**8**). They form distinct peaks with overlap. The overlap was likely caused by two reasons. The first relates to physiological factors including microvascular damage in non-DHE segments. The other is some variability in the segmentation of the DHE and DENSE images, which were performed by two independent observers. In summary, the animal and patient studies showed that the single-shot DENSE sequence is able to provide quantitative maps of both myocardial perfusion and strain in a single scan. In the AMI patients the protocol produced good-to-excellent quality images in 76% of the scans. The limitation was the reduced signal-to-noise ratio and increased artifacts of the images from the T_1 relaxation and resonance frequency shifts introduced by the paramagnetic contrast agent.

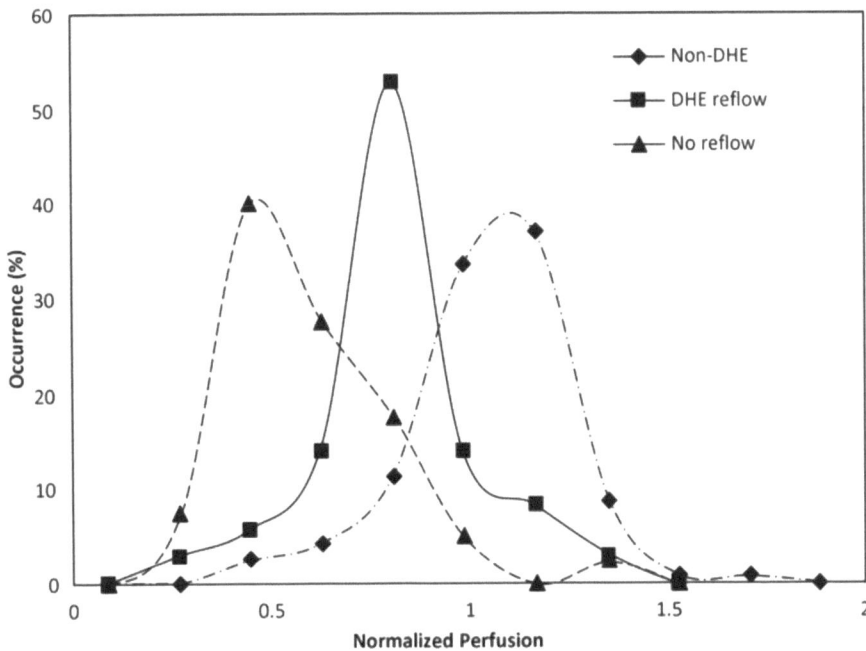

Figure 8: Distribution of normalized perfusion in non-DHE, DHE with reflow and DHE with no-reflow segments in patients. The normalization is relative to remote normal myocardium.

HETEROGENEITY OF INTRAMURAL FUNCTION IN HYPERTROPHIC CARDIOMYOPATHY

This is an example of a clinical study that benefited significantly from the high resolution of displacement-encoded MRI. In this study, Aletras and co-authors used DENSE to evaluate the intramural strain pattern in the myocardium of hypertrophic cardiomyopathy (HCM) patients [37]. In these patients myocardial abnormalities are commonly heterogeneous. Late gadolinium enhancement (LGE) MRI scans reported two types of abnormal patterns: a bright "confluent" and an intermediate intensity abnormality termed "diffuse", each representing different degrees of myocardial scarring. The DENSE protocol was used to study the relation between intramural cardiac function and the extent of fibrosis in HCM, and specifically to determine whether excess collagen or myocardial scarring, as determined by LGE MRI, are the primary mechanisms leading to heterogeneous regional contractile function. In a group of 22 patients with HCM, intramural left ventricular strain, transmural left ventricular function, and regions of myocardial fibrosis/scarring were imaged using DENSE, cine MRI, and LGE. DENSE systolic strain maps were qualitatively and quantitatively compared with LGE images.

The study found that intramural systolic strain by DENSE was significantly depressed within areas of confluent and diffuse LGE but also in the core of the most hypertrophic non-enhanced segment (all $P<0.001$ *versus* non-hypertrophied segments). DENSE demonstrated an unexpected inner rim of largely preserved contractile function and a non-contracting outer wall within hypertrophic segments in 91% of patients. In these HCM patients LGE predicted some but not all of the heterogeneity of intramural contractile abnormalities. This study implies that myocardial scarring or excess interstitial collagen deposition does not fully explain the observed contractile heterogeneity in HCM. Rather, myofibril disarray or other non-fibrotic processes affect systolic function in a large number of patients with HCM.

CAROTID ARTERY WALL STRAIN IMAGING

The spatial resolution advantage of displacement-encoded MRI allows the imaging of circumferential strain in the carotid artery wall, and thereby provides a regional measure of arterial stiffening for further investigation of atherosclerotic plaques in the carotid artery in patients [16]. The wall of conduit arteries undergoes cyclic stretching from the periodic fluctuation of the arterial pressure. The circumferential strain (Ecc) simply measures the percentage of the stretching relative to the point of lowest arterial pressure (diastolic pressure). The stiffness of the arterial wall is derived from strain and blood pressure (BP) measurements.

A comparison study was performed [16] between DENSE and cine based measurements of common carotid artery circumference in normal volunteers at 1.5T (n = 4, all male, age 29 to 37) using a 4 channel carotid coil pair, and at 3T (n = 17, 7 males, 10 females, age 18 to 66) using a single rectangular surface coil. The same scan parameters were used at both field strengths. Some of the imaging parameters were matrix size of 256×192, resolution of 0.60×0.60×4 mm^3, bandwidth of 585 Hz per pixel, 32 k-space lines per heartbeat, and TR/TE = 4.8/2.4 ms. Signal averaging, or phase cycling, of 10 was used and each slice took 6 minutes to complete. Vacuum fixation cushions were used to minimize neck movement during the exam. The circumferential strain from DENSE averaged over the circumference of the artery should match the percentage changes of the circumference by cine imaging. This was proven at both 1.5T and 3.0T (Fig. **9**).

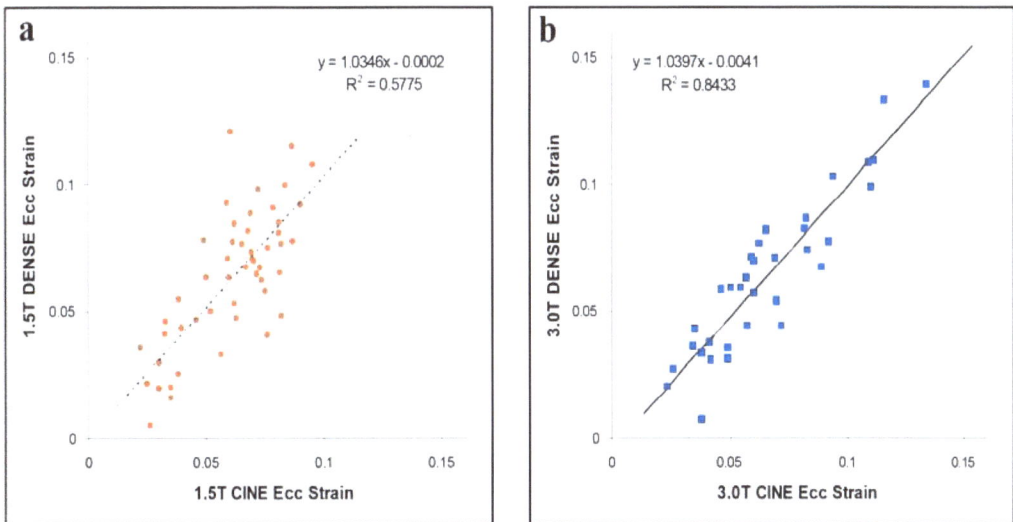

Figure 9: DENSE *vs* cine measurements of circumferential average strain in the common carotid artery wall at (**a**) 1.5T and (**b**) 3.0T.

At 1.5T the group-averaged SNR of the DENSE images was 2.6 in the wall segment bordering the jugular vein, 4.6 in the opposite segment, and 3.4 over the whole circumference. At 3.0T, the average SNR ranged from 1.9 in the segment furthest from the surface coil to 14.9 in the most superficial segment, and 6.3 over the circumference. Even though the 3T single-element surface coil was sub-optimal for carotid imaging, the potential for higher SNR than 1.5T was still clear.

In addition to the circumferentially-averaged strain, the study also looked for evidence of spatial variation around the circumference of the carotid artery. If the spatial variation of strain was only due to measurement noise, then it would be independent of the circumferential average value. If part of the variation was real, then this part would scale with the circumferential average. The data confirmed that the latter was the case in both the 1.5T and 3.0T groups (Fig. **10**). This study also revealed that the segmented k-space image acquisition was susceptible to swallowing-induced artifacts despite the vacuum cushions. A solution to this problem is the single-shot approach, where a number of single-shot images are taken in the same amount of time it would take to acquire the segmented k-space images. These are then averaged to yield a high SNR image. Since each shot produces a complete image, it is much less affected by physiological motion.

Displacement from shot-to-shot are then compensated with rigid body registration. Images with significant displacement after registration are rejected prior to averaging. Fig. (**11**) shows an example where the single-shot approach is clearly superior to the segmented approach. In a preliminary study which included 4 normal volunteers at 1.5T and another 4 at 3.0T, the segmented k-space and single-shot approaches were compared systematically [38]. Both imaging protocols had the same spatial resolution of $0.8{\times}0.8{\times}4$ mm^3 and took 4.8 minutes for each slice. Three slices were acquired above, at and below the carotid bifurcation. The single-shot protocol increased the SNR by 145% at 1.5T and by 66% at 3.0T [38]. However, similar to the single-shot DENSE sequence in the myocardial perfusion-strain study - occasional aliasing artifacts required the operator to exclude some receiver channels manually. It also called for the implementation of parallel imaging to solve this problem.

Distribution of Strain in Carotid Lumen Wall

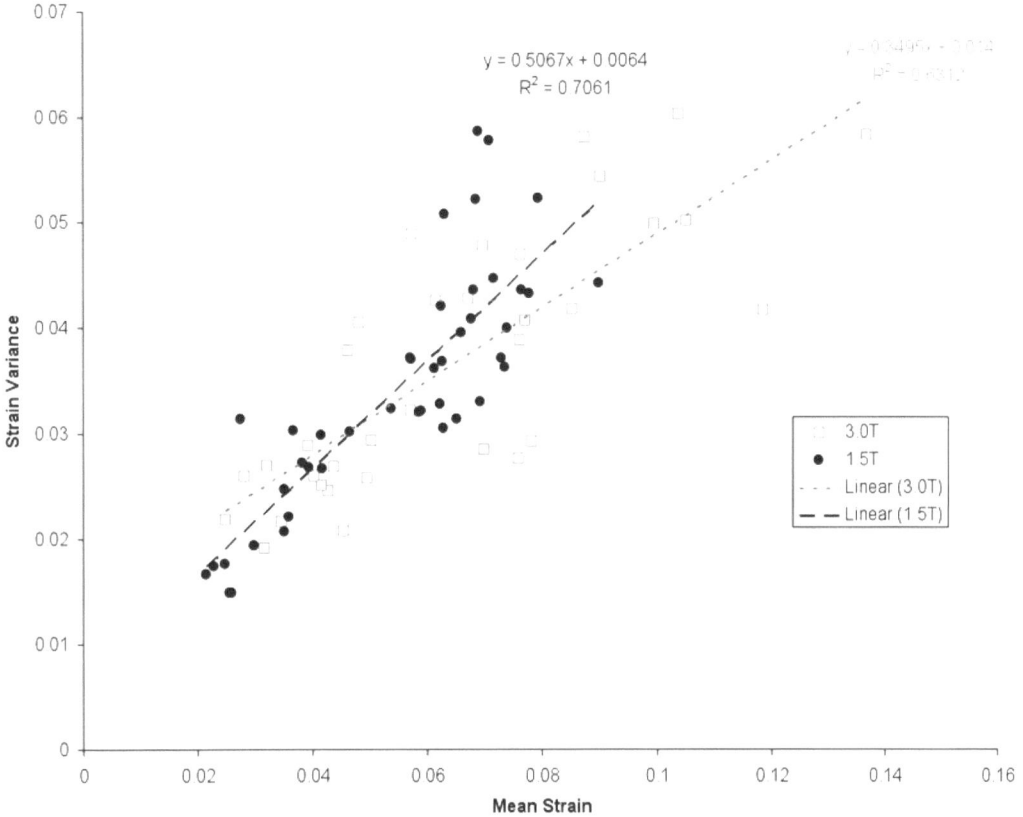

Figure 10: Spatial variation of strain scales with the circumferential mean strain.

The above development also permitted regional measures of carotid wall strain and wall stiffness when taking into account systolic and diastolic blood-pressures. Stiffening of the arterial wall is associated with both the onset of atherosclerosis and later calcification of the plaques [39,40]. Current non-invasive indices of arterial stiffness are either whole-body systemic measures, or lumen size-based average measures (ultrasound and MRI). However, as shown in the example of the carotid strain map of a patient in Fig. (**12**), the strain is reduced only in the volume of the plaque but normal in the remote segments of the wall. Therefore, regional measures of wall strain may potentially improve the sensitivity in the detection of arterial stiffening. In a broader context, although angiography and non-invasive ultrasound can detect stenotic plaques, the angiographically normal occult plaques [41] can only be seen non-invasively with MRI [38]. MRI strain mapping provides a new and relevant piece of information to the multi-contrast approach of MRI plaque detection and characterization.

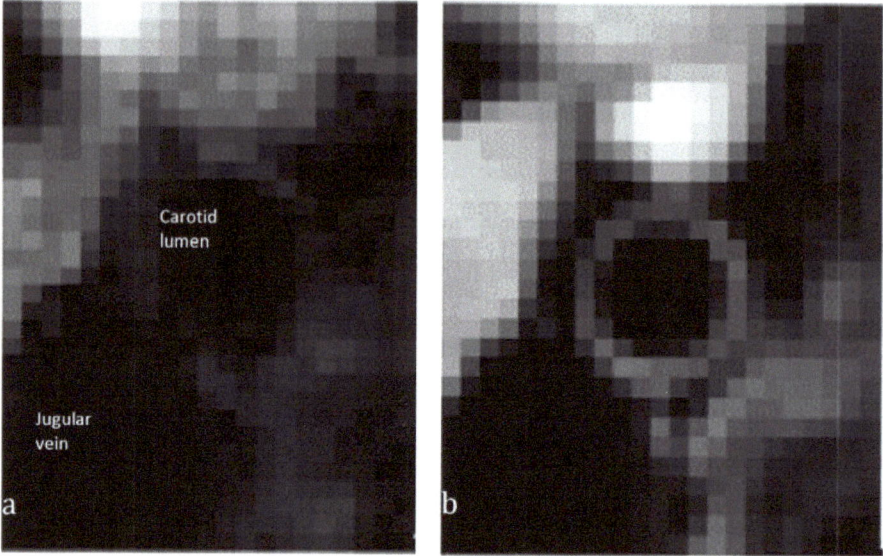

Figure 11: (a) Segmented k-space acquisition of a volunteer with frequent movement. **(b)** Average of motion corrected single-shot images from the same volunteer.

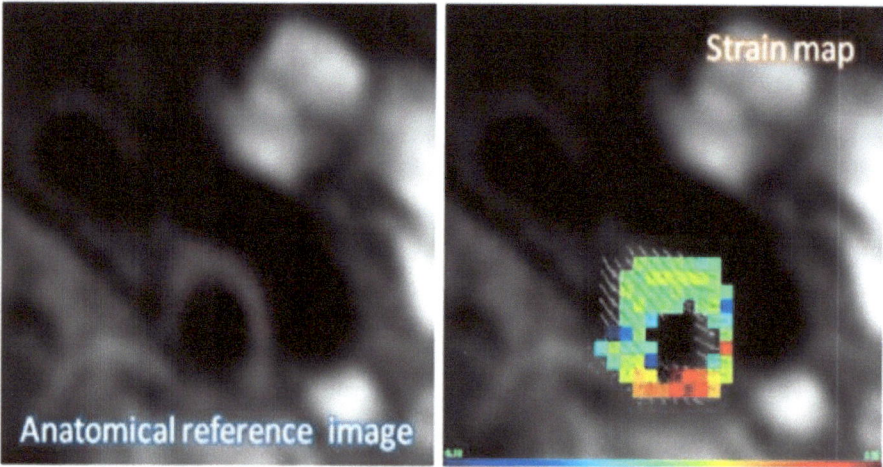

Figure 12: Images of the carotid artery of a patient, T1-weighted Cross section of the internal carotid artery with the plaque outlined in red on the left, and strain map on the right. The small white arrows in the strain map are tissue displacement vectors. The color scale of strain is between -0.3 and 0.3. The plaque has diminished strain, an indication of high stiffness.

CONCLUSION

The magnetic resonance signal contains an angle or phase in addition to its amplitude. Displacement-encoded MRI techniques are able to store the positional information of tissue into the phase of each image pixel, and retain this information over time intervals comparable to the T_1 relaxation time of the spins. These techniques confer the advantages of high spatial resolution and accurate quantification to clinical studies of tissue motion of strain. The T_1 weighting of the displacement-encoded MRI signal has also been explored as a means to quantify the kinetics of Gd-based contrast agents, and thus assessing perfusion in the same scan that obtains functional information. Currently, these methods continue to be developed for clinical and pre-clinical applications.

CONFLICT OF INTEREST

This is to certify that the authors do not have any conflict of interest.

ACKNOWLEDGEMENT

Han Wen is a Principle Investigator at the National Heart, Lung and Blood Institute (NHLBI) of the National Institutes of Health (NIH). The studies are funded in part by the Division of Intramural Research of NHLBI, NIH.

REFERENCES

[1]   Aletras AH, Ding SJ, Balaban R, Wen H. Displacement encoding in cardiac functional MRI. International Society for Magnetic Resonance in Medicine (Abstr) 1998; 1: 281.

[2]   Zerhouni EA, Parish DM, Rogers WJ, Yang A, Shapiro EP. Human heart: tagging with MR imaging--a method for noninvasive assessment of myocardial motion. Radiology 1988; 169: 59-63.

[3]   Axel L, Dougherty L. MR imaging of motion with spatial modulation of magnetization. Radiology 1989; 171: 841-845.

[4]   Constable RT, Rath KM, Sinusas AJ, Gore JC. Development and evaluation of tracking algorithms for cardiac wall motion analysis using phase velocity MR imaging. Magn Reson Med 1994; 32: 33-42.

[5]   Jung B, Zaitsev M, Hennig J, Markl M. Navigator gated high temporal resolution tissue phase mapping of myocardial motion. Magn Reson Med 2006; 55: 937-942.

[6]   Pelc LR, Sayre J, Yun K *et al.* Evaluation of myocardial motion tracking with cine-phase contrast magnetic resonance imaging. Invest Radiol 1994; 29: 1038-1042.

[7]   Guttman MA, Prince JL, McVeigh ER. Tag and contour detection in tagged MR images of the left ventricle. IEEE Trans Med Imaging 1994; 13: 74-88.

[8]   Stuber M, Scheidegger MB, Fischer SE *et al*. Alterations in the local myocardial motion pattern in patients suffering from pressure overload due to aortic stenosis. Circulation 1999; 100: 361-368.

[9]   Meyer FG, Constable RT, Sinusas AJ, Duncan JS. Tracking myocardial deformation using phase contrast MR velocity fields: a stochastic approach. IEEE Trans Med Imaging 1996; 15: 453-465.

[10]   Aletras AH, Ding S, Balaban RS, Wen H. DENSE: displacement encoding with stimulated echoes in cardiac functional MRI. J Magn Reson 1999; 137: 247-252.

[11]   Callaghan PT, Eccles CD, Xia Y. NMR microscopy of dynamic displacements - k-space and q-space imaging. Journal of Physics E-Scientific Instruments 1988; 21: 820-822.

[12]   Tseng WY, Reese TG, Weisskoff RM, Brady TJ, Wedeen VJ. Myocardial fiber shortening in humans: initial results of MR imaging. Radiology 2000; 216: 128-139.

[13]   Aletras AH, Balaban RS, Wen H. High-resolution strain analysis of the human heart with fast-DENSE. J Magn Reson 1999; 140: 41-57.

[14]   Kim D, Gilson WD, Kramer CM, Epstein FH. Myocardial tissue tracking with two-dimensional cine displacement-encoded MR imaging: development and initial evaluation. Radiology 2004; 230: 862-871.

[15]   Wen H, Marsolo KA, Bennett EE *et al*. Adaptive postprocessing techniques for myocardial tissue tracking with displacement-encoded MR imaging. Radiology 2008; 246: 229-240.

[16]   Lin AP, Bennett E, Wisk LE, Gharib M, Fraser SE, Wen H. Circumferential strain in the wall of the common carotid artery: comparing displacement-encoded and cine MRI in volunteers. Magn Reson Med 2008; 60: 8-13.

[17]   Ghiglia DC, Pritt MD. Two-dimensional phase unwrapping: theory, algorithms, and software. New York: John Wiley & Sons, Inc., 1998.

[18]   Wen H. Anatomically guided shaped smoothing in myocardial strain analysis (abstr). Proceedings of European Society of Magnetic Resonance in Medicine and Biology 2005; 22: 469.

[19]   King H, Aubert RE, Herman WH. Global burden of diabetes, 1995-2025: prevalence, numerical estimates, and projections. Diabetes Care 1998; 21: 1414-1431.

[20]   Rubler S, Dlugash J, Yuceoglu YZ, Kumral T, Branwood AW, Grishman A. New type of cardiomyopathy associated with diabetic glomerulosclerosis. Am J Cardiol 1972; 30: 595-602.

[21]   Boudina S, Abel ED. Diabetic cardiomyopathy revisited. Circulation 2007; 115: 3213-3223.

[22]   Fang ZY, Yuda S, Anderson V, Short L, Case C, Marwick TH. Echocardiographic detection of early diabetic myocardial disease. Journal of the American College of Cardiology 2003; 41: 611-617.

[23]   Nakai H, Takeuchi M, Nishikage T, Lang RM, Otsuji Y. Subclinical left ventricular dysfunction in asymptomatic diabetic patients assessed by two-dimensional speckle tracking echocardiography: correlation with diabetic duration. Eur J Echocardiogr 2009; 10: 926-932.

[24]   Ernande L, Rietzschel ER, Bergerot C *et al*. Impaired myocardial radial function in asymptomatic patients with type 2 diabetes mellitus: a speckle-tracking imaging study. J Am Soc Echocardiogr 2010; 23: 1266-1272.

[25]   Ng AC, Delgado V, Bertini M *et al*. Findings from left ventricular strain and strain rate imaging in asymptomatic patients with type 2 diabetes mellitus. Am J Cardiol 2009; 104: 1398-1401.

[26]   Bijnens BH, Cikes M, Claus P, Sutherland GR. Velocity and deformation imaging for the assessment of myocardial dysfunction. Eur J Echocardiogr 2009; 10: 216-226.

[27]   Ernande L, Thibault H, Bergerot C *et al*. Systolic myocardial dysfunction in patients with type 2 diabetes mellitus: identification at MR imaging with cine displacement encoding with stimulated echoes. Radiology 2012; 265: 402-409.

[28]   Shehata ML, Cheng S, Osman NF, Bluemke DA, Lima JA. Myocardial tissue tagging with cardiovascular magnetic resonance. J Cardiovasc Magn Reson 2009; 11: 55.

[29]   Le Y, Kellman P, Taylor E *et al*. Simultaneous myocardial first-pass perfusion and strain imaging with DENSE (Abstr). Journal of Cardiac Magnetic Resonance 2008; 10(1): A96.

[30]   Gatehouse PD, Elkington AG, Ablitt NA, Yang GZ, Pennell DJ, Firmin DN. Accurate assessment of the arterial input function during high-dose myocardial perfusion cardiovascular magnetic resonance. J Magn Reson Imaging 2004; 20: 39-45.

[31]   Kim D, Axel L. Multislice, dual-imaging sequence for increasing the dynamic range of the contrast-enhanced blood signal and CNR of myocardial enhancement at 3T. J Magn Reson Imaging 2006; 23: 81-86.

[32]   Le Y, Stein A, Berry C *et al*. Simultaneous myocardial strain and dark-blood perfusion imaging using a displacement-encoded MRI pulse sequence. Magn Reson Med 2010; 64: 787-798.

[33]   Jerosch-Herold M, Wilke N, Stillman AE. Magnetic resonance quantification of the myocardial perfusion reserve with a Fermi function model for constrained deconvolution. Med Phys 1998; 25: 73-84.

[34]   Svendsen JH, Bjerrum PJ, Haunso S. Myocardial capillary permeability after regional ischemia and reperfusion in the *in vivo* canine heart. Effect of superoxide dismutase. Circ Res 1991; 68: 174-184.

[35]   Heusch G, Schulz R. Perfusion-contraction match and mismatch. Basic Res Cardiol 2001; 96: 1-10.

[36]   Weintraub WS, Hattori S, Agarwal JB, Bodenheimer MM, Banka VS, Helfant RH. The relationship between myocardial blood flow and contraction by myocardial layer in the canine left ventricle during ischemia. Circ Res 1981; 48: 430-438.

[37]   Aletras AH, Tilak GS, Hsu LY, Arai AE. Heterogeneity of intramural function in hypertrophic cardiomyopathy: mechanistic insights from MRI late gadolinium enhancement and high-resolution displacement encoding with stimulated echoes strain maps. Circ Cardiovasc Imaging 2011; 4: 425-434.

[38]   Lin AP. Non-Invasive Imaging of Carotid Arterial Strain Using Displacement-Encoded MRI. California Institute of Technology 2009; PhD Thesis.

[39]   Mattace-Raso FU, van der Cammen TJ, Hofman A *et al*. Arterial stiffness and risk of coronary heart disease and stroke: the Rotterdam Study. Circulation 2006; 113: 657-663.

[40]   van Popele NM, Grobbee DE, Bots ML *et al*. Association between arterial stiffness and atherosclerosis: the Rotterdam Study. Stroke 2001; 32: 454-460.

[41]   Nissen SE, Yock P. Intravascular ultrasound: novel pathophysiological insights and current clinical applications. Circulation 2001; 103: 604-616.

CHAPTER 4

Flow Quantification: 1D to 4D

Christopher J. Francois[*]

Department of Radiology, University of Wisconsin – Madison, 600 Highland Avenue, Madison, WI 53792, USA

Abstract: Flow quantification with magnetic resonance (MR) imaging is an established method for assessing patients with a variety of cardiovascular diseases, particularly valvular heart disease and congenital heart disease. This chapter reviews basic MR physics and clinical applications for flow quantification, from one-directional flow-sensitive MR to time-resolved, three-directional flow-sensitive MR.

Keywords: MR Flow, phase contrast, flow quantification, 4D flow MR, congenital heart disease, valvular heart disease.

INTRODUCTION

Visualization and quantification of blood flow are an essential part of cardiovascular magnetic resonance (MR) imaging studies, with applications as variable as the assessment of valvular regurgitation and stenosis, calculation of pulmonary to systemic circulation shunt ratios, and estimation of pressure gradients. This chapter will begin with a review the basic physics behind how flow is imaged using phase contrast (PC) MR. Subsequently, clinical applications for two-dimensional (2D) and four-dimensional (4D) PC MR will be presented.

A complete review of the physics underlying the generation of flow-sensitive PC MR data is beyond the scope of this chapter. However, a general understanding of the principles of how flow and motion are imaged with MR is essential. P.R. Moran first described the use of MR to image flow in 1982 [1]. This initial description of measuring flow with MR has been modified and improved by

*Address correspondence to Christopher J. Francois: Department of Radiology, University of Wisconsin - Madison, 600 Highland Avenue, Madison, WI, 53792, USA; Tel: 001-608-263-1198; Fax: 001-608-263-0876; E-mail: cfrancois@uwhealth.org

Moran [2] and others [3-9], although the basic techniques used currently to assess blood flow have been widely used for over 30 years.

BASIC PC MR PHYSICS

Briefly, in a constant magnetic field, all protons, whether in stationary or moving tissue, will spin in unison with the same phase (Fig. **1a**). However, when a gradient is applied to the magnetic field, protons will process with different phase depending upon their position within the magnetic field gradient (Fig. **1b**). Protons that are moving through a magnetic field gradient will acquire a phase shift relative to protons in surrounding stationary tissues that is proportional to the velocity at which the protons are moving (Fig. **1b**).

To be able to measure the velocities at which the tissues of interest are moving in one-directional flow sensitive PC MR, it is necessary to acquire two measurements for each voxel within the image to be able to subtract the unknown phase of the background stationary tissues. The first measurement (m_o) serves as a reference scan that is typically flow compensated. The second measurement (m_1) is motion sensitive, or velocity encoded. These two measurements are then subtracted (m_0-m_1) to obtain the final PC MR image. Each of the two measurements, m_0 and m_1, are synchronized to the cardiac cycle through the electrocardiographic signal.

Flow-encoding in one-directional flow sensitive PC MR is achieved by using bipolar gradients that have a net zero area (Fig. **2a**). With a standard bipolar gradient, moving protons will have a residual phase to them relative to stationary tissues. This is used to quantify the phase difference between stationary and moving protons, and therefore measure velocity. To obtain an image with completely refocused spinning protons with the same phase in both stationary and moving tissues, flow compensation is used (Fig. **2b**).

The measured phase differences, ϕ, are proportional to the velocity with which the spins are moving through the slice:

$$\phi = 2\pi\gamma G\Delta\delta v \ \ldots \tag{1}$$

where γ is the gyromagnetic ratio; G, Δ, and δ are related to the gradient amplitudes and times; and v is the velocity of the moving spins. Phase shifts, ϕ, are measured in degrees, from -180° to +180°. The sign of the phase shift corresponds to the direction of flow relative to the slice, either antegrade (+) or retrograde (-). Phase shifts of 0° correspond to tissues that are stationary, with zero velocity.

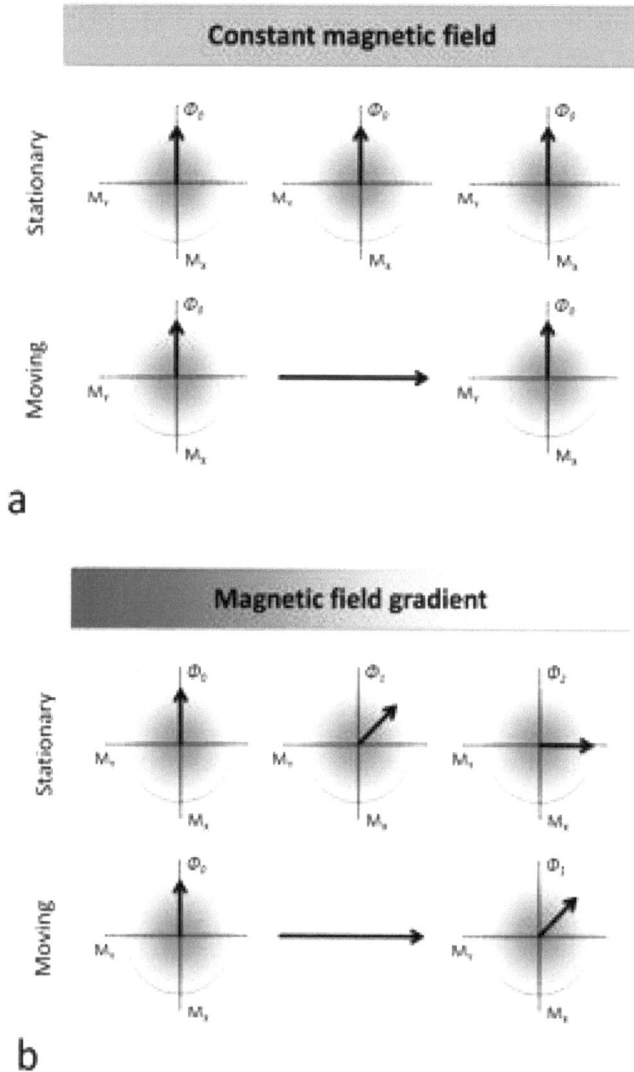

Figure 1: (a) Static and moving tissue in constant magnetic field. **(b)** Static and moving tissue in magnetic field gradient. Arrows indicate the phase of the spin vector with respect to the XY-plane.

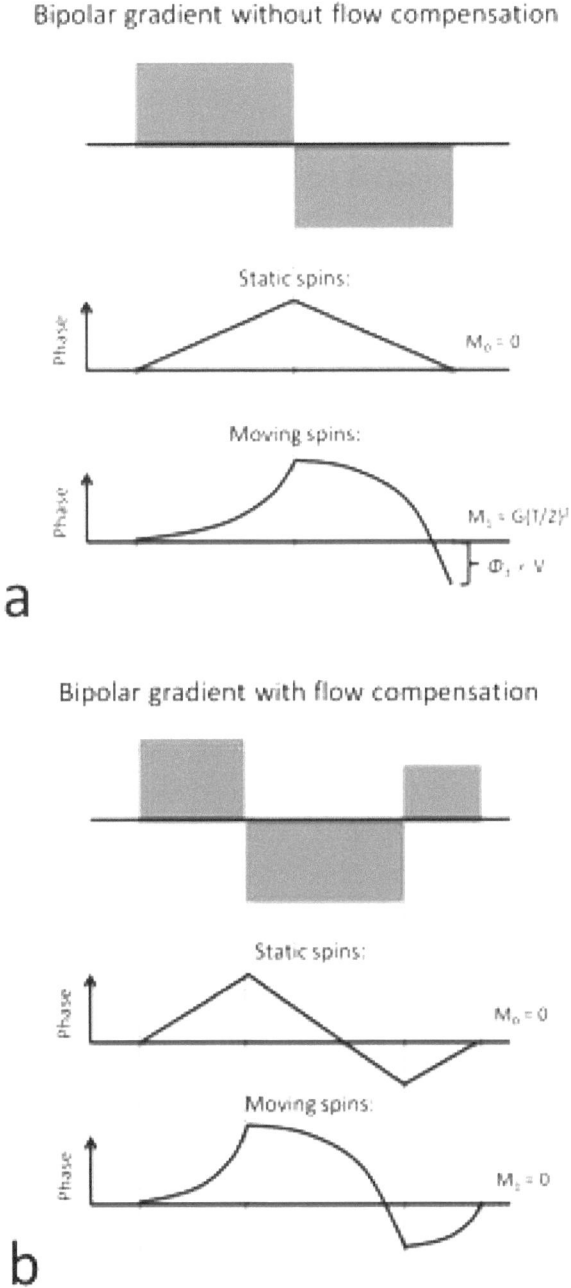

Figure 2: (**a**) Basic bipolar gradient. The residual phase is used to calculate phase difference (Φ) which is proportional to the velocity of the moving spins. (**b**) Bipolar gradient with flow compensation. With flow compensation, both static and moving spins have a zero residual phase difference at the end of the bipolar gradient.

The maximum absolute value of the velocity that can be resolved without aliasing is determined by the velocity encoding sensitivity (VENC). If the velocities are faster than the VENC selected, aliasing will occur and the measured phase shift will be greater than ±180°. On the other hand, it is important to set the VENC as close as possible to the expected maximum velocity to maintain optimal velocity-to-noise-ratio (VNR) performance because it is inversely related to the VENC selected. It can be shown that the VNR is proportional to the ratio of velocity within the image to the VENC [10]:

$$VNR = (\pi/2) \times (v/VENC) \times SNR \quad \ldots \tag{2}$$

In areas with widely variable velocities, variable velocity-encoding [11] or dual velocity-encoding [12] strategies may improve the VNR for areas with slower flow. Equation 2, also reveals that the VNR is proportional to overall SNR of the acquisition. Therefore, what is true for SNR in MR imaging in general also applies to improving VNR in PC MR. As a result, VNR can be improved by increasing the field strength of the acquisition from 1.5T to 3.0T [13] or by performing the acquisition after the administration of gadolinium-based contrast agents [14].

Flow-encoding with PC MR can be done in any of the three orthogonal gradient directions. Although quantification is typically done using flow-encoding in the slice direction (Fig. **3a**), flow-encoding can also be done in the frequency or phase directions to assess flow features within the plane of the image (Fig. **3b**). This can be particularly helpful in determination of flow direction in patients with intra-cardiac shunts (Fig. **4**) in which flow could be either left-to-right or right-to-left.

To obtain time-resolved flow data, the image acquisition in a PC MR is gated to the cardiac cycle. As with other cardiac time-resolved sequences, PC MR can be gated prospectively or retrospectively [15] with respect to the electrocardiographic signal or pulse oximeter tracing. In this fashion, the acquisition of the different lines of k-space for each image is segmented, with a predefined number of k-space lines for the individual time-frames acquired per

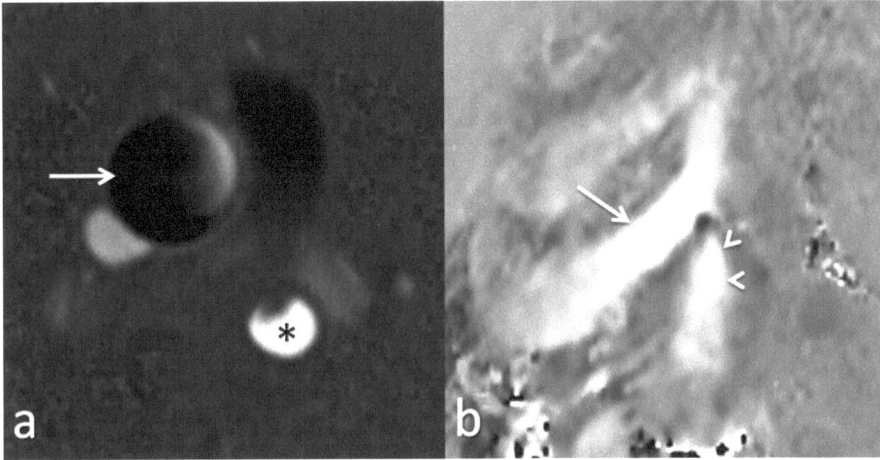

Figure 3: (**a**) 2D PC MR with through-plane flow-encoding. In this example, the signal intensity in the ascending and descending aorta is proportional to the flow through the imaging plane. Because the directions of flow in the ascending and descending aorta are opposite to each other, the signal intensities are also opposite (black in the ascending aorta, arrow, and white in the descending aorta, asterisk). (**b**) 2D PC MR with in-plane flow-encoding. In this example, flow-encoding is in the anterior-posterior direction such that the signal intensity in the left ventricular outflow tract (arrow) during systole is proportional to the velocity of flow leaving the left ventricle. In this patient, this approach also assists with visualization of the mitral regurgitation jet (arrowheads) as well.

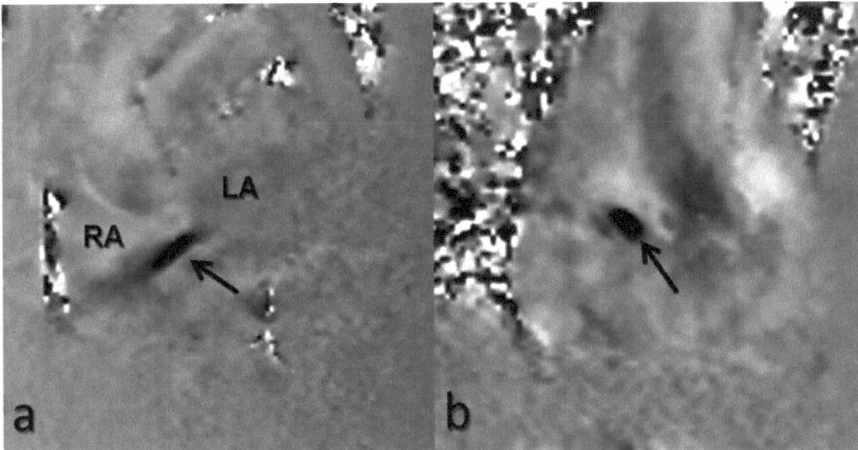

Figure 4: (**a**) 2D PC MR with in-plane flow-encoding in a patient with a secundum atrial septal defect (arrow). Flow-encoding is in the left-right direction, enabling visualization of the flow through the atrial septal defect from the left atrium (LA) to the right atrium (RA). (**b**) 2D PC MR with through-plane flow-encoding in a patient with a secundum atrial septal defect (arrow). Through-plane encoding can be used to calculate the amount of flow through the atrial septal defect during each heart beat.

heart beat. The number of heart beats required to acquire a complete series of time-resolved PC MR data will depend upon the number of k-space lines acquired for each image and the number of lines required to fill k-space, which is determined by the matrix size prescribed. The main advantage of retrospective cardiac gating is that data from throughout the cardiac cycle are available for flow quantification, which is important when diastolic flow is a substantial amount of the overall flow. However, this approach typically results in longer scan times than prospective cardiac gating.

TWO-DIMENSIONAL PC MR

Two-dimensional (2D), 1-directional, velocity encoding images are typically reconstructed with two sets of time-resolved images (Fig. **5a**). Magnitude images are standard gradient echo anatomical images that can be used to segment the vessel(s) of interest. The corresponding phase images provide the velocity information with a grayscale display from white to black, corresponding to the range of velocities from -VENC to +VENC. Flow is determined by integrating the sum of the velocities within the voxels included in the segmented region of interest. When each phase of the cardiac cycle is segmented, flow-time curves (Fig. **5b**) can be evaluated to assess flow velocity and volume, among a variety of additional hemodynamic parameters.

Accuracy of 2D PC MR

As with Doppler ultrasound, errors in velocity measurements using 1-directional velocity encoding can be minimized by orienting the slice of the acquisition perpendicular to the expected direction of flow. In addition, optimization of the flow measurements is achieved by placing the region of interest in the center of the field of view as close to the iso-center of the magnet bore, to ensure maximum homogeneity in the magnetic field. Experiments in phantoms, animal models and human subjects have shown that 2D PC MR is both accurate and reproducible for flow quantification. In human subjects, 2D PC MR measurements can be validated in a rather straight forward manner by comparing the flow through the aorta and pulmonary artery to the stroke volume from the left ventricle and right ventricle, respectively, based on CINE balance steady state free precession acquisitions. Furthermore, in patients without valvular regurgitation or shunts, the flow through the aorta and pulmonary arteries should be essentially the same, taking into account the fact that flow measurements in the aorta above the coronary arteries will be slightly lower. Studies have shown errors of approximately 3-5% for flow quantification and intra- and inter-observer variability of approximately 2-3% [9, 16].

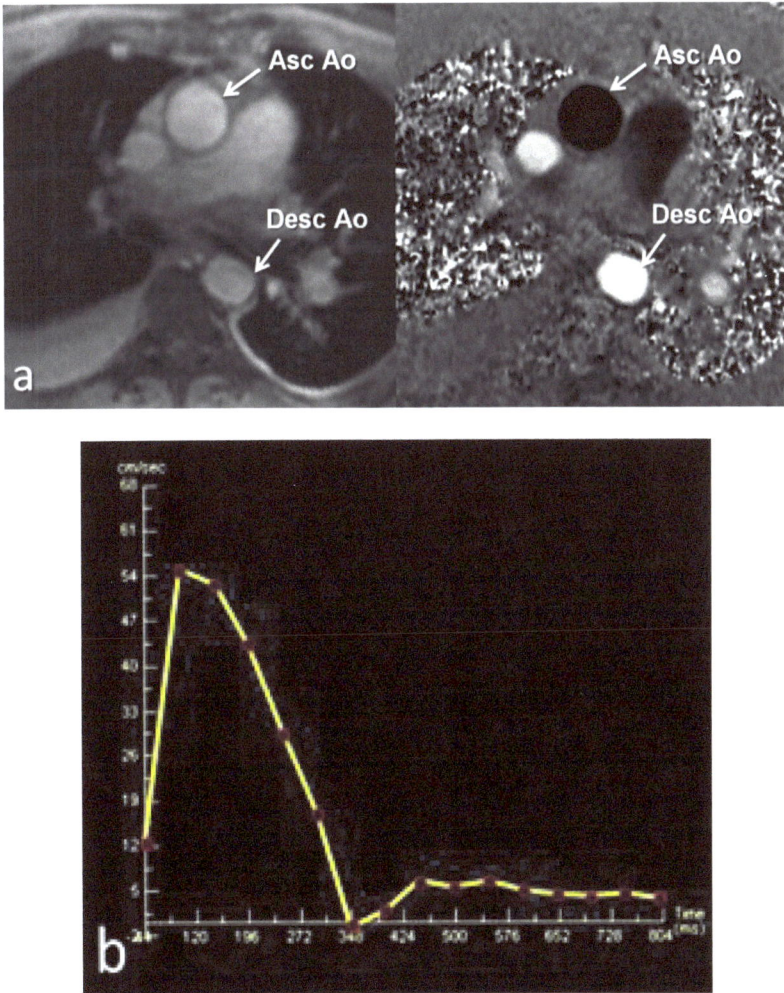

Figure 5: (**a**) Magnitude (left) and phase (right) images from 2D, 1-directional velocity encoded MRI through the ascending aorta. Note that the greyscale values in the ascending aorta (Asc Ao, black) are opposite of those in the descending aorta (Desc Ao, white), indicating that flow is in opposite directions. (**b**) Flow time curve obtained from integration of flow velocities within a region of interest placed over the ascending aorta.

There are multiple sources of error in the observed 2D PC MR signal, which subsequently results in errors in flow measurement [16-18]. In addition to user-related errors secondary to incorrect VENC selection and inappropriate orientation of the slice relative to the direction of flow, there are errors due to MR hardware and sequence acquisition. For example, errors due to imperfections in the MR scanner include concomitant gradients [19], eddy currents [20] and magnetic field gradient non-linearity. These are sources of error that are inherent to the MR scanner and not specific to 2D PC MR. However, an appreciation of these errors is important when considering potential causes for variability in flow quantification measurements. Some of these background errors can be corrected for by optimizing the sequence parameters and acquisition [17, 21]. *A posteriori* correction of these errors can include subtracting the measured flow through known stationary tissue nearby the area of interest from the measured flow through the area of interest. Alternatively, the scan can be repeated using the exact same parameter on a stationary phantom after the patient has gotten off the scanner [22, 23].

Clinical Applications of 2D PC MR

In cardiac MR, 2D PC MR is routinely used clinically to (a) measure peak velocities and flow volumes through the valves in patients with known or suspected valvular heart disease [15, 24], (b) quantify flow volumes in patients with suspected intra- or extra-cardiac shunts [25-27], or (c) estimate pressure drops across stenoses [28-30].

Valvular Heart Disease

The simplest use of 2D PC MR is to measure blood flow velocities through a specified area of interest. For example, in a patient with aortic stenosis, the severity of the stenosis can be quantified by measuring the peak velocity within the stenotic jet [31]. This is done by placing the 2D PC MR imaging plane perpendicular to the aortic root (Fig. **6**), at the expected level of the maximum flow velocity. To minimize errors in determination of the peak velocity, it is important to remember to place the orientation of the 2D PC MR acquisition perpendicular to the stenotic jet. Guidelines for grading the severity of aortic and pulmonic valve stenosis include the peak jet velocity [32]. Aortic valve stenosis is considered mild when the peak velocity is ≤ 3.0 m/s, moderate when the peak velocity is 3.0-4.0 m/s, and severe when the peak velocity is ≥ 4.0 m/s. Similarly, pulmonic valve stenosis is severe when the peak velocity is ≥ 4.0 m/s.

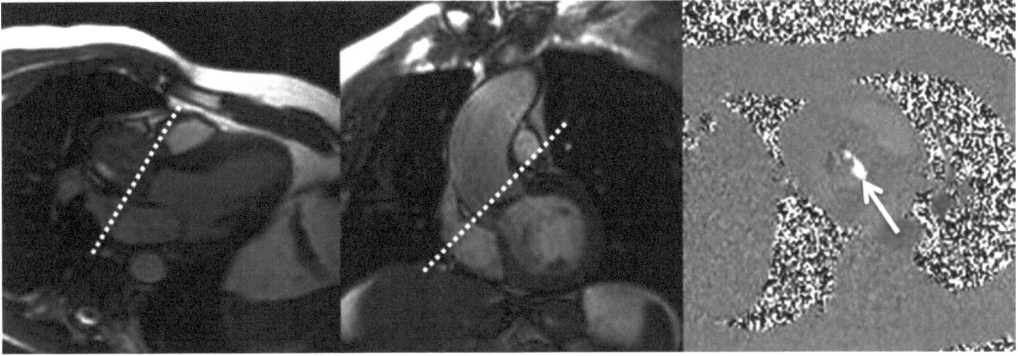

Figure 6: Three-chamber (left) and left ventricular outflow tract (middle) images are used to prescribe the orientation of the 2D PC MR acquisition (dashed lines). 2D PC MR is used to measure the peak velocity resulting from the stenotic bicuspid aortic valve (arrow).

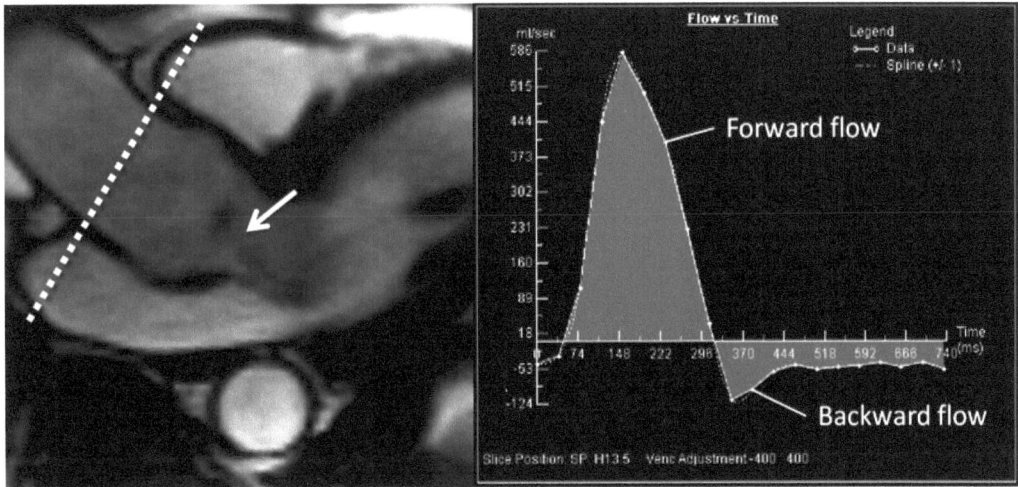

Figure 7: To quantify the severity of aortic regurgitation (arrow), 2D PC MR is performed through the proximal ascending aorta with the orientation perpendicular to the direction of flow (as indicated by the dashed line). From the flow-time curve, the regurgitant fraction is calculated from the ratio of the backward flow to the forward flow. In this case, aortic regurgitation is mild.

By integrating the area under the flow-time curve through a vessel of interest it is possible to measure the total flow through that vessel during the period of interest.

For the aorta and pulmonary artery, the flow within each cardiac cycle corresponds to the stroke volume of the left and right ventricles, respectively, which when multiplied by the subject's heart rate results in the cardiac output. As stated previously, in the absence of valvular regurgitation, the flow through the aorta and pulmonary artery measured with 2D PC MR should equal the cardiac output determined using volumetric methods. If the flow measurements are not equal to the volumetric measurements, then regurgitation should be suspected. The method of quantifying the severity of regurgitation with MR is fairly simple for aortic (Fig. **7**) [33] and pulmonary (Fig. **8**) [34] regurgitation. In analyzing the flow-time curve, the forward flow and backward flow are calculated separately. The severity of aortic regurgitation can be graded from the regurgitant volume per heart beat or based on the ratio of the backward flow to the forward flow. A regurgitant volume of ≥ 60 mL/heartbeat and a regurgitant fraction of ≥ 60% are both considered criteria of severe aortic regurgitation.

Because of the substantial through plane motion of the atrio-ventricular valves (typically greater than 10 mm between end diastole and end systole), calculation of mitral and tricuspid regurgitation is less straight forward. To measure the severity of mitral and tricuspid valve regurgitation, the flow through the great arteries, aorta and pulmonary artery respectively, is compared to the stroke volume determined from the volumetric CINE images.

Q_P/Q_S

2D PC MR is frequently used in patients with known or suspected congenital heart disease to determine whether or not the patient has any sign of intra- or extra-cardiac shunt [35]. In individuals without a shunt, the ratio of flow through the pulmonary artery (Q_P) and through the aorta (Q_S) should be 1.0 - 1.1. 2D PC MR is routinely used to calculate the shunt ratio in patients with known or suspected intra- or extra- cardiac shunts (Figs. **9**, **10**). The use of 2D PC MR to quantify Q_P/Q_S in complex congenital heart disease is particularly important because of the difficulty in quantifying pulmonary artery flow using other methods.

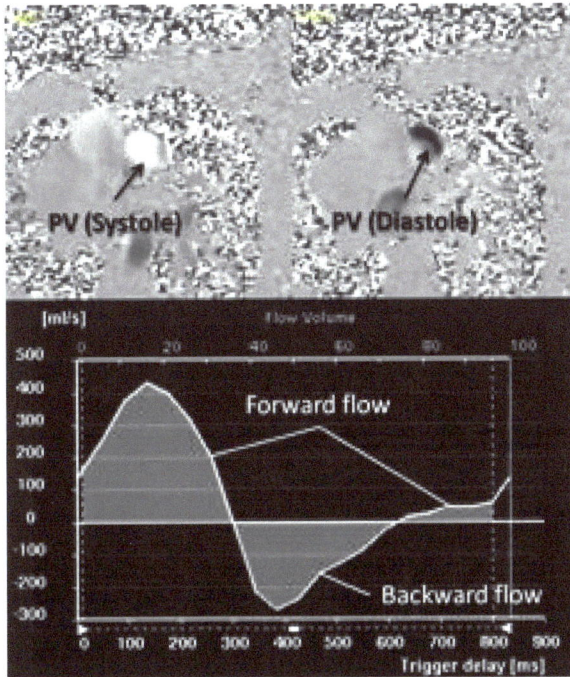

Figure 8: To quantify the severity of pulmonary regurgitation, 2D PC MR is performed through the pulmonary valve (PV) with the orientation perpendicular to the direction of flow. The flow images (top row) from systole and diastole demonstrate the change in signal intensity of flow through the PV from systole (white) to diastole (black), indicating reversal flow direction. From the flow-time curve (bottom image), the regurgitant fraction is calculated from the ratio of the backward flow to the forward flow. In this case, pulmonary regurgitation is moderate.

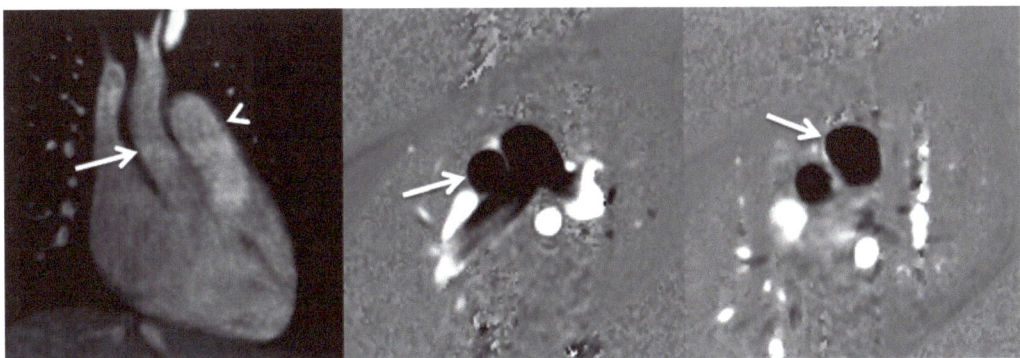

Figure 9: 2D PC MR was used to calculate the left-to-right shunt fraction, or Qp/Qs ratio, in a patient with partial anomalous venous return. The reformatted contrast-enhanced magnetic resonance angiography image on the right illustrates the location of the 2D PC MR acquisitions that were acquired through the ascending aorta (arrow and middle image) and main pulmonary artery (arrowhead and right image) to determine Qp/Qs.

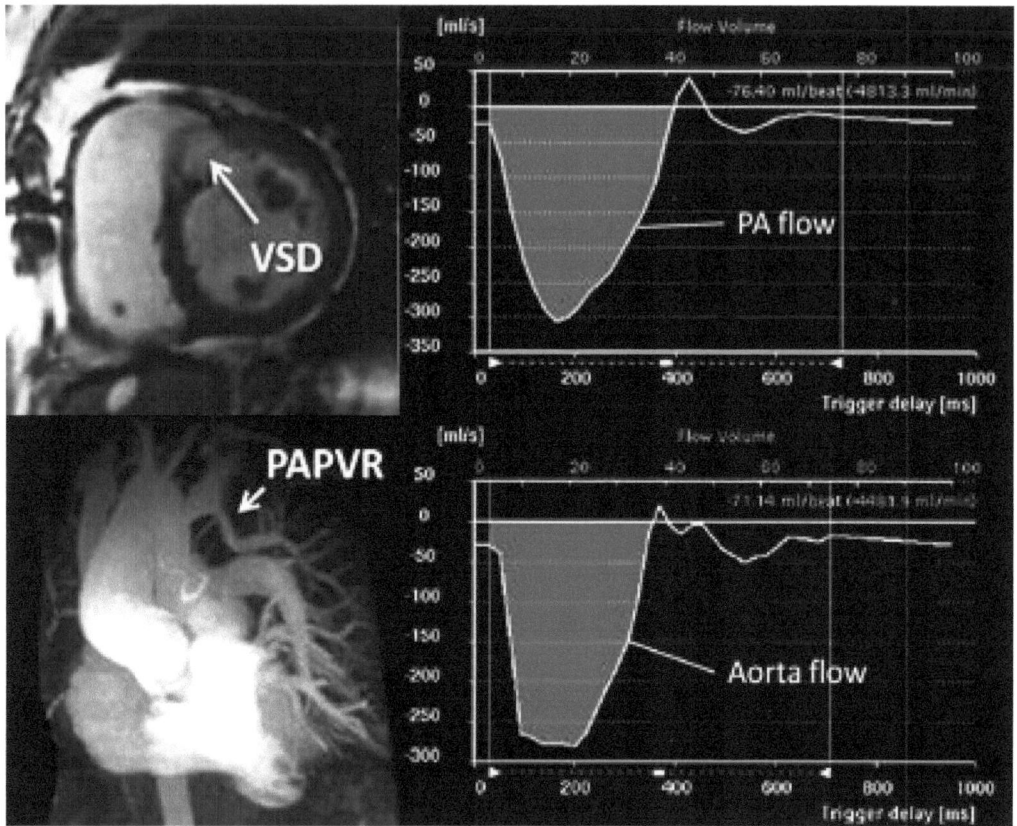

Figure 10: 2D PC MR was used to calculate the left-to-right shunt fraction, or Qp/Qs ratio, in a patient with ventricular septal defect (VSD, top left image) and partial anomalous venous return (PAPVR, bottom left image). Flow-time curves from the 2D PC MR acquisitions that were acquired through the pulmonary artery (PA, top right image) and ascending aorta (bottom right image) are used to determine Qp/Qs. In this case, because flow through the VSD is right-to-left and flow through the PAPVR is left-to-right, the shunts are relatively balanced and results in a Qp/Qs of almost 1 (= 76 mL/beat through PA ÷ 71 mL/beat through aorta).

Pressure Gradients

Similarly, the peak velocity measured through a stenotic vessel can be used to estimate the peak pressure drop across that stenosis using the simplified Bernoulli equation:

$$\Delta P \approx 4(V2 - V1)^2 \quad \ldots \tag{3}$$

*Δ*P is the pressure drop across the stenosis, V1 is the peak velocity proximal to the stenosis and V2 is the peak velocity distal to the stenosis. In general, because V1 is much smaller than V2, Equation 3 is simplified even further, resulting in the following:

$$\Delta P \approx 4V^2 \qquad \dots \tag{4}$$

where V is simply the peak velocity measured distal to the stenosis. This method is typically used to evaluate the severity of stenosis in patients with aortic coarctation (Fig. **11**) or with pulmonary artery stenosis. The simplified Bernoulli equation does make several important assumptions that can affect its accuracy, including the presence of non-viscous, steady and incompressible flow. Including the peak velocity proximal to the stenosis in the calculation of the pressure drop can improve the accuracy in milder stenoses.

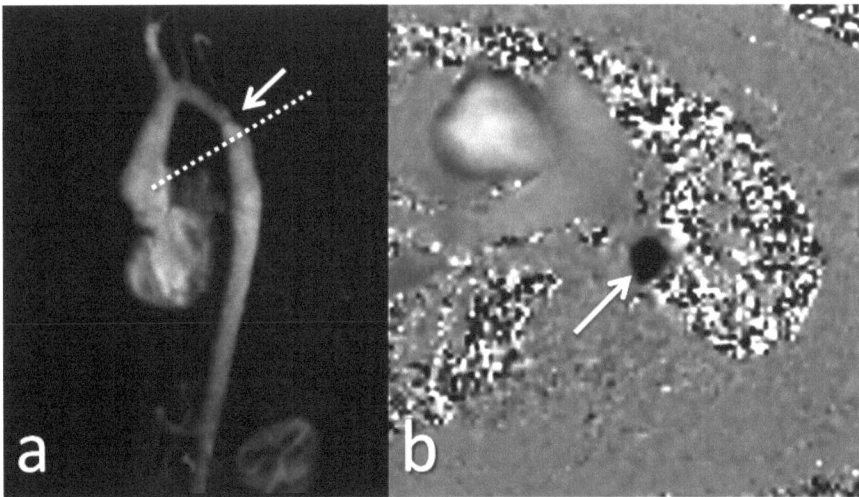

Figure 11: (**a**) Maximum intensity projection image from contrast enhanced magnetic resonance angiography in a patient with repaired coarctation (arrow). (**b**) 2D PC MR image obtained just distal to the coarctation, as indicated by dashed line in (**a**), is used to quantify the peak flow velocity through the coarctation. This can then be used to estimate the pressure gradient across the stenosis using the modified Bernoulli equation.

FOUR-DIMENSIONAL PC MR

Four-dimensional (4D) PC MR is used to describe a three-dimensional (3D), three-directional velocity-encoded, time-resolved acquisition [36-38]. As described previously for 2D PC MR, velocity-encoding can be done in any orthogonal direction. This can be done in one direction or in all three directions simultaneously. In the simplest case, demonstrated in Figs. (**3**, **4**), three-directional velocity encoding can be applied to a 2D acquisition or extended to a 3D, volumetric scan. To be able to resolve the velocity information in all three directions, additional flow-sensitive scans are necessary.

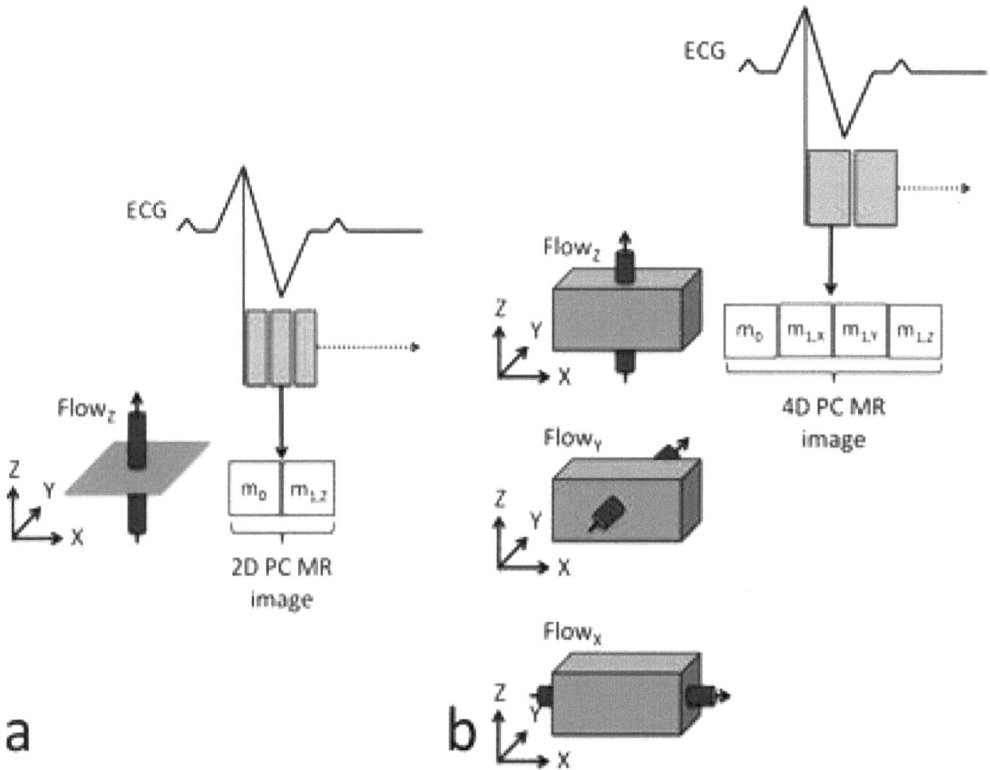

Figure 12: Schematic illustrating differences between 2D PC MR with (**a**) 2-dimensional, 1-directional velocity-encoding and (**b**) 4D PC MR with 3-dimensional, 3-directional velocity-encoding. Compared to 2D PC MR, 4D PC MR requires two additional flow-sensitive scans in the Y and X directions.

As described previously, one-directional velocity-encoding scans uses one reference scan (m_0) and one flow-sensitive scan (m_1) (Fig. **12a**). Initial attempts at acquiring 4D PC MR data acquired reference scans and flow-sensitive scans for each of the flow-encoding directions. It turns out that this is not necessary, and more efficient methods of 4D PC MR flow encoding have been developed, including four-point referenced, four-point balanced and five-point approaches. For a four-point referenced, three-directional velocity-encoding scan (Fig. **12b**), one reference scan (m_0) is followed by three flow-sensitive scans (m_{1X-Z}).

4D PC MR has gained interest because it has the potential to simplify the acquisition of flow data through numerous vessels of interest (Fig. **13**). For example, in patients with complex congenital heart disease, it may be necessary to quantify flow through each of the valves, shunts and great vessels, resulting in the need to prescribe *a priori* $\geq$ 4-6 2D PC acquisitions while the patient is still on the scanner. With 4D PC MR, all of the analysis is performed *a posteriori* after the patient has left the scanner. Furthermore, 4D PC MR can be used to qualitatively and quantitatively evaluate flow characteristics volumetrically, leading to the ability to quantify additional hemodynamic parameters non-invasively in ways that have not been feasible previously.

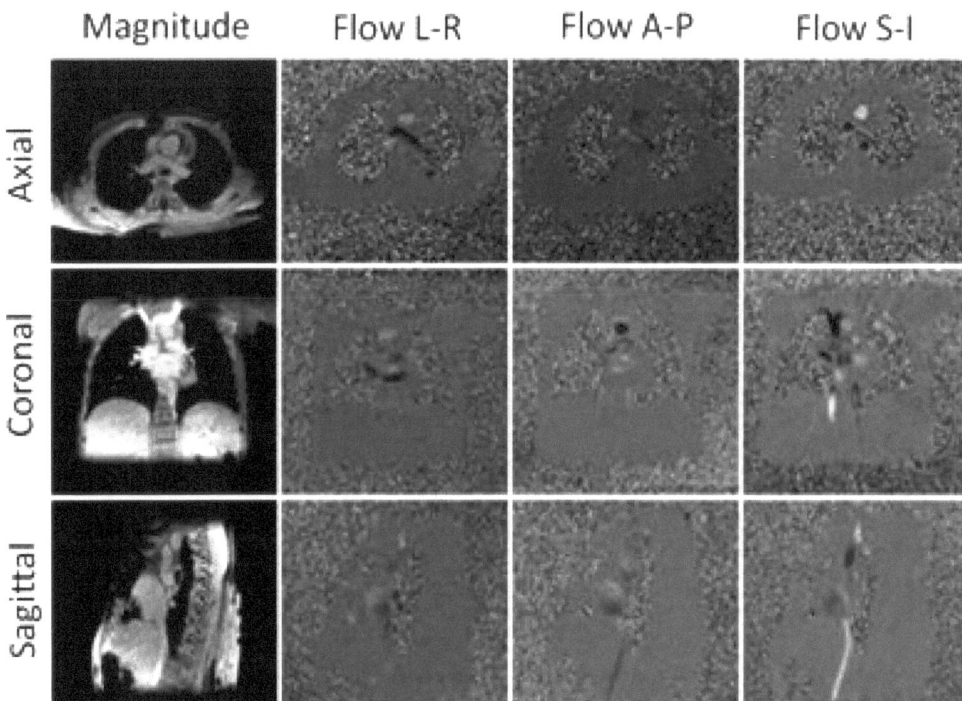

Figure 13: Magnitude and phase (flow) images from 4D PC MR acquisition. 4D PC MR includes 3D volumetric, time-resolved, 3-directional flow sensitive data that can be used to visualize and quantify flow through any region of interest included in the imaging volume.

To enable acquisition of these very large 4D PC MR datasets within a reasonable scan time, various acceleration strategies have been implemented by various groups. For standard Cartesian-based acquisitions [45], parallel imaging and view-sharing techniques have enabled reduction of scan times to less than 10-15 minutes, depending upon the volume of coverage and spatial resolution desired. Non-Cartesian acquisition strategies have also been successfully implemented for 4D PC MR. Of the non-Cartesian k-space trajectories, 3D radial undersampling [12] has been investigated most extensively. The benefits of using 3D radial undersampling, compared to Cartesian-based approaches, include much higher undersampling (and, therefore, greater acceleration factors) without loss of spatial resolution and fewer, tolerable artifacts.

Visualization of 4D PC MR

Currently, there is a paucity of software available to easily visualize 4D PC MR data. Additionally, no standard display for visualizing 4D PC MR flow data exists. As a result, different groups using 4D PC MR use a variety of commercial and home-built software for visualization and analysis of these data. For qualitative assessment of the 3D flow features, a combination of color-coded particle traces, streamlines and velocity vectors are used to determine the direction and complexity of flow through the circulation (Fig. **14**) [36, 38-40].

4D PC MR Clinical Applications

The role of 4D PC MR clinically is still being established. Relatively small, single-center studies have demonstrated its feasibility in a variety of applications, including (A) basic flow quantification [41], including quantification of Q_P/Q_S [42], (B) detection of abnormal flow patterns in congenital heart disease [43, 44] and aortic aneurysms [45-49], and (C) calculation of more advanced hemodynamic parameters [36-38]. 4D PC MR offers an attractive alternative to 2D PC MR for quantification of flow in patients requiring multiple areas to be evaluated because the planes do not have to be prescribed *a priori* (Fig. **15**). Additional small trials have confirmed the utility of 4D PC MR for the visualization of alterations in intra-cardiac and extra-cardiac flow patterns in a

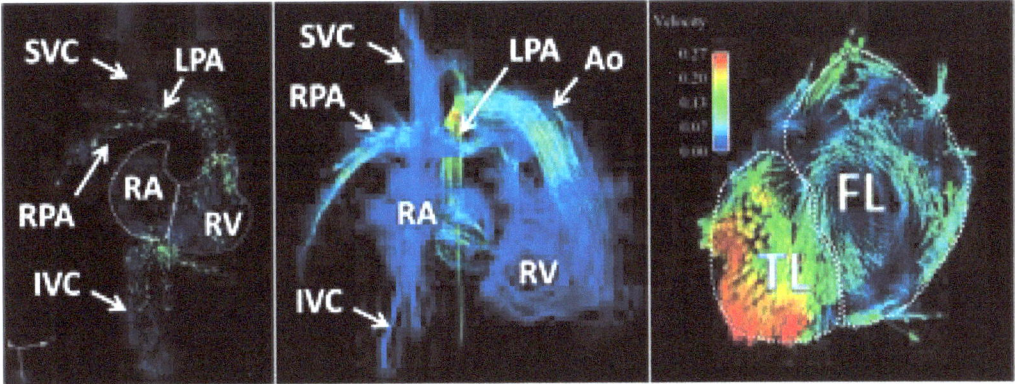

Figure 14: 4D PC MR Visualization. (Left) Particle trace visualization in a patient with a bidirectional Glenn. The short lines in the image represent massless particles emitted from, in this case, throughout the included vasculature. The color coding reflects the velocities of the particles and when visualized over the different phases of the cardiac cycle provide information on directionality of flow. SVC, superior vena cava; IVC, inferior vena cava; RPA, right pulmonary artery; LPA, left pulmonary artery; RA, right atrium; RV, right ventricle. (middle) Pathline visualization in a patient with total cavopulmonary shunt circulation. The lines represent the expected lines that particles are expected to follow at that given instant in time. As in A, the color coding reflects the velocities at that location during that phase of the cardiac cycle. SVC, superior vena cava; IVC, inferior vena cava; RPA, right pulmonary artery; LPA, left pulmonary artery; RA, right atrium; RV, right ventricle; Ao, aorta. (right) Vector visualization in a patient with aortic dissection. Flow within the true-lumen (TL) is directed primarily craniocaudal through the reconstructed image plane. Flow within the false-lumen (FL) is primarily within the plane of the reconstructed image plane, resulting in excess helical flow. Furthermore, the velocities within the FL are much lower than in the TL.

wide range of cardiac and vascular diseases. The future potential strength of this approach to flow imaging is in its ability to derive more complex quantitative hemodynamic parameters. These include parameters used to describe the integrity of the vessel wall, such as wall stress [41, 50, 51] and pulse wave velocity [52, 53], and parameters to describe the flow characteristics, such as vorticity and kinetic energy [54].

CONCLUSION

In conclusion, flow imaging with MRI is a mature, yet evolving, area of cardiac MR. 2D PC MR techniques are well established and used routinely in clinical CMR to assess valvular disease and congenital heart disease. Emerging 4D PC MR techniques offer an opportunity to simplify the acquisition of flow data and provide further insights into our understanding of normal and pathological hemodynamics.

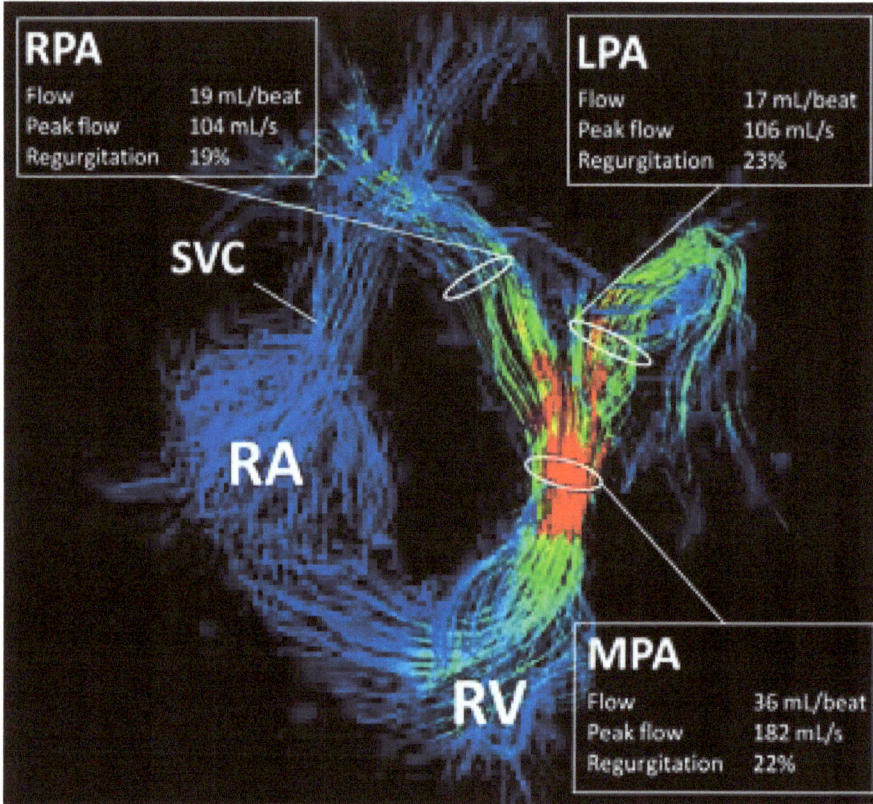

Figure 15: 4D PC MR can be used to retrospectively analyze flow in any area of interest that is included in the imaged volume. Pathline image from 4D PC MR data set in patient with a history of repaired tetralogy of Fallot. In this case, flow is quantified in the main pulmonary artery (MPA), right pulmonary artery (RPA) and left pulmonary artery (LPA). Pathlines are color coded relative to velocity, with highest velocities visible in the MPA due to MPA stenosis. SVC, superior vena cava; RA, right atrium; RV, right ventricle.

CONFLICT OF INTEREST

This is to certify that the authors do not have any conflict of interest.

ACKNOWLEDGEMENT

None declared.

REFERENCES

[1]   Moran PR. A flow velocity zeugmatographic interlace for NMR imaging in humans. Magn Reson Imaging. 1982;1(4):197-203.

[2]   Moran PR, Moran RA, Karstaedt N. Verification and evaluation of internal flow and motion. True magnetic resonance imaging by the phase gradient modulation method. Radiology. 1985 Feb;154(2):433-41.

[3]   Bryant DJ, Payne JA, Firmin DN, Longmore DB. Measurement of flow with NMR imaging using a gradient pulse and phase difference technique. J Comput Assist Tomogr. 1984 Aug;8(4):588-93.

[4]   Nayler GL, Firmin DN, Longmore DB. Blood flow imaging by cine magnetic resonance. J Comput Assist Tomogr. 1986 Sep-Oct;10(5):715-22.

[5]   Dumoulin CL, Souza SP, Darrow RD, Pelc NJ, Adams WJ, Ash SA. Simultaneous acquisition of phase-contrast angiograms and stationary-tissue images with Hadamard encoding of flow-induced phase shifts. J Magn Reson Imaging. 1991 Jul-Aug;1(4):399-404.

[6]   Pelc NJ, Bernstein MA, Shimakawa A, Glover GH. Encoding strategies for three-direction phase-contrast MR imaging of flow. J Magn Reson Imaging. 1991 Jul-Aug;1(4):405-13.

[7]   Bernstein MA, Shimakawa A, Pelc NJ. Minimizing TE in moment-nulled or flow-encoded two- and three-dimensional gradient-echo imaging. J Magn Reson Imaging. 1992 Sep-Oct;2(5):583-8.

[8]   Pelc LR, Pelc NJ, Rayhill SC, Castro LJ, Glover GH, Herfkens RJ, *et al*. Arterial and venous blood flow: noninvasive quantitation with MR imaging. Radiology. 1992 Dec;185(3):809-12.

[9]   Evans AJ, Iwai F, Grist TA, Sostman HD, Hedlund LW, Spritzer CE, *et al*. Magnetic resonance imaging of blood flow with a phase subtraction technique. *In vitro* and *in vivo* validation. Invest Radiol. 1993 Feb;28(2):109-15.

[10]   Conturo TE, Smith GD. Signal-to-noise in phase angle reconstruction: dynamic range extension using phase reference offsets. Magn Reson Med. 1990 Sep;15(3):420-37.

[11]   Buonocore MH. Blood flow measurement using variable velocity encoding in the RR interval. Magn Reson Med. 1993 Jun;29(6):790-5.

[12]   Nett EJ, Johnson KM, Frydrychowicz A, Del Rio AM, Schrauben E, Francois CJ, *et al*. Four-dimensional phase contrast MRI with accelerated dual velocity encoding. J Magn Reson Imaging. 2012 Jun;35(6):1462-71.

[13]   Lotz J, Doker R, Noeske R, Schuttert M, Felix R, Galanski M, *et al*. *In vitro* validation of phase-contrast flow measurements at 3 T in comparison to 1.5 T: precision, accuracy, and signal-to-noise ratios. J Magn Reson Imaging. 2005 May;21(5):604-10.

[14]   Bock J, Frydrychowicz A, Stalder AF, Bley TA, Burkhardt H, Hennig J, *et al*. 4D phase contrast MRI at 3 T: effect of standard and blood-pool contrast agents on SNR, PC-MRA, and blood flow visualization. Magn Reson Med. 2010 Feb;63(2):330-8.

[15]   Sondergaard L, Stahlberg F, Thomsen C, Spraggins TA, Gymoese E, Malmgren L, *et al*. Comparison between retrospective gating and ECG triggering in magnetic resonance velocity mapping. Magn Reson Imaging. 1993;11(4):533-7.

[16]   Lotz J, Meier C, Leppert A, Galanski M. Cardiovascular flow measurement with phase-contrast MR imaging: basic facts and implementation. Radiographics. 2002 May-Jun;22(3):651-71.

[17]   Rolf MP, Hofman MB, Gatehouse PD, Markenroth-Bloch K, Heymans MW, Ebbers T, *et al.* Sequence optimization to reduce velocity offsets in cardiovascular magnetic resonance volume flow quantification--a multi-vendor study. J Cardiovasc Magn Reson. 2011;13:18.

[18]   Gatehouse PD, Rolf MP, Graves MJ, Hofman MB, Totman J, Werner B, *et al.* Flow measurement by cardiovascular magnetic resonance: a multi-centre multi-vendor study of background phase offset errors that can compromise the accuracy of derived regurgitant or shunt flow measurements. J Cardiovasc Magn Reson. 2010;12:5.

[19]   Bernstein MA, Zhou XJ, Polzin JA, King KF, Ganin A, Pelc NJ, *et al.* Concomitant gradient terms in phase contrast MR: analysis and correction. Magn Reson Med. 1998 Feb;39(2):300-8.

[20]   Ahn CB, Cho ZH. Analysis of eddy currents in nuclear magnetic resonance imaging. Magn Reson Med. 1991 Jan;17(1):149-63.

[21]   Morgan VL, Price RR, Lorenz CH. Application of linear optimization techniques to MRI phase contrast blood flow measurements. Magn Reson Imaging. 1996;14(9):1043-51.

[22]   Chernobelsky A, Shubayev O, Comeau CR, Wolff SD. Baseline correction of phase contrast images improves quantification of blood flow in the great vessels. J Cardiovasc Magn Reson. 2007;9(4):681-5.

[23]   Miller TA, Landes AB, Moran AM. Improved accuracy in flow mapping of congenital heart disease using stationary phantom technique. J Cardiovasc Magn Reson. 2009;11:52.

[24]   Sondergaard L, Hildebrandt P, Lindvig K, Thomsen C, Stahlberg F, Kassis E, *et al.* Valve area and cardiac output in aortic stenosis: quantification by magnetic resonance velocity mapping. Am Heart J. 1993 Nov;126(5):1156-64.

[25]   Hundley WG, Li HF, Lange RA, Pfeifer DP, Meshack BM, Willard JE, *et al.* Assessment of left-to-right intracardiac shunting by velocity-encoded, phase-difference magnetic resonance imaging. A comparison with oximetric and indicator dilution techniques. Circulation. 1995 Jun 15;91(12):2955-60.

[26]   Arheden H, Holmqvist C, Thilen U, Hanseus K, Bjorkhem G, Pahlm O, *et al.* Left-to-right cardiac shunts: comparison of measurements obtained with MR velocity mapping and with radionuclide angiography. Radiology. 1999 May;211(2):453-8.

[27]   Beerbaum P, Korperich H, Barth P, Esdorn H, Gieseke J, Meyer H. Noninvasive quantification of left-to-right shunt in pediatric patients: phase-contrast cine magnetic resonance imaging compared with invasive oximetry. Circulation. 2001 May 22;103(20):2476-82.

[28]   Oshinski JN, Parks WJ, Markou CP, Bergman HL, Larson BE, Ku DN, *et al.* Improved measurement of pressure gradients in aortic coarctation by magnetic resonance imaging. J Am Coll Cardiol. 1996 Dec;28(7):1818-26.

[29]   Kilner PJ, Firmin DN, Rees RS, Martinez J, Pennell DJ, Mohiaddin RH, *et al.* Valve and great vessel stenosis: assessment with MR jet velocity mapping. Radiology. 1991 Jan;178(1):229-35.

[30]   Mohiaddin RH, Kilner PJ, Rees S, Longmore DB. Magnetic resonance volume flow and jet velocity mapping in aortic coarctation. J Am Coll Cardiol. 1993 Nov 1;22(5):1515-21.

[31]   Kilner PJ, Manzara CC, Mohiaddin RH, Pennell DJ, Sutton MG, Firmin DN, *et al.* Magnetic resonance jet velocity mapping in mitral and aortic valve stenosis. Circulation. 1993 Apr;87(4):1239-48.

[32]   Bonow RO, Carabello BA, Chatterjee K, de Leon AC, Jr., Faxon DP, Freed MD, *et al.* 2008 Focused update incorporated into the ACC/AHA 2006 guidelines for the management of patients with valvular heart disease: a report of the American College of Cardiology/American Heart Association Task Force on Practice Guidelines (Writing Committee to Revise the 1998 Guidelines for the Management of Patients With Valvular Heart Disease): endorsed by the Society of Cardiovascular Anesthesiologists, Society for Cardiovascular Angiography and Interventions, and Society of Thoracic Surgeons. Circulation. 2008 Oct 7;118(15):e523-661.

[33]   Sondergaard L, Lindvig K, Hildebrandt P, Thomsen C, Stahlberg F, Joen T, *et al.* Quantification of aortic regurgitation by magnetic resonance velocity mapping. Am Heart J. 1993 Apr;125(4):1081-90.

[34]   Wald RM, Redington AN, Pereira A, Provost YL, Paul NS, Oechslin EN, *et al.* Refining the assessment of pulmonary regurgitation in adults after tetralogy of Fallot repair: should we be measuring regurgitant fraction or regurgitant volume? Eur Heart J. 2009 Feb;30(3):356-61.

[35]   Devos DG, Kilner PJ. Calculations of cardiovascular shunts and regurgitation using magnetic resonance ventricular volume and aortic and pulmonary flow measurements. Eur Radiol. 2010 Feb;20(2):410-21.

[36]   Markl M, Frydrychowicz A, Kozerke S, Hope M, Wieben O. 4D flow MRI. J Magn Reson Imaging. 2012 Nov;36(5):1015-36.

[37]   Frydrychowicz A, Francois CJ, Turski PA. Four-dimensional phase contrast magnetic resonance angiography: potential clinical applications. Eur J Radiol. 2011 Oct;80(1):24-35.

[38]   Hope MD, Sedlic T, Dyverfeldt P. Cardiothoracic Magnetic Resonance Flow Imaging. J Thorac Imaging. 2013 May 22.

[39]   Napel S, Lee DH, Frayne R, Rutt BK. Visualizing three-dimensional flow with simulated streamlines and three-dimensional phase-contrast MR imaging. J Magn Reson Imaging. 1992 Mar-Apr;2(2):143-53.

[40]   Buonocore MH. Visualizing blood flow patterns using streamlines, arrows, and particle paths. Magn Reson Med. 1998 Aug;40(2):210-26.

[41]   Stalder AF, Russe MF, Frydrychowicz A, Bock J, Hennig J, Markl M. Quantitative 2D and 3D phase contrast MRI: optimized analysis of blood flow and vessel wall parameters. Magn Reson Med. 2008 Nov;60(5):1218-31.

[42]   Hsiao A, Lustig M, Alley MT, Murphy M, Chan FP, Herfkens RJ, *et al.* Rapid pediatric cardiac assessment of flow and ventricular volume with compressed sensing parallel imaging volumetric cine phase-contrast MRI. AJR Am J Roentgenol. 2012 Mar;198(3):W250-9.

[43]   Kilner PJ, Yang GZ, Wilkes AJ, Mohiaddin RH, Firmin DN, Yacoub MH. Asymmetric redirection of flow through the heart. Nature. 2000 Apr 13;404(6779):759-61.

[44]   Bachler P, Valverde I, Pinochet N, Nordmeyer S, Kuehne T, Crelier G, *et al.* Caval blood flow distribution in patients with Fontan circulation: quantification by using particle traces from 4D flow MR imaging. Radiology. 2013 Apr;267(1):67-75.

[45]   Markl M, Draney MT, Hope MD, Levin JM, Chan FP, Alley MT, *et al.* Time-resolved 3-dimensional velocity mapping in the thoracic aorta: visualization of 3-directional blood

flow patterns in healthy volunteers and patients. J Comput Assist Tomogr. 2004 Jul-Aug;28(4):459-68.

[46]   Hope TA, Markl M, Wigstrom L, Alley MT, Miller DC, Herfkens RJ. Comparison of flow patterns in ascending aortic aneurysms and volunteers using four-dimensional magnetic resonance velocity mapping. J Magn Reson Imaging. 2007 Dec;26(6):1471-9.

[47]   Bogren HG, Buonocore MH. 4D magnetic resonance velocity mapping of blood flow patterns in the aorta in young *vs* elderly normal subjects. J Magn Reson Imaging. 1999 Nov;10(5):861-9.

[48]   Bogren HG, Buonocore MH. Complex flow patterns in the great vessels: a review. Int J Card Imaging. 1999 Apr;15(2):105-13.

[49]   Buonocore MH, Bogren HG. Analysis of flow patterns using MRI. Int J Card Imaging. 1999 Apr;15(2):99-103.

[50]   Frydrychowicz A, Stalder AF, Russe MF, Bock J, Bauer S, Harloff A, *et al.* Three-dimensional analysis of segmental wall shear stress in the aorta by flow-sensitive four-dimensional-MRI. J Magn Reson Imaging. 2009 Jul;30(1):77-84.

[51]   Bieging ET, Frydrychowicz A, Wentland A, Landgraf BR, Johnson KM, Wieben O, *et al. In vivo* three-dimensional MR wall shear stress estimation in ascending aortic dilatation. J Magn Reson Imaging. 2011 Mar;33(3):589-97.

[52]   Markl M, Wallis W, Strecker C, Gladstone BP, Vach W, Harloff A. Analysis of pulse wave velocity in the thoracic aorta by flow-sensitive four-dimensional MRI: reproducibility and correlation with characteristics in patients with aortic atherosclerosis. J Magn Reson Imaging. 2012 May;35(5):1162-8.

[53]   Wentland AL, Wieben O, Francois CJ, Boncyk C, Munoz Del Rio A, Johnson KM, *et al.* Aortic pulse wave velocity measurements with undersampled 4D flow-sensitive MRI: comparison with 2D and algorithm determination. J Magn Reson Imaging. 2013 Apr;37(4):853-9.

[54]   Carlsson M, Heiberg E, Toger J, Arheden H. Quantification of left and right ventricular kinetic energy using four-dimensional intracardiac magnetic resonance imaging flow measurements. Am J Physiol Heart Circ Physiol. 2012 Feb 15;302(4):H893-900.

CHAPTER 5

Spinning to a Different Beat: Non-Proton Cardiac NMR and MRI

Mangala Srinivas[*] and I. Jolanda M. de Vries

Radboud University Nijmegen Medical Center (RUNMC), Department of Tumor Immunology, 278, Nijmegen Center for Molecular Life Sciences (NCMLS), Nijmegen, The Netherlands

Abstract: Non-proton spectroscopy is a powerful tool that allows the assessment of specific and significant metabolites in cardiac tissue, such as key intermediates in energy metabolism. The technique uses spectroscopy, or less often imaging, of nuclei such as ^{31}P, ^{19}F and ^{23}Na. Due to the non-invasive nature of MRS, the technique is also applicable in the clinic, where it is used to assess changes in cardiac metabolism, such as due to a heart infarct. This chapter reviews the main developments in non-proton cardiac MRS and MRI, both clinical and preclinical. Major issues and challenges are also summarized. Finally, the promise of exciting new developments, particularly hyper-polarization, is discussed.

Keywords: ^{19}F, ^{23}Na, ^{31}P, ATP, chemical shift, clinical, energy metabolism, hyperpolarization, lanthanide, metabolism, MRS, spectroscopy, multimodal, NMR, noninvasive, non-proton, preclinical, quantification, sensitivity, spectrum.

INTRODUCTION

Magnetic Resonance Imaging (MRI) is typically carried out on the ^1H nucleus, as this is abundantly present in biological tissues, chiefly in the form of mobile water (H_2O). The proton, or ^1H nucleus, is exquisitely sensitive to the phenomenon of nuclear magnetic resonance (NMR). However, in principle, NMR or MRI can be carried out on certain other nuclei as well. Nuclei such as ^{13}C, ^{23}Na and ^{31}P are present in biological tissues, and often in biologically relevant molecules. Nevertheless, these nuclei present a drop in sensitivity of several orders of magnitude in comparison to standard MRI and NMR (done on ^1H), due to both their lower concentration in tissues and their lower sensitivity to NMR (less

---

Address correspondence to Mangala Srinivas: Radboud University Medical Center, Department of Tumor Immunology, 278, Nijmegen Center for Molecular Life Sciences (NCMLS), Nijmegen, The Netherlands; Tel: +31-(0)24-3610550; Fax: 0031-24-3540339; E-mail: M.Srinivas@ncmls.ru.nl

Christakis Constantinides (Ed)

favourable gyromagnetic ratio; see Table **1** (Adapted from http://en.wikipedia.org/wiki/Composition_of_the_human_body [1]). Thus, imaging of these nuclei is carried out less often, with the exception of ^{23}Na which is described later in the text. Instead, Magnetic Resonance Spectroscopy (MRS) is used, as signal can be acquired from large voxels or even the entire cardiac region. MRS is, in fact, preferable to MRI in some cases, as it allows the specific study of molecules of interest, such as creatine (Cr; ^{1}H), lactate (^{1}H), adenosine triphosphate (ATP; ^{31}P), phosphocreatine (PCr; ^{31}P) and inorganic phosphate (P$_i$, ^{31}P). Externally administered agents, such as ^{13}C-glucose can also be assessed. These metabolites are vital to cardiac metabolism and function. Indeed, cardiac MRS has been described as "opening a window to the metabolism of the heart" [2]. As early as 2001, MRS was already becoming an integral part of clinical MR examinations for a more complete picture of both cardiac morphology and metabolism [3]. MRS offers a noninvasive tool for the study of cardiac metabolism, without the use of radioactive probes and often without the use of any exogenously administered agents.

One further nucleus, ^{19}F nucleus falls into a unique position: It is extremely sensitive to NMR, but biological (endogeneous) ^{19}F does not contribute to the received signal. Thus, exogenous imaging agents must be introduced and these are detected without confounding background signal and at high sensitivity. For these reasons, among others, several applications using ^{19}F NMR, MRI and MRS have been developed. These are discussed in a later section.

MRS allows the differentiation of specific molecules, due to chemical shift differences that arise within them. Chemical shift is typically an undesirable artefact in MRI, for example the "ghosting" due to unsuppressed fat signal in anatomic ^{1}H images. In MRS, chemical shift is a boon, allowing the differentiation of the different forms of ATP (see Fig. **1**). MRS is, or can be, quantitative, allowing inter- and intra-subject comparisons. Both relative and absolute concentration of these metabolites can be measured, although absolute quantification requires an external, known reference. The technique can be used both *in vivo*, and *ex vivo* or *in vitro*. The changes in specific metabolites that occur with myocardial damage are summarized in Table **2** (adapted from (4)), showing the utility of MRS in diagnosis and the assessment of disease.

Table 1: Summary of relative sensitivities of biologically relevant nuclei. The natural abundance is the percentage of the element present as the isotope indicated. Relative concentration in biological tissue indicates the relative amount of each element present. However, it does not indicate how much may actually be available in a mobile state for NMR, for *e.g.*, most of the fluorine is tightly bound in bones and teeth and thus has such a long T_1 that it is essentially unavailable for NMR studies. The relative sensitivity is a constant at a given magnetic field and given an equal number of nuclei; it is dependent on the gyromagnetic ratio which is an inherent property of a nucleus. The effective sensitivity is the product of the preceding three columns, normalised to that of the ^{1}H nucleus (Adapted from http://en.wikipedia.org/wiki/ Composition_of_the_human_body).

Isotope	Natural Abundance (%)	Relative Concentration in Biological Tissue	Relative Sensitivity	Effective Sensitivity
^{13}C	1.108	12	1	10^{-5}
^{1}H	99.98	63	100	1
^{31}P	100	0.14	1	10^{-5}
^{17}O	0.037	24	1	10^{-6}
^{15}N	0.37	0.58	0.1	10^{-8}
^{19}F	100	0.0012	10	10^{-6}

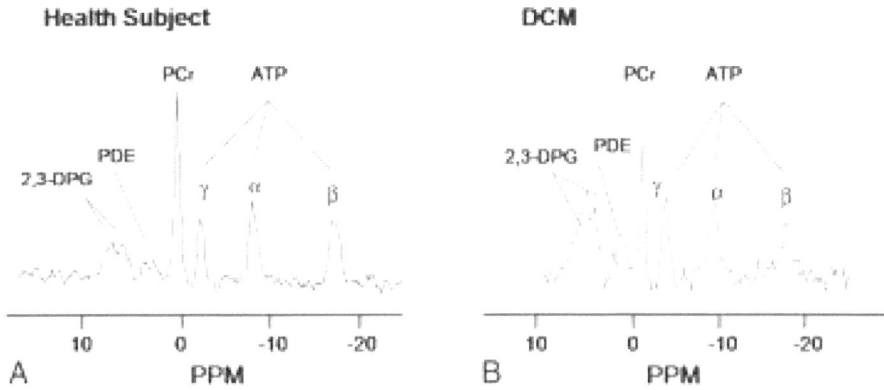

Figure 1: An example of a typical ^{31}P cardiac spectrum from a healthy subject (left) and a subject with heart failure (right). The spectra show the peaks for 2,3-diphosphoglycerate (2,3-DGP), phosphomonoester (PDE), PCr and the there high-energy phosphates in ATP. The ratio of PCr to ATP visibly changes in the unhealthy heart. PPM represents parts per million. Figure reproduced from [5], with permission.

The history of cardiac MR has been well-summarized elsewhere [6, 7]. In brief, ^{31}P spectroscopy was one of the first to be applied to the heart, and remains the most widely used. Phosphorous metabolites, particularly those of ATP and PCr, are key components to cardiac muscle function (Fig. **1**). Fig. (**1**) shows a cardiac

[31]P spectrum of a healthy subject and a patient with heart failure. Typically, the three high energy phosphate atoms in ATP and PCr can be readily identified. Other visible peaks include phosphodiesters and 2,3-diphosphoglycerate (from blood) which can mask the peak due to P_i. The spectra show not only that the various P metabolites can be readily detected and distinguished, but also that the relative concentrations vary with changes in the muscle tissue. This is not surprising, as the metabolism of ATP is essential for muscle function. Phosphorous metabolism is described in detail elsewhere [8, 9]. The importance of Cr and PCr levels has also been shown in transgenic mouse models which over-express the myocardial Cr transporter [10], where these mice developed significant left ventricle dysfunction and hypertrophy, relative to wild-type mice.

Table 2: Summary of changes in specific metabolites that accompany myocardial damage. MRS could potentially differentiate viable, non-viable and stunted (hibernating) tissue based on the differences in their metabolite content. - indicates a decrease, + an increase and a blank indicates no change or high variability. Table adapted with permission [4].

Metabolite	Ischemia	Scar (Nonviable)	Stunning
ATP	-	+	
PCr	-	+	- (possible)
P_i	-		- (possible)
Na	+	+	
Total creatine		+	
deoxymyoglobin	+		

[1]H spectroscopy is also feasible, for example to identify metabolites such as creatinine. However, the water peak can dominate the spectrum, unless properly suppressed. Specific lipids such as triglycerides can also be measured, if the voxel is properly placed to avoid contamination from pericardial fat [8]. The total creatine levels can be measured, as indicated earlier, when both ^{1}H and ^{31}P spectra are acquired. Other nuclei are rarely used, at least in human studies, due to poor sensitivity.

Several studies are often published on similar topics. To avoid undue repetition, reviews are referenced where possible, and otherwise one or two examples have been selected to showcase the technique or results.

PRECLINICAL WORK

Preclinical studies are frequently done on isolated, perfused murine or rodent hearts. This allows the detailed study of metabolite levels through MRS or even NMR in various animal models of disease, including transgenic animals. A standard technique for isolating animal hearts has been described, with an accompanying video of the procedure [11]. Alternatively, rather more drastic means such as open-chest ^{31}P MRS have been developed [12]. Here the anterior chest wall was removed, and high-resolution spectra were obtained within 12 minutes. Such experiments are necessarily terminal.

Rapid intracellular Na^+ flux occurs in myocardial tissue during ischemia [13]. However, sodium is present in both the intracellular and extracellular components, and the extracellular concentration is much higher. Intraveneous paramagnetic shift reagents are used to differentiate these components. These compounds, typically chelates of lanthanides such as dysprosium [14] (Dy) or Thulium (Tm), which are confined to the blood stream and cause a localized chemical shift (Fig. **2**). Thus, the intracellular and extracellular components can be differentiated. The utility of these measurements have been studied extensively in animal models; the reader is directed to a comprehensive review article that covers the utility of ^{23}Na MRI or MRS for the determination of the extent of non-viable tissue after a heart infarct [15]. Cellular damage, caused by an infarct, typically results in membrane damage and poor ion homeostasis, further compounded by any accompanying edema. Thus, it is readily detected using ^{23}Na MRS. In particular, both total myocardial Na ion levels and extracellular myocardial Na ion levels increase in edema, and this can be detected using MRI. A recent study combined ^{31}P MRS, ^{23}Na CSI and contrast-enhanced MRI to study myocardial edema in an *ex vivo* rat heart model (Fig. **3**) [16]. This study confirms that extracellular myocardial ^{23}Na is a viable endogeneous marker to distinguish between edema, and acute and chronic myocardial infarct.

^{23}Na studies have been carried out in mouse, rat, dog, rabbits [18] and pig models [19], as well as in humans. Thus, the role of sodium in ischemia is very well-characterized. Imaging can also be fast; for example, a fast gradient echo sequence in rabbits yielded ^{23}Na images in minutes [18]. The changes in ^{23}Na signal intensity before, during and after coronary occlusion are clearly visible. ^{23}Na MRS has also been used to follow allogeneic and syngeneic heart transplants in rats over a period of up to 29 days post-transplant [20]. [23]Na levels increased steadily prior to rejection of allogeneic hearts at days 4 to 5 post-transplant. Sodium levels were sharply elevated after rejection. Thus, this study showed that ^{23}Na MRS was able to detect rejection, even at the early stages. The total sodium content can also be measured using [23]Na MRI [21]. This technique has been validated using *ex vivo* chemical analyses on tissue samples.

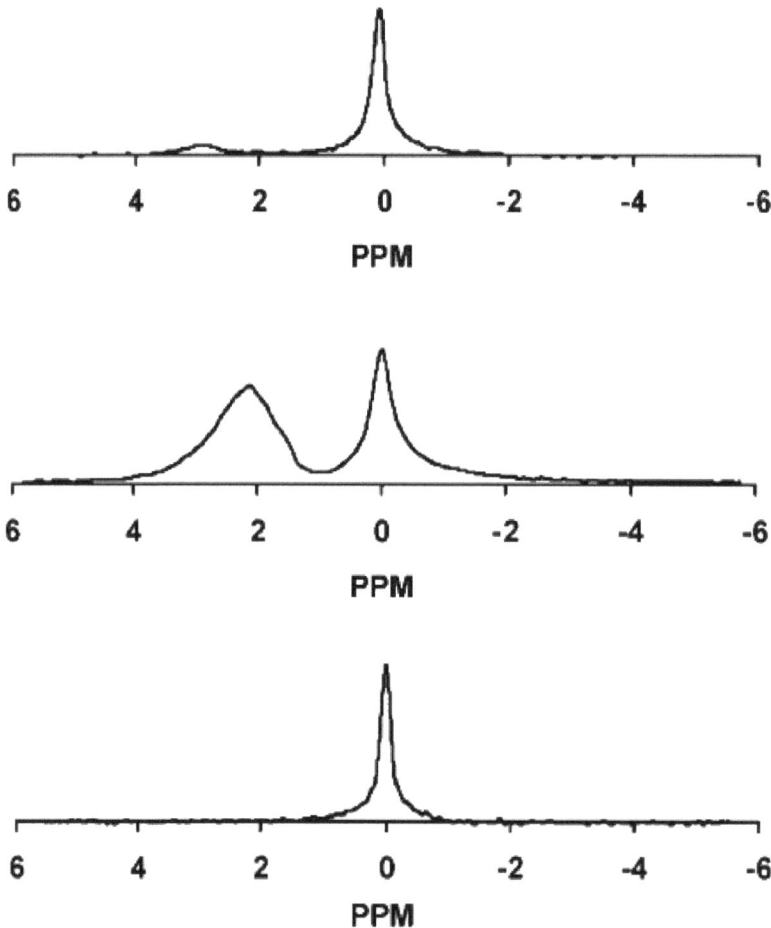

Figure 2: Lanthanide chelates cause a localised chemical shift in the blood. The shift was carried out using a thulium (Tm) chelate and [23]Na spectra are shown before (bottom) and after the shift (upper panels; middle panel is a non-localized voxel and the top panel is localised). Figure reproduced with permission from [17].

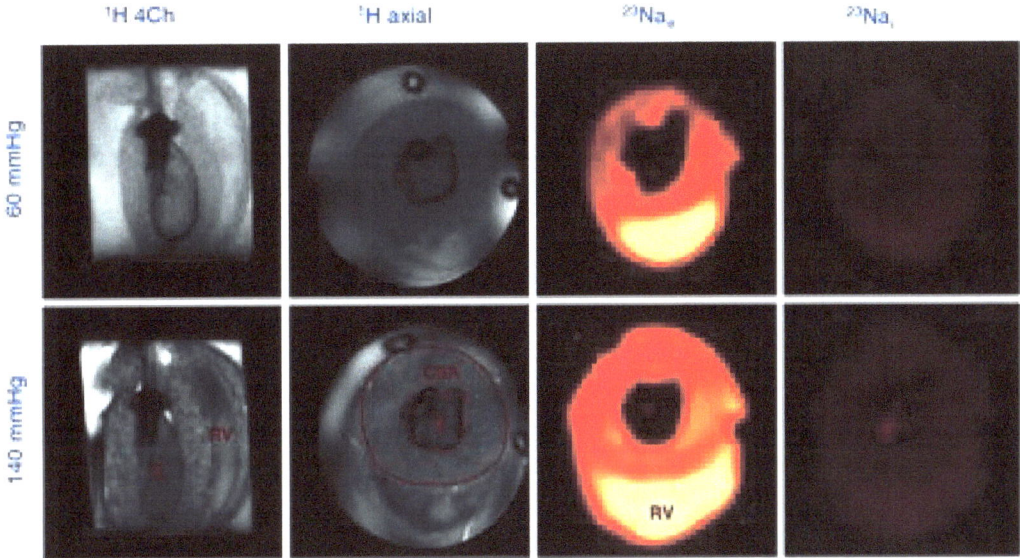

Figure 3: An example of a ^{23}Na image of a isolated, perfused rat heart at 60 and 140 mmHg in an edema model. Longitudinal and axial views are shown with the corresponding extracellular and intracellular Na ion levels (^{23}Na$_e$ and ^{23}Na$_i$ respectively). ^{23}Na CSI was used to acquire the images; signal is visibly stronger in the extracellular compartment due to the higher concentration (at least an order of magnitude difference). *B* labels the balloon in the left ventricle and *CSA* is the cross sectional area of the LV. Figure reproduced from open-access publication [16].

Contrast agents, such as super-paramagnetic iron oxide (SPIO) which are used for ^{1}H MRI, can also be applied to non-proton MRI. For example, iron oxides have been used to suppress the Na$^+$ signal from blood in canine hearts *in vivo* [22]. This allowed better visualization of the myocardial Na$^+$ signal before and after infarct.

Other ions that have been studied include ^{87}Rb and ^{7}Li, typically using MRS on isolated hearts, for example [23]. This study showed that cation flux is temperature dependant, when studied in perfused rat hearts. ^{35}Cl and ^{59}Co have also be studied using NMR in perfused rat hearts [24]. Other nuclei have also been studied in animal models. For instance, ^{87}Rb and ^{31}P MRS have been used to study cardiac K$^+$-ATP channels [25]. ^{87}Rb is commonly used as an NMR-sensitive substitute for K. ^{133}Cs is another interesting ion: It acts as an analogue of K$^+$ in biological tissues. However, Cs occurs exclusively in the NMR-active form, and it naturally shows a chemical shift for the intra- and extracellular components. Thus, it is an ideal substitute for K in animal models. It has been used to quantify ion transport in perfused rat hearts [26].

Interestingly, one study in 1988, concluded that there are two distinct cardiac intracellular compartments of ATP, and only one can be detected using ^{31}P MRS [27]. This conclusion was based on discrepancies between the ATP content determined by NMR and that determined using chemical analyses, which was significantly higher (nearly two-fold higher at 22.4 ± 0.7 μmol/g dry weight). The authors suggest that only free ATP in the cytosol is detected using NMR, and this is depleted more rapidly than non-cytosolic ATP during ischaemia. Regardless, ^{31}P MRS has proved its utility in the assessment of cardiac energy metabolism.

CLINICAL WORK

Clinical work has focused on ^{31}P spectroscopy. MRS has become a standard technique for measuring myocardial metabolism in a non-invasive manner. In particular, disruptions in cardiac energy metabolism can be indicative of various heart problems. This includes relatively common conditions such as heart infarcts, as well as less common conditions such as the inherited, X-linked Fabry disease [28]. Patients with this disease show characteristically impaired PCr and ATP levels relative to normal subjects. Examples of a ^{31}P CSI image, overlaid on an anatomic scan from individuals with the inherited condition and a healthy control are shown in Fig. (**4**) [29]. It is conceivable that spectroscopy can be used to diagnose or understand other genetic conditions, given that suitable markers are found.

It was suggested in 1997, based on theoretical calculations, that clinical [23]Na MRI should be feasible at 1.5T [30]. The same authors calculated that [37]K MRI would not be feasible, due to sensitivity and concentration restrictions. The authors calculated that [23]Na MRI should be feasible with 7 mm isotropic resolution with a signal to noise ration of over 10 and an acquisition time of about 15 minutes. This is in close agreement with actual clinical data, published just 3 years later [31]. Much of the clinical non-proton cardiac MRI has focused on [23]Na, due to its high sensitivity, high concentration and significance in cardiac tissue [32]. Using specialized acquisition techniques, such as modified k-space filling, it is possible to acquire images with a resolution of 10 mm (or better) and a signal to noise ratio of 10 within 20 minutes, with ECG-gating [31]. High-resolution ^{1}H images can also be used to enhance low resolution non-proton images using specialized algorithms. This has been shown for [23]Na images [33].

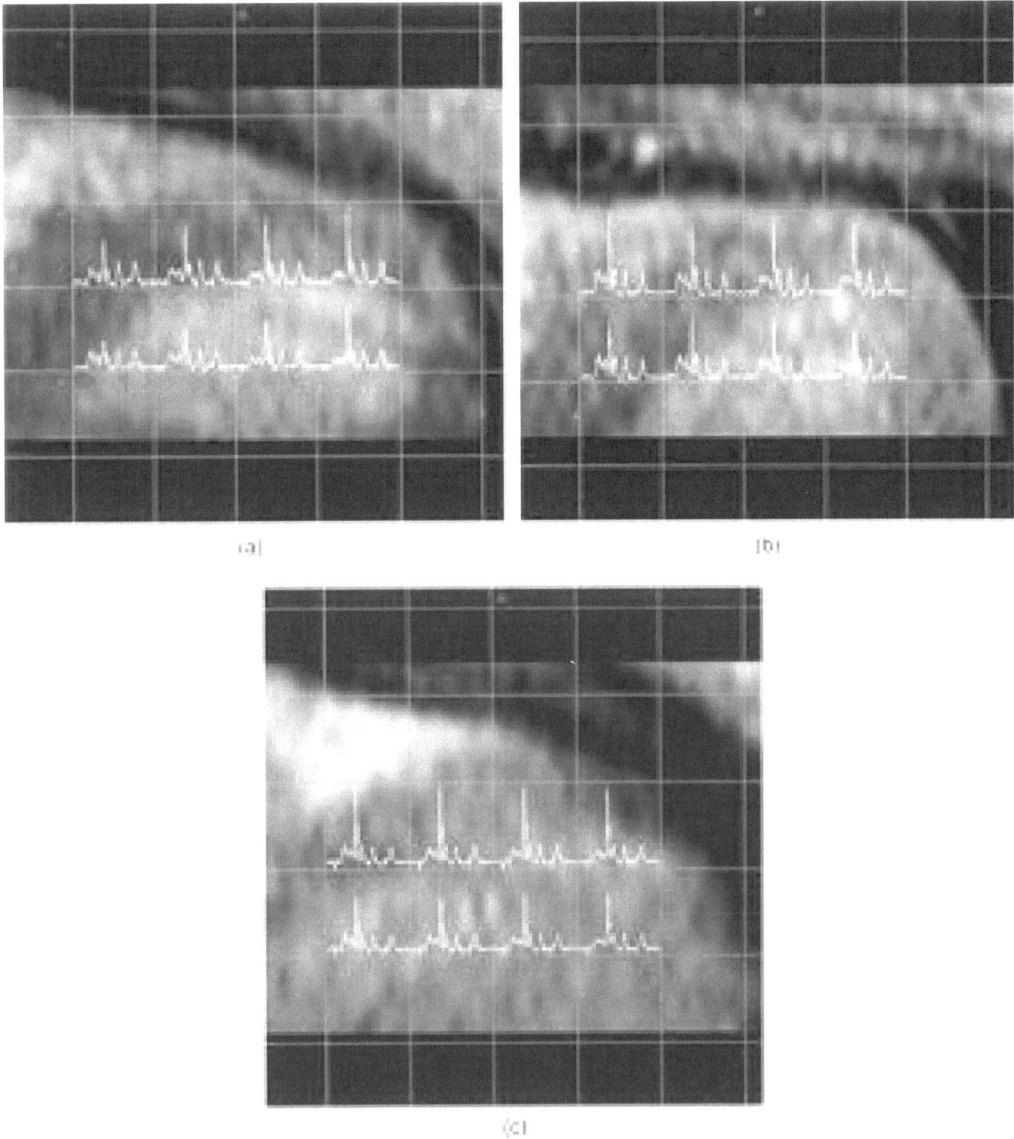

Figure 4: An example of a 2D ^{31}P CSI acquisition overlaid on a ^{1}H scan. Panels (**a**) and (**b**) show spectra of patients with hereditary hemochromatosis (HCC), which affects the PCr/β-ATP ratio. Panel (**c**) shows the corresponding spectrum from a healthy control. This study was carried out on a 1.5T whole body scanner, with ECG-gating, and a spectral voxel size of 64ml. The time for the CSI acquisition was under 10 minutes. Figure reproduced with permission [29].

Interestingly, it has been found that the PCr/ATP ratio can become abnormal even without clinically-significant coronary artery obstruction (determined using standard angiograms) [34]. Women who were hospitalised for chest pain, but without angiographically significant coronary artery obstruction, were subjected to ^{31}P cardiac MRS before, during and after an isometric handgrip exercise at 30% of their full grip strength. Their PCr/ATP ratio was significantly lower than in healthy controls. The authors suggest that the most likely cause is microvascular coronary artery disease. This study indicates that ^{31}P may, in fact, be superior to standard (and more invasive) techniques in some cases.

MRS is also well-suited to study the effect of drugs or other treatments. A new drug was tested in heart failure patients, by taking ^{31}P spectra of their left ventricles to look for any effect on the PCr/ATP ratio [35], together with standard measures of cardiac function such as exercise testing and echocardiography. This example illustrates how powerful the ability to detect local concentrations of specific metabolites can be.

The non-invasive nature of MRS, particularly where no exogenous agents are introduced, allows the extensive use of the technique in healthy volunteers. For example, ^{31}P MRS in healthy volunteers showed that there is a significant decrease in PCr and ATP levels in subjects over 40 years of age. Interestingly, the same study found no differences based on gender [36]. The ability to carry out such studies is one major advantage of non-invasive spectroscopy.

^{19}F MRS and MRI

^{19}F is a rather unique nucleus for MRS or MRI, as it is present in biological tissues in relatively large concentrations, but this endogenous signal does not result in background. This is because the fluorides in bones and teeth have very long T_1 relaxation times and cannot be imaged *in vivo*. Thus, only exogeneously administered ^{19}F is detected. ^{19}F itself has very high sensitivity, second only to ^{1}H, and a very large chemical shift range. This makes the nucleus ideal for NMR, and it has been used for a wide range of applications relevant to cardiac study. ^{19}F MRI has been in the spotlight lately as a technique for quantitative *in vivo* cell tracking, and is currently in clinical trials for imaging cell therapy [37]. ^{19}F MRI and MRS are also used for measuring oxygen tension *in vivo*, as the T_1 of ^{19}F as some molecules, particularly perfluorocarbons, can be sensitive to oxygen concentration. The F-C bond itself is extremely stable and is not metabolized *in vivo*, although fluorinated byproducts can be reactive. Relevant to this chapter, ^{19}F MRI and MRS have been used to measure oxygen tension in the heart, pH, Ca^{2+} concentrations (through a change in chemical shift) and to image immune cells in organ rejection. In particular, due to the lack of background endogeneous signal, ^{19}F signal from both MRS and MRI can be used for absolute quantification when an external reference is present. In general, the versatility of fluorinated compounds, the wide range of the ^{19}F chemical shift and the lack of *in vivo* background allow for a range of applications, including the measurement of oxygen tension and specific ion concentrations, and cell tracking. *Ex vivo* NMR, *in vivo* MRS and MRI have all been carried out.

Ion and pH

Ca^{2+} concentrations can be measured using ^{19}F shift reagents, similar to that for Na^+. ^{19}F chelators are introduced that undergo a measurable chemical shift upon binding Ca ions. The technique can only be carried out in perfused organs, as the chelators would be toxic *in vivo*. Changes in Ca^{2+} levels can be indicative of cell damage, and thus such measurements can be predictive. Fig. (**5**) shows the changes in Ca^{2+} levels in a perfused rat heart before and during ischemia [38]. The ^{19}F spectra show two peaks, for the fluorinated chelator with and without bound Ca^{2+}. The chelator used here (5F-BAPTA: 1,2-bis(2-amino-5-fluorophenoxy) ethane-N,N,N',N'-tetraacetic acid) shows two distinct peaks, for the bound and free forms. The ratio of the intensity of these peaks can be used to calculate Ca ion concentration. Global ischemia resulted in a 3-fold rise in Ca^{2+} concentration, with a return to basal levels after 10-15 minutes of reperfusion (figure reproduced from [38]). Another early study using 5F-BAPTA to measure intracellular Ca^{2+} concentrations showed that Ca ion levels increased preceding lethal myocardial injury brought about by ischemia, in perfused rat hearts [39]. The first study showing the simultaneous measurement of different ion concentrations and pH was done in the perfused ferret heart using 5F-BAPTA [40].

5F-BAPTA has also been used to distinguish free, cytosolic and intracellular Ca^{2+} levels, specifically that in the sarcoplasmic reticulum [41] in excised rabbit hearts.

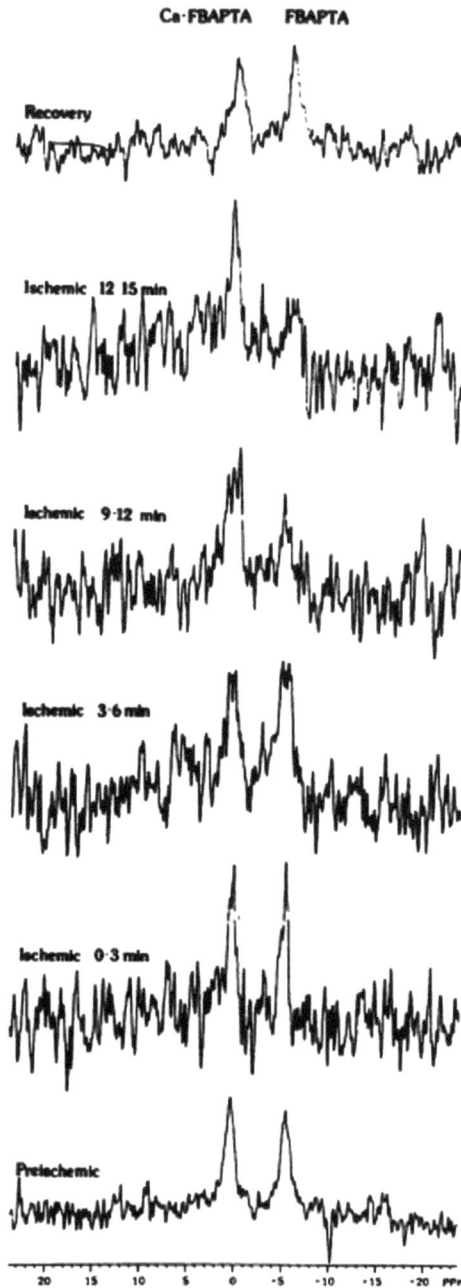

Figure 5: Measurement of Ca^{2+} levels in an *ex vivo* heart using ^{19}F NMR. The fluorous chelator, 5F-BAPTA, shows distinct peaks for the Ca^{2+}-bound and non-bound forms. The ratio of these peaks can be used to assess Ca ion concentration. Spectra are shown during reperfusion after ischemia. Figure reproduced with permission from [38].

Thus, it is possible to use ^{19}F agents to measure multi-compartmental Ca^{2+} levels simultaneously. Similar results have been obtained on Ca^{2+} levels in cardiac myocytes [42]. In a similar fashion, intracellular pH can be measured using fluorinated compounds that undergo a pH-dependant chemical shift and are able to cross cell membranes. For example, fluorinated vitamin B analogues have been developed and applied to this purpose [43]. 6-fluoropyridoxol has also been used to measure pH in both the intra- and extracellular compartments simultaneously with a time resolution of 2 min in perfused hearts [44]. The ^{19}F agent showed two distinct peaks in the intracellular and extracellular region respectively. ^{31}P NMR and pH electrodes were used to validate the results. In general, the applicability of such agents to *in vivo* use is limited due to toxicity and delivery issues.

However, it is important to keep in mind that cellular ion homeostatis is extremely complex, and changes in the concentration of one ion (even due to chelation) may impact that of another. Intracellular (cytosolic, free) Mg^+ concentrations have been measured using fluorinated chelators in cultured chick heart cells [45]. It was found that Mg ion concentration measurements could be confounded by inherent cell homeostasis mechanisms, in this case Na-coupled Mg ion counter-transport. Thus, extracellular Na^+ concentrations were lowered. However, it was found that Mg ion concentration could also increase due to increasing intracellular Ca^{2+} concentration, which occurs due to low extracellular Na^+. Finally, perfusion with low Na^+, Mg^+-free buffers also triggered an increase in intracellular Mg ion concentration. Hence, the intracellular regulation of Mg ion concentration is very complex, and can be affected by the buffers used, as well as other factors, such as the effect of chelation. Such factors can complicate NMR-based ion concentration measurements, and must be taken into account when designing experiments.

Note that most studies using ^{19}F NMR to measure the concentration of other ions, are restricted to perfused hearts and *in vitro* studies due to the toxicity of the fluorinated compound used, particularly trifluoroacetic acid. Perfluorocarbons are significantly less toxic and can be used *in vivo*, including in humans [46], as discussed in the following sections.

Oxygen Tension

Some fluorinated compounds, particularly perfluorocarbons such as perfluorooctyl bromide or perfluorodecalin, can dissolve oxygen. The compounds are also inert and generally not toxic, although they have very poor solubility in aqueous media. Their ability to dissolve oxygen led to much of the early research in injectable perfluorocarbon emulsions as clinical blood substitute in the 1980's. However, these emulsions were eventually either withdrawn or discontinued for clinical development, primarily due to problems with stability of the insoluble perfluorocarbon in aqueous format. However, interest in fluorine emulsions has rekindled due to their increasing using as cell labels for MR-based cell tracking [37]. Otherwise, current techniques to measure *in vivo* oxygen tension include inserted electrodes, or PET; electrodes, in particular, are invasive and are now frequently replaced by imaging techniques, particularly in humans.

Oxygen tension measurements have also been carried out using ^{19}F agents. Although this has been done *in vivo* for tumours, it has primarily been carried out on perfused hearts. The hearts are typically excised after intraveneous injection of the perfluorocarbon emulsion. For example, perfluorooctyl bromide has been used to determine oxygen tension in excised hearts which were either normally perfused or ischemic. The ^{19}F T_1 of the compound is oxygen-sensitive, and showed significant differences in these cases [47]. Perfluorocarbon emulsions can also be applied to study myocardial vascular space, using an intravascular agent. In one study, the data were validated using standard radiotracers showing the validity of the ^{19}F data [48]. Similarly, ^{19}F NMR studies can be readily combined with NMR of other nuclei to acquire more comprehensive data. For example, ^{23}Na and ^{31}P levels can both be measured, and intracellular ^{23}Na and ^{31}P levels were measured using ^{39}K and ^{19}F NMR respectively [49].

It has also been shown that the ^{19}F T_1 is linearly related to oxygen tension, given a constant temperature; and to temperature, given a constant oxygen partial pressure in the range 27-50°C [50]. However, the different ^{19}F resonances in the agent (perfluoro-tributylamine) respond uniquely to these parameters, and thus assessment of two more resonances can be used to measure pO$_2$ and temperature simultaneously and unambiguously. This was demonstrated both *in vivo* in a murine tumor model and *ex vivo* in a perfused rat heart. However, this kind of data may be limited to specific perfluorocarbons. Early studies using the same perfluorocarbon emulsion for oxygen tension measurements found that the loss of oxygen occurred as quickly as 40 seconds after the onset of global ischemia in perfused hearts [51]. Furthermore, ^{19}F MRI was used to confirm that the perfluorocarbon was indeed distributed throughout the heart, thus validating the hypoxia measurements.

Other Applications

Recent studies in transplant rejection have used injectable perfluorocarbon agents that are non-specifically taken up by phagocytic immune cells (monocytes and machrophages), which then accumulate at the active immune site resulting in a detectable ^{19}F signal in MR images. Cell tracking using ^{19}F MRI has been done in mice with commercially available perfluorocarbon agents [52]. Perfluorocarbons have also been used to detect and quantify angiogenesis in plaque development [53] in rabbits on high cholesterol diets. Perfluorocarbon emulsions targeted to integrin accumulated in neovasculature within valve leaflets and could be imaged at 3T. The technique can potentially be used to evaluate patients for aortic valve disease. Other similar studies involving MR agents (primarily ^{1}H) to detect atherosclerosis are described elsewhere [54]. Another application of ^{19}F NMR has been to study protein properties *in situ*. This requires the synthesis and introduction of a fluorinated (and functional) analogue of the relevant protein for detection. For example, *in vitro* tests have been carried out with proteins such as cardiac troponin-C [55], a contractile regulatory protein. It is also possible to use a ^{19}F-fluorinated glucose analogue to study glucose metabolism, analogous to the ^{18}F-glucose PET studies that are routinely used both clinically and pre-clinically. ^{19}F MRS is less sensitive than ^{18}F PET, but the technique does not require radioactive tracers.

Fluorinated glucose analogues have been used to study glucose metabolism in the heart using ^{19}F NMR in the past [56], although now the technique has been replaced by ^{18}F PET which has much higher sensitivity and is routinely used both in the clinic and in preclinical studies.

The first *in vivo* ^{19}F MR images were acquired several decades ago in rats with 50% of their blood volume replaced by a perfluorocarbon emulsion [57]. This allowed imaging of the cardiovascular system with a spatial resolution of 1 mm within 10 minutes of imaging time. The heart and other major organs could be readily defined in the images. However, the sensitivity and resolution of ^{19}F MRI is poor compared to data obtained using T_1 contrast agents, such as Gd chelates, which is now the standard technique for MR-based angiography.

Some early applications of ^{19}F agents have now largely been replaced by other techniques, due to poor sensitivity. Thus, much of the current research in ^{19}F MRI focuses on cell tracking and *in vivo* hypoxia measurements, where the technique is particularly advantageous.

MAJOR CHALLENGES

The major challenges facing cardiac MRS are those related to spectroscopy in general, and those specific to the cardiac region. For example, placement of the voxel with precision is vital to avoid contamination from skeletal muscle and pericardial fat. This is true for all spectroscopy applications, but particularly for cardiac MRS, where skeletal muscle contamination can obscure ^{31}P signal from the cardiac muscle. Furthermore 2,3-diphosphoglycerate (2,3-DPG) is found in blood, and its elicited signal this can mask or contaminate the signal from P_i in cardiac tissue. Thus high-resolution (^{1}H) anatomic scans are essential for the positioning of the spectroscopy voxel prior to MRS. In some cases, adjustments such as shimming may also be carried over from the original ^{1}H setting. Voxels are typically positioned in the anterior myocardium or intra-ventricular septum [5] and made as large as possible. Positioning must be done in 3D with precision. Various pulse sequences exist for this, described elsewhere [4]. Spectral localization with optimum point spread function (SLOOP) is one of the more common techniques.

Acquisitions are typically gated to cardiac and/or respiratory cycles, to minimize motion artifacts. Internal motion, from the circulating blood can also play a role, particularly if the relevant metabolites are also present in the blood. It is possible to correct for motion using specific imaging techniques, such as navigator echoes, which are also commonly used in ^{1}H MRI. Multiple navigator echoes have been used to track motion of the heart due to respiration in real-time, and the resulting displacement information applied to calculate the spectroscopic volume [58]. This technique consistently improved data fitting in healthy volunteers, without adding to the scan time.

Another major issue facing MRS is the difficulty in comparing data across different subjects, especially when acquired in different locations. It has been shown that the inter-subject variability can be as high as 20%, even when healthy volunteers were studied twice using the same setup [59]. The same study also found that there was no significant difference between observers of the same data. However, it is necessary to implement standardized protocols for obtaining data, including the acquisition protocols and positioning of the relevant voxels. In particular, this becomes more essential as MRI scanners move to higher fields with better sensitivity and resolution, thus also becoming more sensitive to errors. The types of coils and sequences are discussed in detail elsewhere [8]. In brief, nucleus-specific coils and a broadband radiofrequency transmitter are necessary.

Low signal to noise, indistinct or overlapping peaks and strong artifacts are problems with MRS, particularly *in vivo* where imaging time is limited and motion and contaminants (such as non-cardiac muscle or fat) are present. Various solutions have been proposed, such as improvements in coil design and better acquisition techniques [60, 61]. However, it is feasible to carry out MRS with standard, commercially available sequences. For example, ^{31}P 2D CSI was carried out successfully using a voxel size of $40\times40\times100$ mm^3 in patients with cardiomyopathy [62].

Finally, long scan times can be difficult, especially for cardiac patients. Averaging is necessary for these non-proton scans; typical settings for ^{31}P cardiac MRS at 1.5T, are voxel sizes of 20-70 ml and an acquisition times of 20-40 minutes [9].

FUTURE POSSIBILITIES

The non-invasive nature of MRI and MRS has not yet been fully exploited. In part, the techniques are hampered by their high cost, relatively long imaging times and poor sensitivity. Higher magnetic fields, better gradients, faster acquisition parameters and better hardware will contribute to improvements in these areas. These improvements may allow the eventual replacement of the invasive techniques in current use by MRS. For example, coronary angiography is a relatively invasive technique, which requires the use of a cardiac catheter to inject a dye for detection using X-rays. The technique is used to assess plaque build-up. Coronary angiography is also used to detect cardiac allograft vasculopathy, which is a complication of heart transplants and results in a rapid development of coronary disease. It has been shown using ^{31}P CSI in patients that the PCr/ATP ratio may be indicative of developing cardiac allograft vasculopathy, and this technique may serve as a non-invasive substitute for coronary angiography [63].

Other techniques that are currently limited to preclinical models may also eventually prove applicable in the clinic. In particular, the large sensitivity gains brought about by hyperpolarization can make these techniques clinically feasible. For instance, a recent study used hyperpolarized ^{13}C-pyruvate in rats to measure intracellular pH in healthy and diseased rat hearts [64]. Hyperpolarised reagents yield several orders of magnitude improvements in signal, although the effect is very short-lived. In this study, isolated rat hearts were perfused with the hyperpolarised pyruvate before and immediately after ischaemia. [13]C spectra were obtained to detect the formation of CO_2 and HCO_3^-, and the ratio of these two metabolites was used to calculate the pH. The researchers were also able to use this technique *in vivo* to estimate the intracellular cardiac pH in healthy, living rats. Hyperpolarization technology is an area of intense research for various fields, and rapid developments are being made including clinical MRI of hyperpolarized agents [65].

Finally, multimodal imaging, that is imaging using different modalities to gain different types of information on a subject, is being carried out together with cardiac MRS, even in humans. For example, a recent study used a combination of positron emission tomography (PET), MRI and ^{31}P MRS to assess the relationship between hepatic triglyceride content and myocardial metabolism in type 2 diabetes patients [66]. Here, PET was carried out using ^{15}O-tagged water, ^{11}C-palmitate and an ^{18}F-tagged glucose analogue. These metabolites measured perfusion, glucose uptake, and cardiac fatty acid metabolism respectively.

Standard MRI was used to measure left ventricular function, ^{1}H MRS for hepatic triglyceride content and ^{31}P MRS for phosphate metabolism. This example demonstrates how the non-invasive nature of MRI and MRS allows them to be readily combined with other techniques.

CONCLUSION

In summary, non-proton MRI and particularly MRS offer many advantages and insights into specific areas of cardiac metabolism. These techniques are readily combined with proton (anatomic MRI), as well as other imaging modalities. In particular, exciting developments such as hyper-polarization, may pave the way for more extensive use of non-proton MRS and MRI in the near future.

CONFLICT OF INTEREST

This is to certify that the authors do not have any conflict of interest.

ACKNOWLEDGEMENTS

This work was supported by The Netherlands Institute of Regenerative Medicine (NIRM, FES0908), the EU FP7 program ENCITE (HEALTH-F5-2008-201842), and The Netherlands Organization for Scientific Research (VENI 700.10.409 and VIDI 917.76.363).

REFERENCES

[1]   Villafranca JJ, Raushel FM. Biophysical applications of NMR to phosphoryl transfer enzymes and metal nuclei of metalloproteins. Annu Rev Biophys Bioeng. 1980; 9: 363-92.

[2]   Horn M. Cardiac magnetic resonance spectroscopy: a window for studying physiology. Methods Mol Med. 2006; 124: 225-48.

[3]   Pohost GM, Meduri A, Razmi RM, Rathi VK, Doyle M. Cardiac MR spectroscopy in the new millennium. Rays. 2001 Jan-Mar; 26(1): 93-107.

[4]   Hudsmith LE, Neubauer S. Magnetic resonance spectroscopy in myocardial disease. JACC Cardiovasc Imaging. 2009 Jan; 2(1): 87-96.

[5]   Holloway CJ, Suttie J, Dass S, Neubauer S. Clinical cardiac magnetic resonance spectroscopy. Prog Cardiovasc Dis. 2011 Nov-Dec; 54(3): 320-7.

[6]   Pohost GM. The history of cardiovascular magnetic resonance. JACC Cardiovasc Imaging. 2008 Sep; 1(5): 672-8.

[7]   Neubauer S. Cardiac magnetic resonance spectroscopy. Curr Cardiol Rep. 2003 Jan; 5(1): 75-82.

[8]   Bottomley PA. NMR Spectroscopy of the Human Heart. eMagRes [serial on the Internet]. 2009.

[9]   Neubauer S. Metabolic imaging with cardiac magnetic resonance spectroscopy. Heart Metab. 2009; 44: 17-20.

[10]   Wallis J, Lygate CA, Fischer A, ten Hove M, Schneider JE, Sebag-Montefiore L, *et al.* Supranormal myocardial creatine and phosphocreatine concentrations lead to cardiac hypertrophy and heart failure: insights from creatine transporter-overexpressing transgenic mice. Circulation. 2005 Nov 15; 112(20): 3131-9.

[11]   Kolwicz SC, Jr., Tian R. Assessment of cardiac function and energetics in isolated mouse hearts using 31P NMR spectroscopy. J Vis Exp. 2010(42).

[12]   Lee J, Hu Q, Nakamura Y, Wang X, Zhang X, Zhu X, *et al.* Open-chest 31P magnetic resonance spectroscopy of mouse heart at 4.7 Tesla. J Magn Reson Imaging. 2006 Dec; 24(6): 1269-76.

[13]   Imahashi K, Kusuoka H, Hashimoto K, Yoshioka J, Yamaguchi H, Nishimura T. Intracellular sodium accumulation during ischemia as the substrate for reperfusion injury. Circ Res. 1999 Jun 25; 84(12): 1401-6.

[14]   Gaszner B, Simor T, Hild G, Elgavish GA. The effects of the NMR shift-reagents Dy(PPP)2, Dy(TTHA) and Tm(DOTP) on developed pressure in isolated perfused rat hearts. The role of shift-reagent calcium complexes. J Mol Cell Cardiol. 2001 Nov; 33(11): 1945-56.

[15]   Horn M. 23Na magnetic resonance imaging for the determination of myocardial viability: the status and the challenges. Curr Vasc Pharmacol. 2004 Oct; 2(4): 329-33.

[16]   Aguor EN, van de Kolk CW, Arslan F, Nederhoff MG, Doevendans PA, Pasterkamp G, *et al.* 23Na chemical shift imaging and Gd enhancement of myocardial edema. Int J Cardiovasc Imaging. 2013 Feb; 29(2): 343-54.

[17]   Ronen I, Kim SG. Measurement of intravascular Na(+) during increased CBF using (23)Na NMR with a shift reagent. NMR Biomed. 2001 Nov-Dec; 14(7-8): 448-52.

[18]   Kim RJ, Lima JA, Chen EL, Reeder SB, Klocke FJ, Zerhouni EA, *et al.* Fast 23Na magnetic resonance imaging of acute reperfused myocardial infarction. Potential to assess myocardial viability. Circulation. 1997 Apr 1; 95(7): 1877-85.

[19]   Balschi JA. 23Na NMR demonstrates prolonged increase of intracellular sodium following transient regional ischemia in the *in situ* pig heart. Basic Res Cardiol. 1999 Feb; 94(1): 60-9.

[20]   Waldrop SM, Alexander DZ, Lowry R, Winn KJ, Pearson TC, Constantinidis I. Analysis of allogeneic and syngeneic rat heart transplants using 23Na magnetic resonance spectroscopy. Biochem Biophys Res Commun. 1996 Jun 14; 223(2): 379-83.

[21]   Constantinides CD, Kraitchman DL, O'Brien KO, Boada FE, Gillen J, Bottomley PA. Noninvasive quantification of total sodium concentrations in acute reperfused myocardial infarction using 23Na MRI. Magn Reson Med. 2001 Dec; 46(6): 1144-51.

[22]   Constantinides CD, Rogers J, Herzka DA, Boada FE, Bolar D, Kraitchman D, *et al.* Superparamagnetic iron oxide MION as a contrast agent for sodium MRI in myocardial infarction. Magn Reson Med. 2001 Dec; 46(6): 1164-8.

[23]   Gruwel ML, Kuzio B, Xiang B, Deslauriers R, Kupriyanov VV. Temperature dependence of monovalent cation fluxes in isolated rat hearts: a magnetic resonance study. Biochim Biophys Acta. 1998 Dec 9; 1415(1): 41-55.

[24] Jelicks LA, Gupta RK. Multinuclear NMR studies of the Langendorff perfused rat heart. J Biol Chem. 1989 Sep 15; 264(26): 15230-5.

[25] Jilkina O, Kuzio B, Rendell J, Xiang B, Kupriyanov VV. K+ transport and energetics in Kir6.2(-/-) mouse hearts assessed by 87Rb and 31P magnetic resonance and optical spectroscopy. J Mol Cell Cardiol. 2006 Nov; 41(5): 893-901.

[26] Schornack PA, Song SK, Ling CS, Hotchkiss R, Ackerman JJ. Quantification of ion transport in perfused rat heart: 133Cs+ as an NMR active K+ analog. Am J Physiol. 1997 May; 272(5 Pt 1): C1618-34.

[27] Takami H, Furuya E, Tagawa K, Seo Y, Murakami M, Watari H, *et al.* NMR-invisible ATP in rat heart and its change in ischemia. J Biochem. 1988 Jul; 104(1): 35-9.

[28] Machann W, Breunig F, Weidemann F, Sandstede J, Hahn D, Kostler H, *et al.* Cardiac energy metabolism is disturbed in Fabry disease and improves with enzyme replacement therapy using recombinant human galactosidase A. Eur J Heart Fail. 2011 Mar; 13(3): 278-83.

[29] Schocke MF, Zoller H, Vogel W, Wolf C, Kremser C, Steinboeck P, *et al.* Cardiac phosphorus-31 two-dimensional chemical shift imaging in patients with hereditary hemochromatosis. Magn Reson Imaging. 2004 May; 22(4): 515-21.

[30] Parrish TB, Fieno DS, Fitzgerald SW, Judd RM. Theoretical basis for sodium and potassium MRI of the human heart at 1.5 T. Magn Reson Med. 1997 Oct; 38(4): 653-61.

[31] Jerecic R, Bock M, Wacker C, Bauer W, Schad LR. 23Na-MRI of the human heart using a 3D radial projection technique. Biomed Tech (Berl). 2002; 47 Suppl 1 Pt 1: 458-9.

[32] van Emous JG, Nederhoff MG, Ruigrok TJ, van Echteld CJ. The role of the Na+ channel in the accumulation of intracellular Na+ during myocardial ischemia: consequences for post-ischemic recovery. J Mol Cell Cardiol. 1997 Jan; 29(1): 85-96.

[33] Constantinides CD, Weiss RG, Lee R, Bolar D, Bottomley PA. Restoration of low resolution metabolic images with a priori anatomic information: 23Na MRI in myocardial infarction. Magn Reson Imaging. 2000 May; 18(4): 461-71.

[34] Buchthal SD, den Hollander JA, Merz CN, Rogers WJ, Pepine CJ, Reichek N, *et al.* Abnormal myocardial phosphorus-31 nuclear magnetic resonance spectroscopy in women with chest pain but normal coronary angiograms. N Engl J Med. 2000 Mar 23; 342(12): 829-35.

[35] Fragasso G, Perseghin G, De Cobelli F, Esposito A, Palloshi A, Lattuada G, *et al.* Effects of metabolic modulation by trimetazidine on left ventricular function and phosphocreatine/adenosine triphosphate ratio in patients with heart failure. Eur Heart J. 2006 Apr; 27(8): 942-8.

[36] Kostler H, Landschutz W, Koeppe S, Seyfarth T, Lipke C, Sandstede J, *et al.* Age and gender dependence of human cardiac phosphorus metabolites determined by SLOOP 31P MR spectroscopy. Magn Reson Med. 2006 Oct; 56(4): 907-11.

[37] Srinivas M, Heerschap A, Ahrens ET, Figdor CG, de Vries IJ. (19)F MRI for quantitative *in vivo* cell tracking. Trends Biotechnol. 2010 Jul; 28(7): 363-70.

[38] E Murphy LL, B Raju, C Steenbergen, J T Gerig, P Singh, R E London. Measurement of cytosolic calcium using 19F NMR. Environ Health Perspect. 1990 March; 84: 95-8.

[39] Steenbergen C, Murphy E, Watts JA, London RE. Correlation between cytosolic free calcium, contracture, ATP, and irreversible ischemic injury in perfused rat heart. Circ Res. 1990 Jan; 66(1): 135-46.

[40]   Kirschenlohr HL, Metcalfe JC, Morris PG, Rodrigo GC, Smith GA. Ca2+ transient, Mg2+, and pH measurements in the cardiac cycle by 19F NMR. Proc Natl Acad Sci U S A. 1988 Dec; 85(23): 9017-21.

[41]   Yanagida S, Luo CS, Balschi JA, Pohost GM, Pike MM. Simultaneous multicompartment intracellular Ca2+ measurements in the perfused heart using 19F NMR spectroscopy. Magn Reson Med. 1996 May; 35(5): 640-7.

[42]   Gupta RK, Wittenberg BA. 19F nuclear magnetic resonance studies of free calcium in heart cells. Biophys J. 1993 Dec; 65(6): 2547-58.

[43]   He S, Mason RP, Hunjan S, Mehta VD, Arora V, Katipally R, *et al.* Development of novel 19F NMR pH indicators: synthesis and evaluation of a series of fluorinated vitamin B6 analogues. Bioorg Med Chem. 1998 Sep; 6(9): 1631-9.

[44]   Hunjan S, Mason RP, Mehta VD, Kulkarni PV, Aravind S, Arora V, *et al.* Simultaneous intracellular and extracellular pH measurement in the heart by 19F NMR of 6-fluoropyridoxol. Magn Reson Med. 1998 Apr; 39(4): 551-6.

[45]   Rotevatn S, Murphy E, Levy LA, Raju B, Lieberman M, London RE. Cytosolic free magnesium concentration in cultured chick heart cells. Am J Physiol. 1989 Jul; 257(1 Pt 1): C141-6.

[46]   Ramasamy R, Zhao P, Gitomer WL, Sherry AD, Malloy CR. Determination of chloride potential in perfused rat hearts by nuclear magnetic resonance spectroscopy. Am J Physiol. 1992 Dec; 263(6 Pt 2): H1958-62.

[47]   Shukla HP, Mason RP, Bansal N, Antich PP. Regional myocardial oxygen tension: 19F MRI of sequestered perfluorocarbon. Magn Reson Med. 1996 Jun; 35(6): 827-33.

[48]   Rottman GA, Judd RM, Yin FC. Validation of 19F-magnetic resonance determination of myocardial blood volume. Magn Reson Med. 1995 Oct; 34(4): 628-31.

[49]   Yanagida S, Luo CS, Doyle M, Pohost GM, Pike MM. Nuclear magnetic resonance studies of cationic and energetic alterations with oxidant stress in the perfused heart. Modulation with pyruvate and lactate. Circ Res. 1995 Oct; 77(4): 773-83.

[50]   Mason RP, Shukla H, Antich PP. *In vivo* oxygen tension and temperature: simultaneous determination using 19F NMR spectroscopy of perfluorocarbon. Magn Reson Med. 1993 Mar; 29(3): 296-302.

[51]   Mason RP, Jeffrey FM, Malloy CR, Babcock EE, Antich PP. A noninvasive assessment of myocardial oxygen tension: 19F NMR spectroscopy of sequestered perfluorocarbon emulsion. Magn Reson Med. 1992 Oct; 27(2): 310-7.

[52]   Hitchens TK, Ye Q, Eytan DF, Janjic JM, Ahrens ET, Ho C. 19F MRI detection of acute allograft rejection with *in vivo* perfluorocarbon labeling of immune cells. Magn Reson Med. 2011 Apr; 65(4): 1144-53.

[53]   Waters EA, Chen J, Allen JS, Zhang H, Lanza GM, Wickline SA. Detection and quantification of angiogenesis in experimental valve disease with integrin-targeted nanoparticles and 19-fluorine MRI/MRS. J Cardiovasc Magn Reson. 2008; 10: 43.

[54]   Mulder WJ, Strijkers GJ, Vucic E, Cormode DP, Nicolay K, Fayad ZA. Magnetic resonance molecular imaging contrast agents and their application in atherosclerosis. Top Magn Reson Imaging. 2007 Oct; 18(5): 409-17.

[55]   Wang X, Mercier P, Letourneau PJ, Sykes BD. Effects of Phe-to-Trp mutation and fluorotryptophan incorporation on the solution structure of cardiac troponin C, and analysis of its suitability as a potential probe for *in situ* NMR studies. Protein Sci. 2005 Sep; 14(9): 2447-60.

[56]   Nakada T, Kwee IL, Card PJ, Matwiyoff NA, Griffey BV, Griffey RH. Fluorine-19 NMR imaging of glucose metabolism. Magn Reson Med. 1988 Mar; 6(3): 307-13.

[57]   Joseph PM, Fishman JE, Mukherji B, Sloviter HA. *In vivo* 19F NMR imaging of the cardiovascular system. J Comput Assist Tomogr. 1985 Nov-Dec; 9(6): 1012-9.

[58]   Kozerke S, Schar M, Lamb HJ, Boesiger P. Volume tracking cardiac 31P spectroscopy. Magn Reson Med. 2002 Aug; 48(2): 380-4.

[59]   Tyler DJ, Emmanuel Y, Cochlin LE, Hudsmith LE, Holloway CJ, Neubauer S, *et al.* Reproducibility of 31P cardiac magnetic resonance spectroscopy at 3 T. NMR Biomed. 2009 May; 22(4): 405-13.

[60]   Gabr RE, Ouwerkerk R, Bottomley PA. Quantifying *in vivo* MR spectra with circles. J Magn Reson. 2006 Mar; 179(1): 152-63.

[61]   Robson MD, Tyler DJ, Neubauer S. Ultrashort TE chemical shift imaging (UTE-CSI). Magn Reson Med. 2005 Feb; 53(2): 267-74.

[62]   Hansch A, Rzanny R, Heyne JP, Leder U, Reichenbach JR, Kaiser WA. Noninvasive measurements of cardiac high-energy phosphate metabolites in dilated cardiomyopathy by using 31P spectroscopic chemical shift imaging. Eur Radiol. 2005 Feb; 15(2): 319-23.

[63]   Caus T, Kober F, Marin P, Mouly-Bandini A, Quilici J, Metras D, *et al.* Non-invasive diagnostic of cardiac allograft vasculopathy by 31P magnetic resonance chemical shift imaging. Eur J Cardiothorac Surg. 2006 Jan; 29(1): 45-9.

[64]   Schroeder MA, Swietach P, Atherton HJ, Gallagher FA, Lee P, Radda GK, *et al.* Measuring intracellular pH in the heart using hyperpolarized carbon dioxide and bicarbonate: a 13C and 31P magnetic resonance spectroscopy study. Cardiovasc Res. 2010 Apr 1; 86(1): 82-91.

[65]   Kirby M, Svenningsen S, Owrangi A, Wheatley A, Farag A, Ouriadov A, *et al.* Hyperpolarized 3He and 129Xe MR imaging in healthy volunteers and patients with chronic obstructive pulmonary disease. Radiology. 2012 Nov; 265(2): 600-10.

[66]   Rijzewijk LJ, Jonker JT, van der Meer RW, Lubberink M, de Jong HW, Romijn JA, *et al.* Effects of hepatic triglyceride content on myocardial metabolism in type 2 diabetes. J Am Coll Cardiol. 2010 Jul 13; 56(3): 225-33.

CHAPTER 6

Technical Advances - Fast Imaging Acquisition Techniques

Jürgen E. Schneider[*]

BHF Experimental MR Unit, Radcliffe Department of Medicine - Division of Cardiovascular Medicine, University of Oxford, Oxford, UK

Abstract: Cardiac magnetic resonance (CMR) is an imaging modality that allows for a non-invasive assessment of anatomy, function, structure, viability and metabolism in hearts of patients and of small animal models (*e.g.*, mice and rats) with cardiovascular disease. Dedicated techniques to accelerate the inherently slow MR imaging process have resulted in a shift of paradigm in clinical CMR. The application of fast imaging techniques in preclinical CMR research lags far behind the clinical standard. The aim of this chapter is to review the challenges and advances in fast preclinical CMR. More specifically, parallel imaging, and reconstruction based techniques, including k-t-BLAST, k-t-PCA and Compressed Sensing will be discussed and examples for each application will be provided. We conclude that there is indeed a need for accelerating preclinical CMR, to increase the amount of information obtainable from each animal, to reduce the number animals used in preclinical research and to make an inherently expensive imaging modality more cost-efficient.

Keywords: Heart, myocardium, cardiovascular disease, phased-array, parallel imaging, compressed sensing, k-t BLAST, k-t PCA, cardiac function, T_1-mapping, LGE, Fast imaging acquisition techniques, CMR.

INTRODUCTION

Mice and rats are the most commonly used animal models in basic cardiovascular research. Surgical (*i.e.*, transient or permanent occlusion of the left coronary artery (LCA), or transverse aortic constriction (TAC)) and transgenic techniques (*i.e.*, deletion, alteration or over-expression of specific genes and gene products) allow not only for mimicking conditions found in patients with heart disease, but more importantly, help to answer fundamental questions in cardiology that would be unethical to obtain in humans. Magnetic resonance imaging (MRI) and

---

*Address correspondence to Jürgen E. Schneider: British Heart Foundation Experimental Magnetic Resonance Unit (BMRU), Wellcome Trust Centre for Human Genetics, Roosevelt Drive, Oxford OX3 7BN, UK; Tel: +44 1865 287762; Fax: +44 1865 287763; E-mail: jurgen.schneider@cardiov.ox.ac.uk

magnetic resonance spectroscopy (MRS) are non-invasive and radiation-free phenotyping tools, which utilize intrinsic contrast mechanisms without the need for external tracer reagents, and are capable of acquiring true three-dimensional (3D) volumes. More specifically, cardiac magnetic resonance (CMR) is used clinically to provide accurate multi-parametric and quantitative information on the heart, such as: left- and right ventricular volumes and mass to characterize global cardiac function; transmural wall motion (*i.e.*, myocardial tissue displacements, velocities and/or strain) to assess regional cardiac function; the amount of reversibly and irreversibly damaged tissue in, for example, post myocardial infarction to characterize viability; or on myocardial blood flow and perfusion reserve. Over the past decade, advances in MR hardware and acquisition techniques paved the way for clinical CMR to become a well-established diagnosis tool, which has found its way into clinical routine use in many centers and hospitals around the world. In particular, dedicated techniques to accelerate the inherently slow MR imaging process resulted in a shift of paradigm as they allowed for individual scans to be completed within a single breath-hold. This increased both applicability and accuracy of the technique. It also facilitated the development of the 'One-Stop-Shop' [1-4], whereby the multi-parametric information is obtained within one examination typically not exceeding 1 h, which is acceptable for most patients.

Various CMR techniques have also been reported in surgically or genetically modified rodent models of human heart disease (*e.g.,* see for example [5-7] for reviews). However, the progress in pre-clinical CMR, and in particular in acceleration techniques, lags far behind the clinical standard. There are multiple reasons for this: firstly, technical challenges associated with the small animals are significant: approximately 10-times higher physiological rates (heart rates of approximately 500-600 beats per minute, corresponding to a cardiac cycle length of 100-120 ms and respiratory rates of 60-120 breaths per minute are typically observed in anaesthetized mice), combined with the miniature size of the murine heart (compared to humans, the left ventricular volume in mice is about 2000-times smaller with typical end-diastolic volumes (EDV) of ~50-100 μl) require high temporal and spatial resolution. While dedicated MR-systems, comprising of ultra-high field magnets (*i.e.*, magnetic field strengths of 7 T and more), optimized radio-frequency (RF) coils and gradient systems are typically used in pre-clinical CMR to meet the requirements, the small geometries of these set-ups make hardware solutions - otherwise readily available on clinical MR-scanners - very challenging. This is the second main reason, which particularly hampers the progress in scan-time reduction, and will be discussed in more detail below. Finally, given the significantly smaller size of the pre-clinical market compared to the clinical sector (it is estimated that there are less than 1,000 pre-clinical MR-systems worldwide, which compares to 25,000 clinical MR-systems [8]), it is not surprising that only a fraction of the clinical developmental efforts are being spent to advance preclinical CMR.

The aim of this book chapter is to provide an overview of the advances in the development of fast preclinical CMR imaging techniques on rodents. While large animal models, such as pigs or dogs are also being used in cardiovascular research, their body size and physiological characteristics makes them suitable for CMR investigation using the clinical setup.

In this context, the term 'fast' has two different meanings: it can either refer to the timing of an MR sequence, which is ultimately characterized by the echo (TE) and repetition times (TR). Achieving short TE's and TR's primarily requires high-performance gradient systems with rapid switching times (< 200 µs), high duty cycles and strengths (≥ 600 mT/m), which are readily available nowadays. Clinically important constraints, which may affect pulse-sequence speed, such as gradient induced peripheral nerve stimulations, play no major role in small animal imaging, and are therefore neglected in this discussion. Given the time-scale of cardiac and respiratory motion in mice, mentioned above, short TE/TR are inherently desirable.

It is the second meaning of the term 'fast', which is of relevance to this chapter. The MR acquisition process is inherently slow, as one pixel line of the image is typically obtained within one TR[1]. The sequence needs to be repeated *N*-times to measure all data required to reconstruct the full two-dimensional image. Relaxation times, particularly the longitudinal (*i.e.*, T_1-relaxation) time adds another physical constraint affecting, for example, the rate with which a sequence

---

[1]This statement is simplified and does not apply to multi-echo sequences or single-shot methods.

can be repeated in order to obtain a specific contrast and / or sufficient signal-to-noise ratio (SNR). Thus, we will focus on techniques that provide overall scan-time reduction without impacting on the accuracy of the measured parameter. Long scan times can not only constrain the applicability of pre-clinical CMR, particularly in hemodynamically compromised mice and rats (due to their increased sensitivity to general anesthesia), but also limit the number of functional or tissue characterizing parameters available in one imaging session. Therefore, speeding up the acquisition process will increase the information that can be obtained from the same specimen, reduce the number of animals required for preclinical research, and ultimately, make an inherently expensive imaging modality more cost-effective.

Acceleration of the MR acquisition process can broadly be achieved either by using dedicated hardware combined with special post-processing (*i.e.*, 'Parallel Imaging'), or by sophisticated reconstruction techniques alone (for example, by 'Compressed Sensing'). The aim of this chapter is to review both approaches, and to discuss their relevance and impact on preclinical CMR.

HARDWARE BASED APPROACHES

Background

Magnetic resonance experiments on rodent hearts are typically performed using a single RF-coil, which is used for both transmitting and receiving the MRI / MRS signals. Quadrature-driven volume coils, such as birdcage resonators, which have been optimized in geometry (*i.e.*, resonator length and diameter) [9-11], provide the best compromise between B_1-field homogeneity and sensitivity, while surface RF-coils (operated in linear or in quadrature mode) have the advantage of high sensitivity in close proximity to the coil, but a rapidly decaying B_1-profile [12-14]. An arrangement consisting of a volume RF-coil for transmitting and a small surface receive coil aims to combine the advantages of both designs [15, 16]. Roemer *et al.* proposed the concept of replacing a single (receive) coil with multiple, smaller and independent surface coils (*i.e.*, phased-array) more than two decades ago [17]. While this design was initially aimed to increase the signal-to-noise ratio (SNR) at simultaneously large field-of-view (FOV) coverage and no increase of experimental time [17], it also laid the foundation for the development of acceleration techniques. Phased-coil arrays not only became fairly quickly standard on clinical MR systems at magnetic field strengths of 1.5 - 3 Tesla, but they had major impact on cardiological diagnostics by enabling scan-time reductions that made cardiac MR applicable in clinical routine as mentioned above [18-20]. However, it was not until mid-2000 that the first conference papers reported on 2- and 4-element phased coil arrays for murine CMR (*e.g.,* [21-23]). While coil-arrays are now readily commercially available for cardiac MR in mice and rats, many studies published today still use a single volume transmit-receive RF-coil[2]. Several reasons can explain this finding: (1) unlike clinical MR-systems, where 32 receive channels are typical (*e.g.,* [24, 25]), many (older) pre-clinical MR-systems are only equipped with a single receive channel; upgrading a pre-clinical MR-system with multi-receive capability represents a significant investment; (2) space-constraints add complexity to the setup/animal preparation when using coil-arrays (which need to be placed as close as possible to the heart), and may therefore impact on workflow and on throughput; (3) the higher static magnetic field found at pre-clinical MR-systems, and smaller array geometries render it not only technically more challenging to build well-isolated (*i.e.,* decoupled) coil-arrays, but also to benefit from this technology: decreasing the coil-sizes, low filling factors and high Larmor frequencies can potentially result in a domination of the coil noise, which adversely affects the SNR. The latter two arguments in particular hint at the limits of this technology. While phased arrays consisting of 128 elements have been reported for CMR in humans at 3 Tesla [26, 27], the array-size for murine CMR at ultra-high magnetic fields is somewhat more modest with typically two to four elements. Up to 8-elements have been reported for the application on mouse hearts [4] an example is shown in Fig. (**1**). It worthwhile to note that an alternative approach to increase throughput was proposed by M. Henkelman and his group who used multiple RF-coils to image several mice in parallel rather than to accelerate the acquisition process of a single mouse [28]. This required replication of the animal monitoring [29] and, specifically for cardiac imaging, retrospective gating techniques [30] to individually reconstruct the functional image data for each mouse. Technical

---

[2]A PubMed search revealed that the overwhelming majority of publications on mouse cardiac MR in 2012 still used a transmit-receive coil arrangement.

challenges and animal welfare legislation may, however, limit the general applicability of this approach.

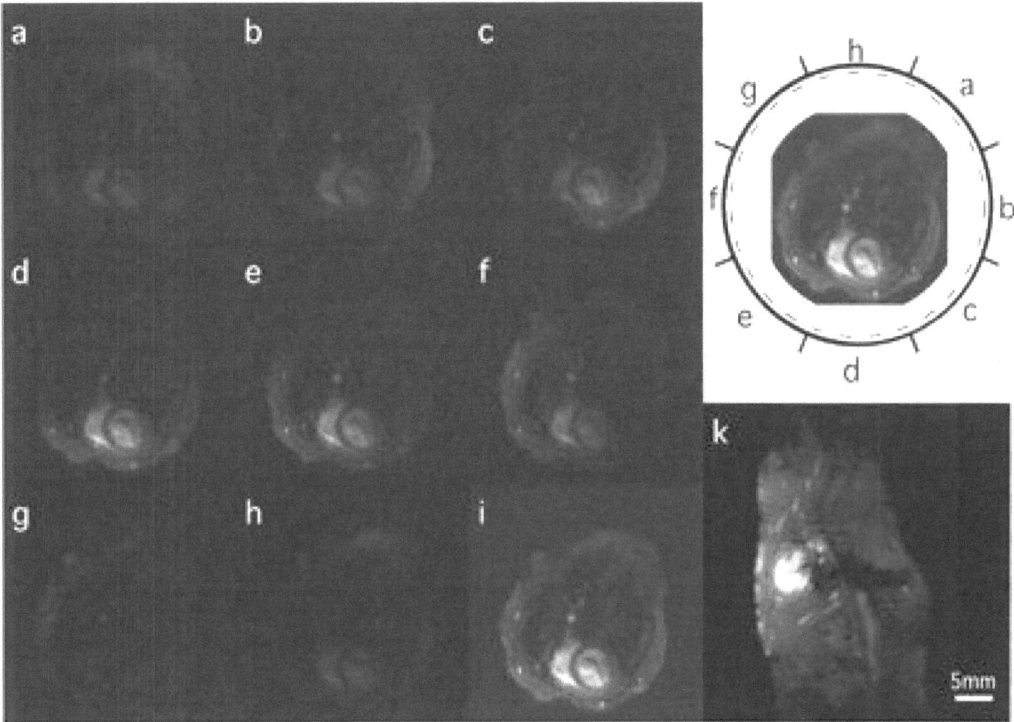

Figure 1: a-h: Axial gradient echo images from a mouse heart *in vivo* obtained with the individual coil elements of an 8-channel volume array [31]. The sum-of-squares combined axial (**i**) and sagittal (**k**) images illustrating excellent sensitivity covering the entire heart in each relevant direction for the off-centered positioned mouse. The schematic in panel j depicts the location of the individual coil elements (shown in Fig. **1a-h**) relative to the mouse (indicated by the grey circle); the dashed black line represents the inner tube of the probe head, and the solid black circle illustrates the coil-array. (Adapted from [4] - reproduced with permission from John Wiley and Sons).

Not surprisingly, and as demonstrated in Fig. (**1**), most of the signal in the cardiac region arises from the anteriorly located coil-elements. Nevertheless, the posterior coil-elements still contribute constructively and are beneficial, particularly for the posterior wall. This was also demonstrated quantitatively in reference [4]. A more detailed characterization of this design revealed that approximately only half of the SNR was obtained in the iso-centre of this volume-array compared to a quadrature driven birdcage coil [31]. While alternative coil designs may provide some improvements in SNR performance [32], fundamental challenges and potential limits of the phased-array approach for applications using ultra-high field small-bore MR systems still persist.

Parallel Imaging

Multiple receive-coils not only boost the SNR, but can also be used to accelerate the MR scan. This is known as *Parallel Imaging* or *Parallel Acquisition Technique*, the basics of which are described extensively in the literature (see for example [33-38] for methodological description and clinical applications). In brief, the data are under-sampled in the phase-encoding direction during the acquisition process (top left panel in Fig. **2**), which leads to aliasing in this direction (bottom left panel in Fig. **2**). The missing data are subsequently restored from the information based on the spatial variations in the coil-array. This restoration can be performed in k-space or in the image domain as illustrated in the right half of Fig. (**2**). The most commonly used methods in the (pre-) clinical setting nowadays are *SENSE* (*i.e.*, Sensitivity Encoding [39]), which operates in the image space, or *GRAPPA* (*i.e.*, Generalized Auto-calibrating Partially Parallel Acquisitions [40]), which performs the reconstruction in k-space. SENSE requires knowledge of the sensitivity profiles of the individual coil elements and uses the framework of linear algebra to reconstruct the fully sampled image [39]. Conversely, GRAPPA requires *auto-calibration lines*, which are typically acquired prior to the under-sampled scan to calculate the contributions of the individual coil elements to a total sensitivity based on their spatial positions. The missing information is then recovered in k-space for each coil-image separately prior to combining the individual images. Thus, image reconstruction (*i.e.*, anti-aliasing) and SNR optimization (*i.e.*, coil combination) are performed separately, potentially providing improved results [40]. It has been demonstrated that the SENSE reconstruction is superior to GRAPPA with respect to SNR performance and image quality, whenever the coil sensitivity maps can be determined in a precise fashion. However, there are many real-life situations, in which it is difficult to obtain accurate knowledge of the complex sensitivities of component coil sensitivities, including motion, or in low SNR regions. In these cases, GRAPPA is particularly beneficial and should be used [40, 41]. It is clinical

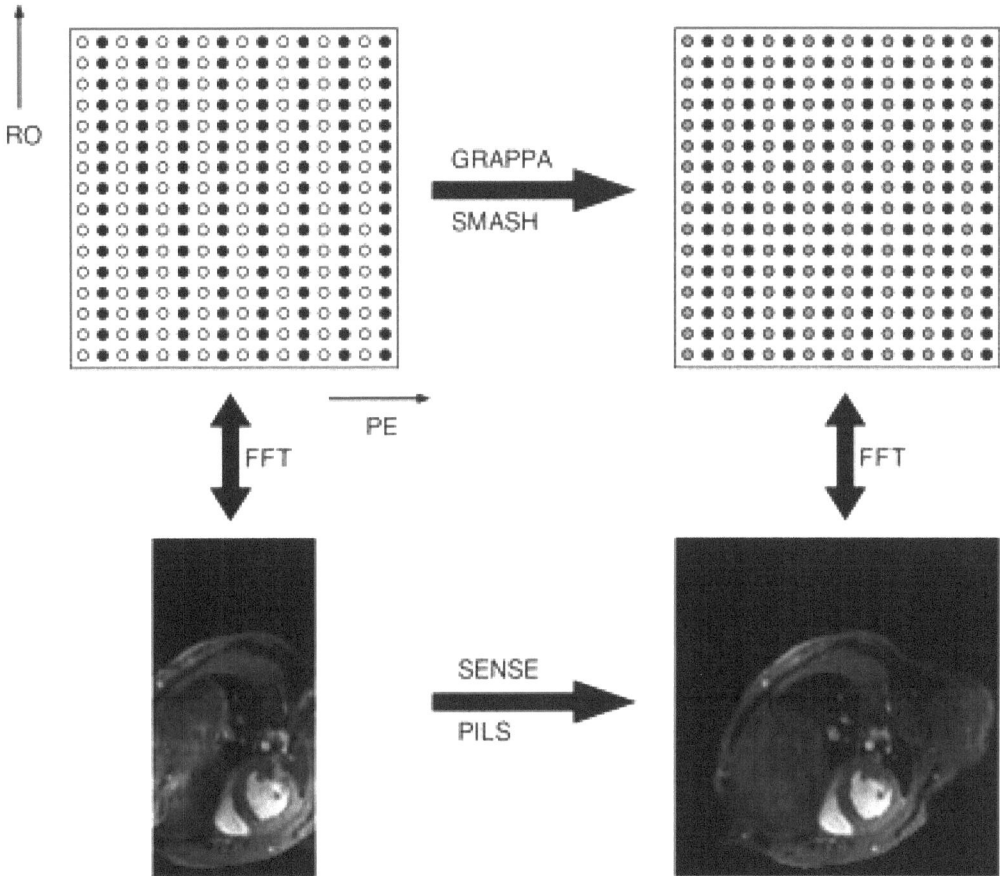

Figure 2: Parallel imaging on a mouse heart using an acceleration factor 2: under-sampling is achieved by acquiring only every second k-space line (black filled circles in top left panel) resulting in an aliased image (bottom left panel). The missing k-space lines (open circles in top left panel) can be calculated prior to Fourier transform based on the information from the multi-receiver coil array using SMASH (*i.e.*, Simultaneous Acquisition of Spatial Harmonics [45]) or GRAPPA (grey filled circles in top right panel). Conversely, image domain techniques (such as SENSE or PILS [46]) require coil sensitivity maps to reconstruct the full from the aliased image. RO denotes the frequency encoding (readout), and PE the phase encoding direction, respectively.

practice, especially in cardiac imaging, to acquire the images with a field-of-view, which is smaller than the object size, resulting in partially aliased images. It has been shown that, in these cases, GRAPPA is able to generate virtually artifact-free image reconstructions, while the SENSE reconstruction suffers from artifacts [42, 43]. This artifact is also known as the 'SENSE ghost' [43].

An *R*-fold under-sampled acquisition results in a reduced signal-to-noise ratio SNR_{Acc} compared to the fully sampled image (SNR_{Full}) according to:

$$SNR_{Acc} = \frac{SNR_{Full}}{g \cdot \sqrt{R}} \tag{1}$$

Equation (1) was initially derived for the SENSE reconstruction, and gives an upper limit for the SNR, which is characterized by the square root of the under-sampling factor [39]. An additional reduction in SNR is caused by the geometry factor *g*, which is always ≥1 and which describes the ability to separate aliased pixels for a given coil configuration [39]. Notably, an equivalent *g*-factor expression has been derived for the GRAPPA reconstruction [44].

Applications

Parallel imaging in particular facilitated the application of CMR in clinical routine as individual scans can be completed within a single breath-hold of 15-20 s, which is well tolerated by most patients. More recently, the combination with non-cartesian (*i.e.,* radial) imaging techniques allowed for capturing dynamic processes such as the beating heart and (R1.6 blood flow in real-time [47-49]), eliminating the need for cardiac triggering and enabling free-breathing.

Conversely, very few studies in preclinical CMR have used parallel imaging to accelerate the acquisition for the reasons outlined above. We were first to demonstrate the feasibility and the benefits of parallel imaging for left-ventricular (LV) function assessment in rats at 9.4 T using a four-element array [50]. In this study, two high-resolution data sets were acquired in an interleaved fashion (to minimize the influence of anesthesia), *i.e.*, one consisting of eight averages and using a large volume coil, while the second one used the four-element coil array without averaging. Two-, three-, and four-fold under-sampled data sets were generated retrospectively from the phased array data, and subjected to a temporal GRAPPA ('*TGRAPPA*') reconstruction [51]. Despite the significantly reduced SNR of the four-fold accelerated cine images shown in Fig. (**3**), excellent agreement was obtained in LV functional parameters (*i.e.*, left-ventricular mass, volumes and ejection fraction) between the volume coil and the four-fold under-sampled datasets. Importantly, it took less than three minutes to acquire the stack of cine-images, consisting of 24 to 30 frames and eight to nine contiguous slices, covering the entire left ventricle. This represents a factor of 20-30 compared to conventionally conducted functional studies in rats, which are based on volume coils [50].

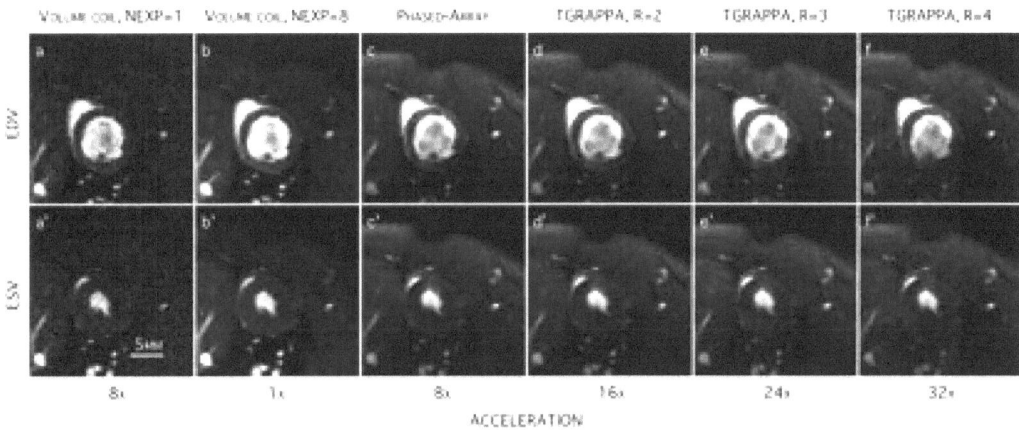

Figure 3: Mid-ventricular end-diastolic (top row) and end-systolic frames (bottom row) out of a cine-train of 30 images in short-axis orientation. The data were acquired with the (3a,a') volume coil - one average, (3b,b') volume coil - eight averages) and (3c,c') coil-array sum-of-square reconstruction - one average. From the data set acquired for Fig. (**3c,c'**), accelerated data sets with (Fig. **3d,d'**) $R = 2$, (Fig. **3e,e'**) $R = 3$, and (Fig. **3f,f'**) $R = 4$ were generated, followed by a TGRAPPA reconstruction. Pixel size is 100×100 μm in-plane; slice thickness: 1.5 mm. (Taken from [50] - reproduced with permission from John Wiley and Sons).

The first proof-of-principle, parallel imaging application in murine hearts was performed by Ramirez *et al.*, using SENSE reconstruction first [23], and later, more comprehensively, using GRAPPA reconstruction [52]. The main purpose of this study was to investigate the feasibility of multiple-mouse MRI mentioned before, and retrospectively gated cine-MRI was used as a showcase. Two mice were placed simultaneously next to each other in a 7 T - 30 cm bore animal scanner, with a two-element phased-coil array dedicated to each animal. In this study, three-fold accelerated scans yielded an SNR in the heart that was equivalent to the SNR obtained in a fully sampled scan using a commercial mouse birdcage coil [52]. Schneider *et al.* were first to comprehensively investigate the benefits of parallel imaging for cardiac MRI in mice on a 9.4 T MR system [4]. This study used an 8-channel volume phased-array mentioned before, and combined parallel imaging (*i.e.*, GRAPPA and TGRAPPA) with cine-MRI to quantify global cardiac function, a T_1-mapping sequence to assess longitudinal relaxation times, and a high-resolution, 3D late gadolinium enhanced (LGE) imaging sequence to determine infarct sizes, respectively. Measurement of the longitudinal relaxation time T_1 in normal and diseased myocardium has recently become highly relevant in clinical CMR, as T_1-maps provide objective and absolute-quantitative diagnostic information, and do not require a reference ROI (see for example [53-55] for applications). Conventional T_1-mapping, based on inversion or on saturation recovery techniques are time-consuming. Look-Locker-type [56], segmented [11] and snapshot-based [57] techniques have been used in the past to reduce the scan time. T_1-mapping is for example used in preclinical research to measure myocardial blood-flow, and requires the acquisition of two T_1-maps, *i.e.*, one with slice-selective and one with global inversion [15, 58, 59]. Thus, this technique would benefit considerably from acceleration techniques.

We demonstrated quantitatively in mice that a threefold acceleration of the data acquisition is generally possible in mice without compromising the accuracy of any of the measured parameters [4]. Examples for accelerated T_1-maps and LGE images are shown in Figs. (**4, 5**). Furthermore, Table **1** lists the T_1-times for three different tissues (*i.e.*, liver, skeletal muscle and myocardium), obtained from fully sampled and two-, three- and fourfold under-sampled acquisitions, respectively. Statistical analysis yielded no statistically significant difference between the different T_1 values for each tissue type, and demonstrated the validity of this approach.

Table 1: **T_1-Relaxation Time Measurements (mean ± SD - taken from [4], reproduced with permission from John Wiley and Sons)**

T_1/[s]	R=1	R=2	R=3	R=4
LV Myocardium	1.00 ± 0.07	1.03 ± 0.09	0.99 ± 0.11	1.05 ± 0.19
Skeletal Muscle	1.34 ± 0.10	1.41 ± 0.09	1.38 ± 0.12	1.48 ± 0.18
Liver	1.03 ± 0.06	1.02 ± 0.09	0.98 ± 0.09	1.06 ± 0.16

Contrast-enhance MRI to measure infarct size was also demonstrated to benefit from scan-time reduction [4]. This technique is based on the difference in T_1-relaxation time between normal and injured myocardium post-contrast application. Choosing the time between the inversion pulse and readout appropriately (*i.e.*, TI~400 ms, see [60] for more details) nulls the signal of remote the myocardium, and provides hyper-intense signal from the injured area of the ventricle. The TI time between an inversion pulse is the time-limiting factor in this scan, and even small acceleration factors can translate into considerable time savings as demonstrated in Fig. (**5**).

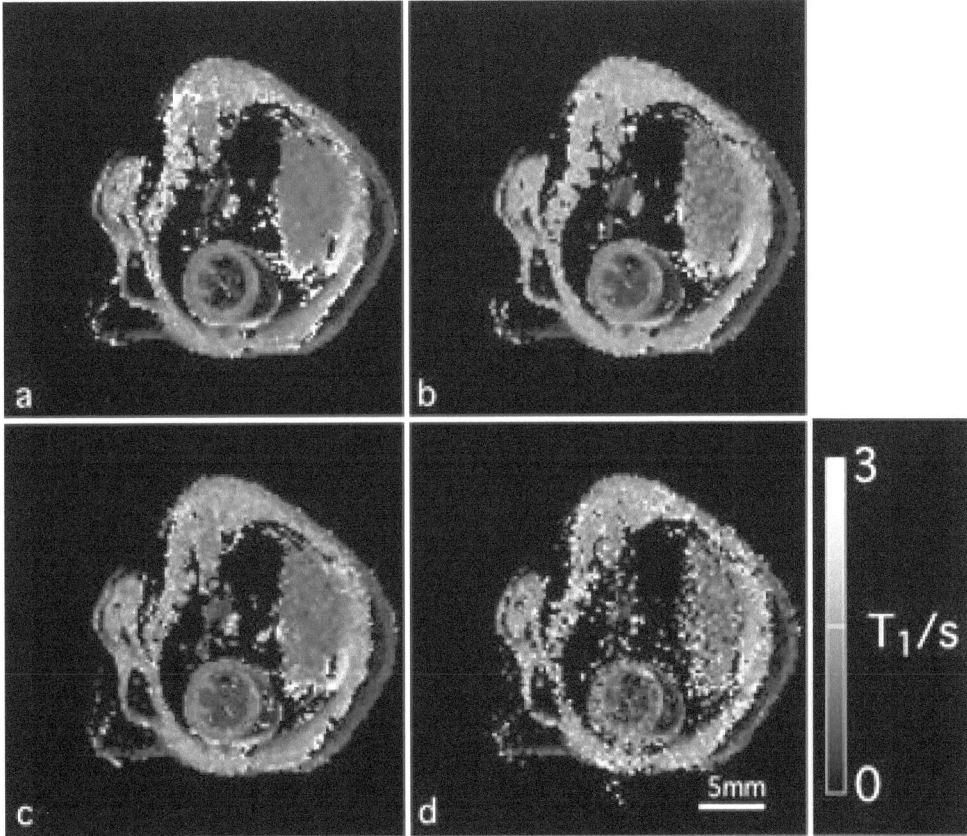

Figure 4: T_1-parameter maps in a mid-ventricular short-axis slice across a moue heart for acceleration factors (**a**) R = 1, (**b**) R = 2, (**c**) R = 3, and (**d**) R = 4, respectively. The maps were masked in the range 0-3 sec to remove outliers from the fit. Twenty-four auto-calibration lines were used to reconstruct the missing information from the undersampled datasets. T_1-values for various tissue types are listed in Table **1**. (Taken from [4] - reproduced with permission from John Wiley and Sons).

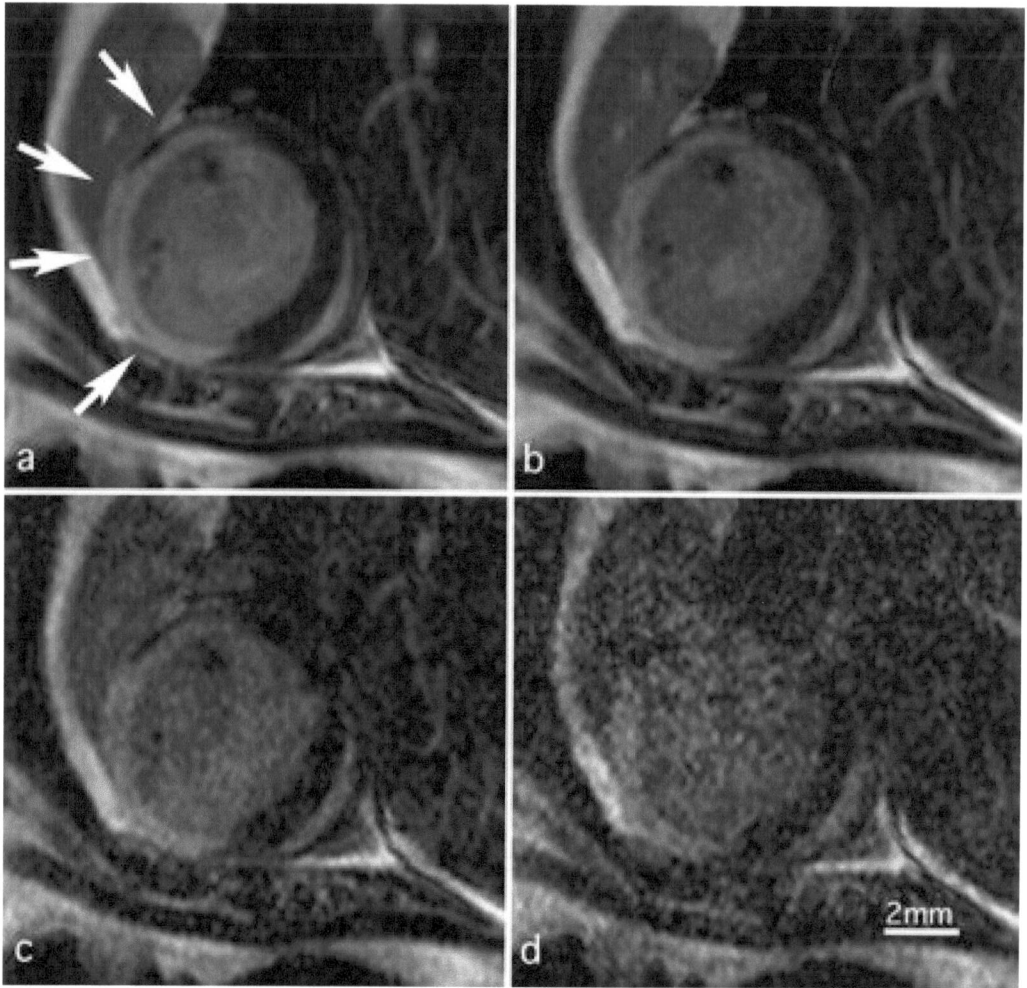

Figure 5: Contrast-enhanced mid-ventricular short-axis slice across a mouse heart out of 3D stack for acceleration factors (**a**) R = 1, (**b**) R = 2 and (**c**) R = 3, respectively. The arrows in Fig. (**5a**) indicate the infarcted area. The required scan times (which also depended on the ratio heart to respiratory rate) were: R = 1: 1189 ± 85 s; R = 2: 626 ± 44 s; R = 3: 401 ± 47 s; and R = 4: 317 ± 40 s, respectively. (Taken from [4] - reproduced with permission from John Wiley and Sons).

Parallel imaging (*i.e.*, SENSE) has also been used to speed-up the acquisition of retrospectively gated murine LV-functional imaging [61], and of 3D Time-of-Flight (ToF) MR angiography in supra-aortic vessels of atherosclerotic mice [62]. Importantly, the scan time reduction achieved with parallel imaging (*i.e.*, GRAPPA) facilitated two novel developments in murine cardiac MRI, which have not been possible before. Firstly, the rapid acquisition of functional cine-MRI data allowed for the first time full left-ventricular coverage in mice under intravenous infusion of dobutamine. Previous studies derived left-ventricular peak filling and ejection rates for a single, mid-ventricular slice [63] for technical reasons: the maximum intravenous (iv) administrable volume for an adult mouse, which has a total blood volume of approximately 2 ml, and is limited to 200 µl. Infusion volumes in excess of 200 µl can cause adverse physiological effect, and have thus to be avoided. In this study, maximum inotropic stimulation was obtained using 16 ng/g body wt/min, which translated to an infusion rate of 27.8 µl/g body weight/h. The maximal iv volume is therefore reached after ~15 min in a mouse with a body weight of 30 g. Allowing for a stabilization period of 5-7 min [64] leaves only 8-10 min for the imaging protocol. Therefore, full left-ventricular coverage without sacrificing spatial and temporal resolution in the cine images is only feasible if dedicated acceleration techniques are being used. More importantly, Schneider *et al.* also showed in this pilot study a difference between contractility parameters calculated from a single slice or from the whole LV volume.

The second application facilitated by parallel imaging was first pass perfusion imaging in the mouse heart [65, 66]. Again, the high rate and the miniature size of the mouse heart require both spatial and temporal resolution to adequately resolve and depict the arrival of the contrast bolus in the blood pool and the myocardium. Coolen *et al.* used a four-element phased-array coil, an acceleration factor of ~1.6 and GRAPPA reconstruction to capture the first pass of the Gd-DTPA contrast bolus through the mouse heart [65]. Using a segmented gradient echo sequence with saturation module, they showed that a sampling rate of 3 heart beats per image - corresponding to a temporal resolution of 300 - 400 ms - was sufficient to adequately resolve contrast arrival [65]. An image series demonstrating first-pass perfusion in a healthy mouse heart and intensity-time curves for blood and myocardium are shown in Fig. (**6**). While this study only performed semi-quantitative analysis of the perfusion data by calculating the slope of the contrast arrival in myocardium normalized to the equivalent slope of the LV blood pool, Coolen *et al.* demonstrated in mice with permanent ligation of the left coronary artery not only that, unsurprisingly, these values were significantly reduced in infarcted compared to remote myocardium, but also that the remote myocardium in the infarcted mice had significantly reduced perfusion than the myocardium of healthy control mice. In a follow-up study by the same group, van Nierop *et al.* refined the experimental design and analysis to provide absolute perfusion values in four segments of a mid-ventricular slice and assessed repeatability of this technique [66]. Specifically, this study reported perfusion values obtained at two measurements on the same animals but separated by one week of 7.3 ± 0.9 and 7.2 ± 0.6 mL min^{-1} g^{-1}, respectively. The between-session coefficient of variation was found to be only 6%, indicating excellent repeatability. For comparison, the inter-animal coefficient of variation was 11 and 8% for the separate experiments [66].

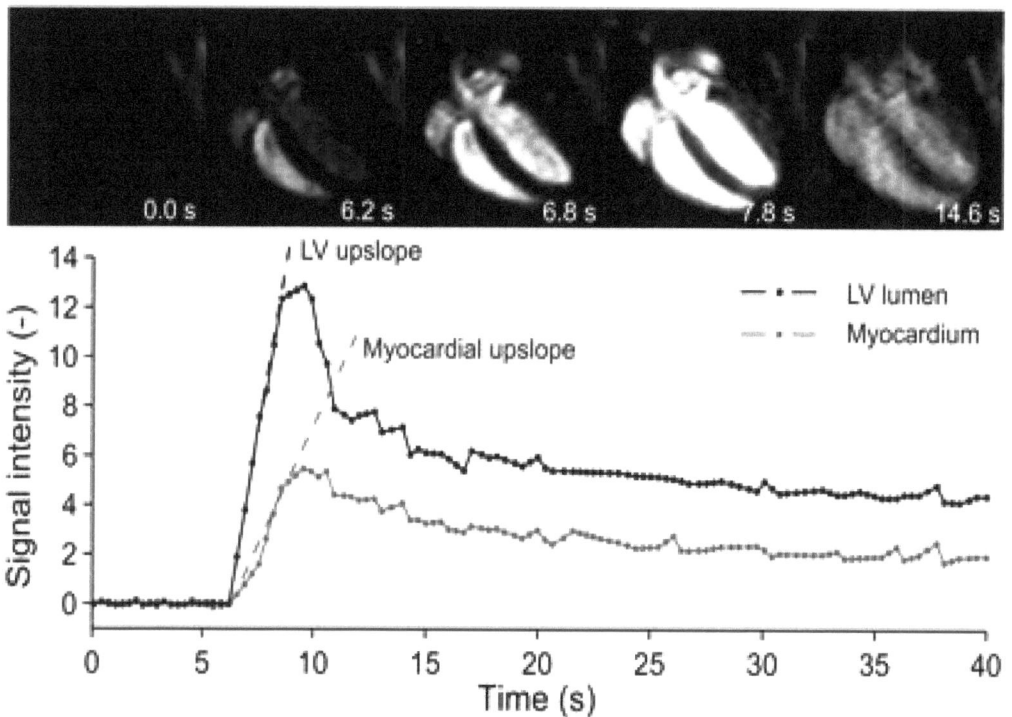

Figure 6: **(a)** Representative image series demonstrating first-pass perfusion in a healthy mouse heart, illustrating the arrival of the contrast agent contrast agent in the right (t = 6.2 s) and left ventricle (t = 6.8 s), influx of the contrast agent in the LV myocardial wall (t = 7.8 s), followed by dilution and washout (t = 14.6 s). **(b)** Intensity-time curves from the LV lumen and myocardial wall before, during and after first pass of the contrast agent. Signal intensities were referenced to baseline intensity values. The initial myocardial up-slope (normalized to the LV lumen up-slope) can be used to calculate semi-quantitative perfusion values. (Courtesy of BJ van Nierop and GJ Strijkers, Eindhoven University of Technology, The Netherlands).

RECONSTRUCTION BASED METHODS

The acceleration of the MR imaging process by parallel imaging as described in the previous section requires that the MR console is equipped with multiple receiver channels. This represents an additional and not insignificant expense, and may therefore not always be available, particularly on older MR systems. In addition, the upper limit for accelerating the acquisition, which is given by the number of RF-coils of the phased array used for receiving the signals, is quite low for reasons outlined above. In real experiments however, only gains in speed were achieved that remained well below this upper limit, as exemplified in the three studies [4, 65, 66]. The aim of this section is to describe three different acceleration techniques, namely *k-t* BLAST, *k-t* PCA and Compressed Sensing, all of which have been used to predominantly speed-up dynamic imaging processes in murine hearts. These methods utilize correlations, which are present in the dynamic data to recover the missing information, and are as such entirely based on sophisticated reconstruction techniques. While several alternative acceleration methods in this category have been developed, for example partial Fourier imaging [67, 68], reduced-field-of-view methods [69], UNFOLD [70, 71], keyhole [72, 73] or view-sharing techniques (*e.g.,* [74-76]), which have not played a major role for cardiac MR in rodents, and will therefore only be listed.

k-t BLAST

a) Method: k-t BLAST (*i.e.,* Broad-use Linear Acquisition Speed-up Technique) was proposed by Tsao *et al.* to dynamically image areas that exhibit quasi-periodic motion, including the heart, the lungs, the abdomen, and the brain under periodic stimulation [77]. *k-t* BLAST represents an advancement of the original BLAST paper [78], and exploits spatio-temporal correlations in the acquired MR signal. Each dynamic acquisition comprises of a low-spatial/high-temporal resolution training data set, followed by the under-sampled (*i.e.,* only every n^{th} phase encoding step is acquired), high-resolution data. A Fourier transform of the under-sampled data into space-frequency (*x-f*) domain results in periodic replication of the object signals, mapping signals from several locations into one target voxel. The task of the reconstruction is to determine the individual signal intensities of the aliased voxels. In essence, this is achieved by splitting the signal at each location into a baseline value and a fluctuation around this baseline. Thus, the reconstruction involves the calculation of the baseline value from the under-sampled data, and the fluctuations from the training data set on a voxel-by-voxel basis to obtain the object signals in x-f space. A final Fourier transform along f yields the object signals in x-t space, which corresponds to a series of images over time t [77]. It should be noted that k-t BLAST and k-t SENSE are closely related, except for the fact that k-t SENSE additionally takes the sensitivities of the individual coil of a phased array into consideration. The k-t SENSE approach has the additional advantage that complimentary information from the multiple receive coils can be used to aid the unaliasing process [77]. Furthermore, it is also worth to mention that in case of k-t SENSE, the achievable accelerating factor can exceed the upper limit (given by the number of receivers) of conventional parallel imaging as the described reconstruction methods make a smooth transition from the over-determined to the underdetermined case [77].

b) Application: Typical scan time reduction, obtained clinically with k-t BLAST, are in the order of five-fold [79]. Only one study has reported on the application of k-t BLAST on functional (cine) imaging in mouse hearts [80]. Marshall *et al.* compared standard cardiac cine imaging with threefold under-sampled k-t BLAST acquisition in healthy mice and one animal with myocardial infarct (MI). Analysis of left-ventricular volumes and mass for fully-sampled and accelerated acquisition of these pilot data showed a trend towards overestimation of ESV, LV mass, and an underestimation of end-diastolic volume [80]. Nevertheless, this study illustrated the feasibility of k-t BLAST as a means to reduce scan time of preclinical CMR in mice.

k-t PCA

a) Method: k-t PCA (*i.e.*, Principal Component Analysis) is a generalization of the k-t BLAST approach, and is more suitable for situations, in which significant aliasing in the x-f space is present. The reconstruction problem in k-t BLAST is inherently underdetermined as there are fewer equations than unknowns, while constraining the reconstruction in this case with the principal component analysis (PCA) results in an over-determined reconstruction problem, if the number of principal components is chosen sufficiently low. Thus, this approach allows for the use of higher acceleration factors [81]. In its basic form, *k-t* PCA does not require any specific hardware, but like *k-t* SENSE, can incorporate additional information from the multiple receiver coils to resolve the aliasing (*i.e.*, *k-t* PCA/SENSE).

b) Application: Pedersen *et al.* used *k-t* PCA and *k-t* PCA/SENSE in their methods paper to acquire eight-fold undersampled myocardial perfusion data in a pig, and demonstrated significantly reduced relative root-mean-square (RMS) errors of PCA-constraint reconstruction compared to *k-t* BLAST / *k-t* SENSE [81]. This approach was subsequently applied to mice to acquire first-pass perfusion data in mouse hearts on a clinical 3T MR system [82]. Like in the parallel imaging accelerated application [65, 66], perfusion MRI was applied to a single, mid-ventricular slice, but achieved an improved spatial (*i.e.*, $0.2 \times 0.2 \times 1.5 mm^3$) and temporal resolution (acquisition window length of 43 ms). Hence, this approach allowed for a sampling rate of one image per cardiac cycle. The perfusion values obtained in this study for control mice were 7.3 ± 1.5 mL g^{-1} min^{-1} [82], and were therefore in good agreement with the values quoted above, obtained with parallel imaging [66].

Compressed Sensing (CS)

Due to the time-consuming data acquisition process in MRI and MRS, Compressed Sensing (CS) is becoming increasingly more important as a means to reduce acquisition time [83-85]. Both the inherently slow MR acquisition process and the fact that MR images are naturally compressible, make this modality highly suitable for this acceleration technique. There is an increasing wealth of literature on this topic (see for example [86, 87] for overviews). We therefore aim to provide only a brief recapitulation of the methodological background in this section and to focus on the application of CS for preclinical CMR.

a) Method: Conventional data sampling in MRI obeys the Nyquist criterion, which states that the sampling rate must be at least twice the highest frequency present in the data. Otherwise, the Fourier reconstructions exhibit aliasing artifacts as shown in Fig. (**2**). Conversely, CS is a reconstruction technique that facilitates the reconstruction of signals from a number of acquisitions well below the Nyquist limit in any measurement basis. To make this possible, CS requires that three conditions hold true:

(1) <u>Sparsity</u>: The desired image has a sparse representation in a known transform domain, *i.e.*, that the signal is compressible. Notably, the signal is not required to be sparse in the displayed domain, but it is sufficient to know a transformation into a basis in which it has a sparse representation. Wavelet transforms or finite difference operators have been shown to promote sparsity. Furthermore, sparsity is not limited to the spatial domain only as dynamic images can also be sparse in the temporal dimension (see for example [88, 89]). In particular, cine-MRI is suitable for the application of CS as the quasi-periodicity of cardiac images has a sparse temporal Fourier transform [87]. Sparsity can for example be found in the temporal domain using the dynamic image series of the beating heart. Although each timeframe of the cine-train in the image domain $\{x_i\}$ may not be sparse, we have shown that the information content in every acquired cardiac phase relative to the temporal average over all timeframes is much lower than the required information for every single frame. Thus, a difference operator T transforms the image series $\{x_i\}$ in a series $\{s_i\}$ with sparse members. T can be obtained from the temporal average image A, which is calculated by summing all cine-frames, and by normalizing to the number of frames N for each slice:

$$A = \frac{1}{N} \sum_{J=1}^{N} x_j \qquad\qquad (2)$$

Subtracting A from each individual image space $\{x_i\}$ leads to a series $\{s_i\}$ of sparse representations. The $\{s_i\}$ contain only the temporal information and, thus, meet the CS condition of sparsity, as illustrated graphically in Fig. (7) [90].

(2) <u>Incoherence</u>: The aliasing artifacts due to k-space under-sampling are incoherent (noise like) in that transform domain. However, uniform random sampling patterns do not take the energy distribution of MR images in k-space in consideration, where most energy is concentrated in the center and rapidly decays away towards the edges of k- space. Thus, variable-density sampling with denser sampling close to the center of k-space, matching the energy distribution in

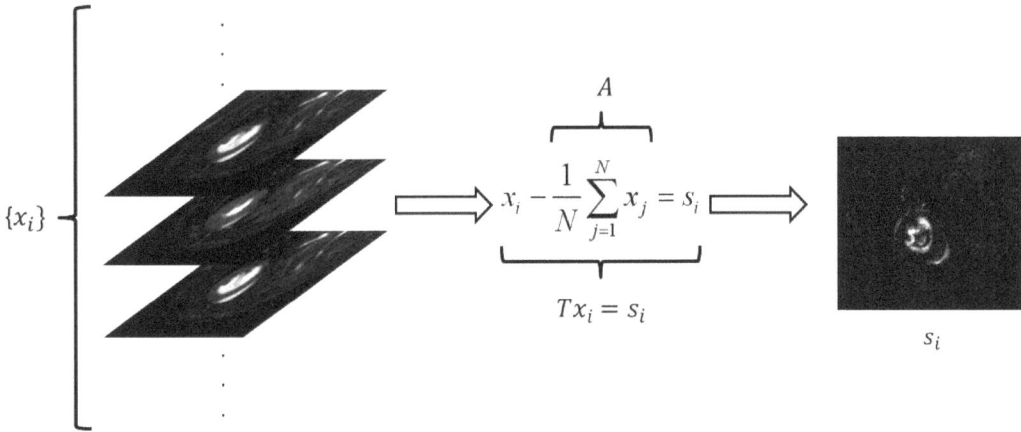

Figure 7: Transformation operator T: an average image A for the entire image series $\{x_i\}$ is first calculated on a slice-by-slice basis. Sparse representations of individual cardiac phases $\{s_i\}$ are subsequently generated by subtracting the average image from each frame in the cine-train. (Taken from [90] - reproduced with permission from John Wiley and Sons).

k-space and partially mimicking the incoherence properties of pure random sampling are preferable [83]. A simple way to evaluate the incoherence generated by a particular sampling scheme is to calculate the sidelobe-to-peak ratio of the Point Spread Function (PSF) and/or the size of the sidelobes of the Transform Point Spread Function (TPSF) in the transform domain [83]. Fig. (**8**) shows an example of a pseudo-random sampling scheme, which was derived based on computer simulations to provide a miminum side lobe-to-peak ratio of the PSF [90].

(3) <u>Non-linear reconstruction:</u> A nonlinear reconstruction is used to enforce both sparsity of the image representation and consistency with the acquired data [83]. This can be achieved by solving the constrained optimization problem [86]:

$$min\{\|Tx\|_1\}, \text{ subject to } \|Rx - k\|_2 \leq \varepsilon. \tag{3}$$

Here, T represents a transformation from pixel space x to a sparse representation. R denotes a partial Fourier transform corresponding to a particular under-sampling scheme, k are the measured *k*-space data, and ε considers the noise contained in k. It has been shown that minimization of the ℓ_1-norm promotes sparsity, while the additional constraint $\|\cdot\|_2 \leq \varepsilon$ enforces data consistency [87].

Eq. 3 implies that from all possible reconstructions, which are consistent with the data, the one whose coefficient sequence has minimal ℓ_1-norm is chosen. It can be proven that when Tx is sufficiently sparse, the recovery *via* ℓ_1-minimization yields the exact solution [86]. It should also be noted that there are alternative ways to the ℓ_1-minimization to recover sparse solutions, such as for example greedy algorithms [91].

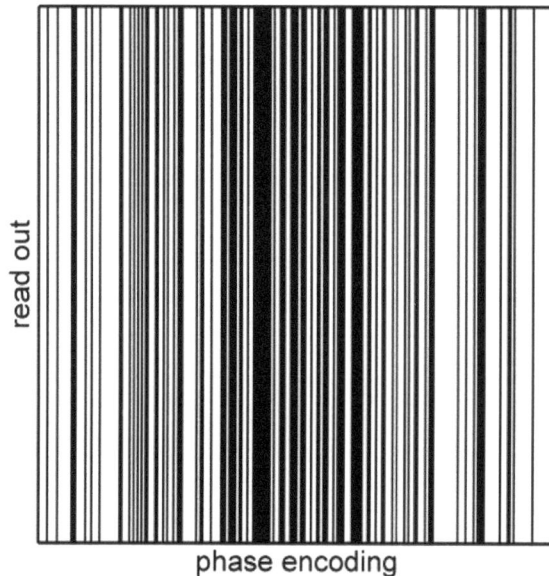

Figure 8: Random sampling scheme for CS reconstruction. Black lines resemble acquired data, and white lines / band illustrate missing data. The steps are chosen by random numbers according to a Gaussian function to minimize the sidelobe-to-peak ratio of the point spread function as suggested by Lustig *et al.* [83]. The maximum of the distribution is located at the center of *k*-space where most of the energy of the MR-image in k-space is concentrated. (Taken from [90] - reproduced with permission from John Wiley and Sons).

(b) Applications: As mentioned above, cine-MRI is particularly suitable for the application of CS. We were first to use CS for speeding up LV-functional assessment in mice [90]. Each cine-frame was randomly under-sampled in the phase encoding direction using a Gaussian weighting function. Fig. (**9**) shows a histogram of every measured phase encoding step of all time frames, illustrating the underlying Gaussian distribution of the *k*-space weighting.

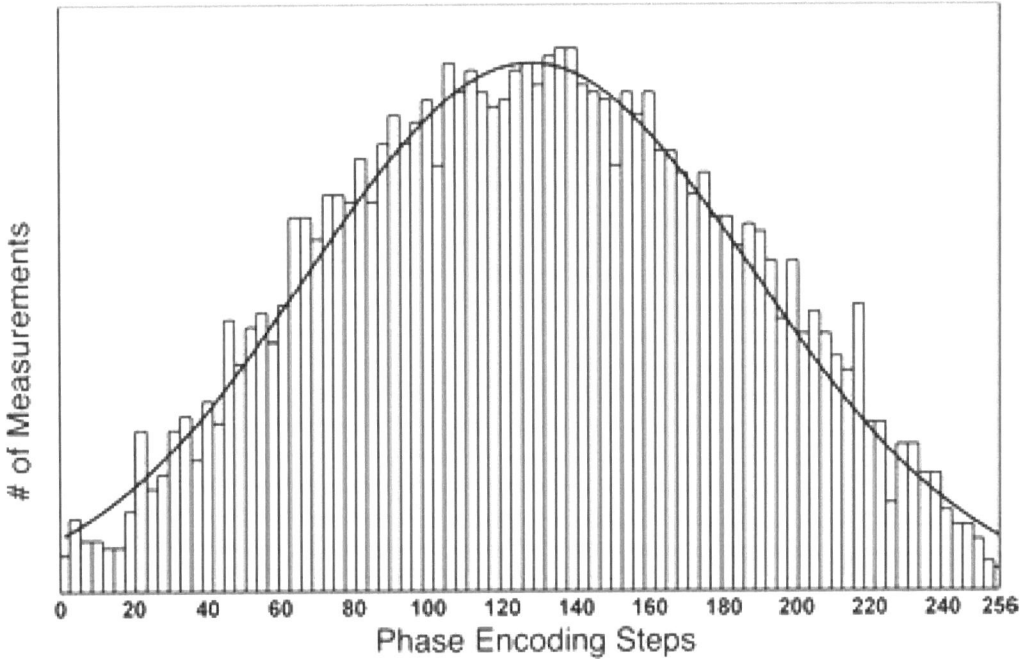

Figure 9: Histogram of all phase-encoding steps over the full cycle of all acquired N timeframes per slice. Each individual sampling scheme represents a random choice of phase encodings steps weighted according to a Gaussian distribution. (Taken from [90] - reproduced with permission from John Wiley and Sons).

Sparsity was generated in the temporal domain using the difference operator shown in Fig. (**7**). A modified version of an algorithm proposed by Ma *et al.* was applied to each sparse representation of each frame [92], followed by adding the temporal average.

In Fig. (**10**), fully, 2- and 3-fold under-sampled mid-ventricular short-axis views, acquired in a normal mouse in end-diastole (top row, panels a-c) and in end-systole (middle row, panels a'-c'), are shown. The bottom row (panels d-f) shows corresponding end-diastolic 4-chamber-long-axis views. While the epicardial border appeared less well-defined in the 3-fold accelerated datasets (Fig. **10c, c'**), and an increased artifact level was visible in the liver and skeletal muscle of the long-axis view (arrows in Fig. **10f**), neither had a detrimental effect on the quantification of the left ventricular volumes and mass. In fact, statistical analysis of retrospectively under-sampled cine-data obtained in sham-operated and in chronically infarcted mice showed no significant difference in any of the functional indices for up to three-fold acceleration (Table **2**), while for four-fold acceleration, only the stroke volume (which is the amount of blood ejected from the left ventricle in one cardiac cycle) was significantly reduced in the sham group compared to the fully sampled data. The three-fold accelerated data also allowed for an accurate assessment of infarct size [93]. In general, infarct size can be obtained from non-contrast enhanced cine-MRI data by relating the akinetic section to the entire left-ventricular circumference [5, 94]. The ability to accurately determine volumes, mass and infarct size from CS-accelerated cine-images makes this reconstruction method a powerful technique.

Table 2: **Left-ventricular functional indices obtained in normal mouse hearts (mean ± SD, n = 5).**

	LV-Mass/[mg]	EDV/[µl]	ESV/[µl]	SV/[µl]	EF/[%]
Conventional	74.7 ± 2.6	60.4 ± 9.0	23.3 ± 5.5	37.1 ± 4.1	61.8 ± 4.4
3× CS	76.1 ± 6.9	59.0 ± 7.9	23.7 ± 6.4	35.4 ± 2.0	60.5 ± 5.9

Motaal *et al.* combined self-gated fast low-angle shot (FLASH) acquisition and compressed sensing reconstruction to obtain very high-frame-rate cine-movies within reasonable scan times [95]. These data can be used to assess diastolic function in rodent models of cardiovascular disease [96, 97]. For this, the stochastic nature of the retrospective triggering acquisition scheme was utilized to produce a randomly under-sampled *k-t* space filling and to facilitate compressed sensing reconstruction and, thus, acceleration. Given the statistical nature of *k*-space filling and binning of cardiac time, a fully sampled, reference acquisition requires long scan times (*i.e.*, ~ 10 min for one slice) to ensure that all *k* lines are measured at least once and averaging is homogeneous in k space. In this study, under-sampled cine movies (*i.e.*, 90 frames) were generated from the first 2.5 and 1.5 minutes of the full data acquisitions (corresponding to an approximate under-sampling factor of two and three, respectively) and subjected to a compressed sensing reconstruction. The authors demonstrated by quantitatively analyzing left ventricular functional parameters (in this case end-systolic and end-diastolic lumen surface areas), and early-to-late filling-rate ratio as a parameter to evaluate diastolic function, an excellent agreement between standard and accelerated data sets. Thus, the reduction in scan time achieved by CS will facilitate the application of this method to cover the entire ventricle, which might otherwise be impossible/impractical in diseased animal due to the prolonged experimental times.

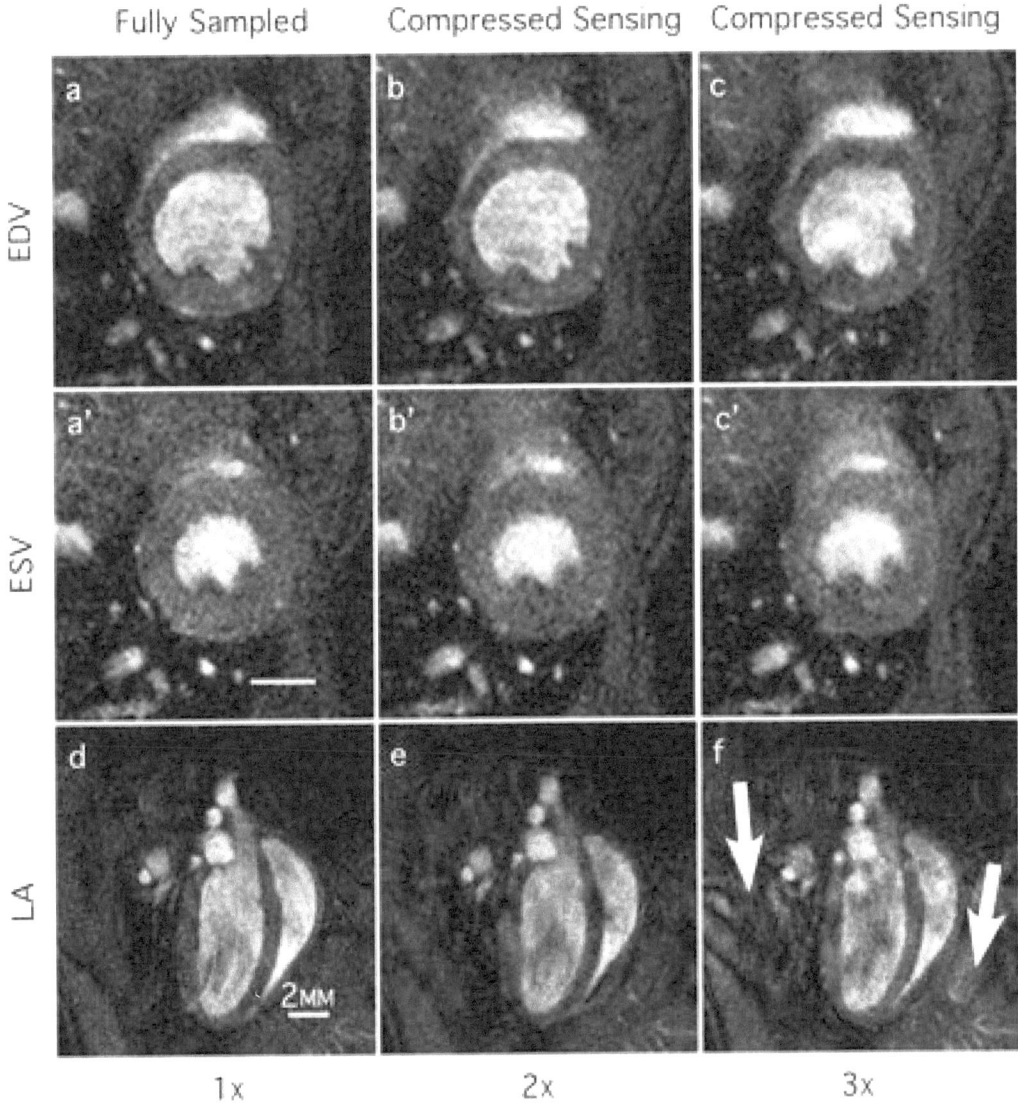

Figure 10: Mid-ventricular short- axis views in (**a-c**) end-diastole (ED) and in (**a'-c'**) end-systole (ES); (**d-f**) corresponding end-diastolic 4-chamber-longaxis (LA) views. The data were acquired with under-sampling factors 1-3. The arrows in panel f indicate an increased artifact in the liver and skeletal muscle. (Adapted from [90] - reproduced with permission from John Wiley and Sons).

Another example for the application of CS is on the acceleration of T_1-relaxation time measurements. In this context, dynamic contrast-enhanced MRI (DCE-MRI) using Manganese (Mn^{2+}) Enhanced MRI (also referred to as *MEMRI*) can be used to assess myocardial viability and perfusion by probing potentially altered Ca^{2+} homeostasis. Mn^{2+} is a T_1-shortening contrast agent, and a linear relationship between relaxation rate ($R_1=1/T_1$) and the (Mn^{2+}) concentration in myocardial tissue has been demonstrated over a relatively wide range [98]. As mentioned above, T_1 mapping methods are generally time consuming, and therefore benefit particularly from fast/accelerated imaging. Li *et al.* exploited the sparsity of the signals in the T_1 recovery direction, based on physics consideration of magnetization recovery, to remove the aliasing artifact associated with under-sampling [99]. A saturation recovery Look-Locker sequence was used to map T_1 in the myocardium [100]. In order to evaluate the reconstruction accuracy for various experimental conditions, simulations were performed prior to the validation in phantom studies. The optimized, two-fold accelerated method was then applied *in vivo* to longitudinally monitor the change in myocardial T_1 following the administration of $MnCl_2$-with a temporal resolution of < 80 s.

FUTURE DEVELOPMENTS

Parallel Imaging and Compressed Sensing are fundamentally different methods to speed-up the acquisition process as outlined above. Therefore, both techniques can also be combined to further accelerate MR imaging. While initial reports on parallel imaging and Compressed Sensing for CMR techniques in humans have recently been published (for example [101, 102]), we were first to use this approach to accelerate cine-MRI in murine models of cardiovascular disease [103]. In this pilot work, data were retrospectively under-sampled and subjected to a hybrid image reconstruction consisting of two consecutive steps: first, a CS-algorithm exploiting spatio-temporal sparsity as proposed by Lustig *et al.* [104] was utilized to generate an up to 4-fold under-sampled *k*-space. This was then followed by TGRAPPA-reconstruction [51] to obtain fully sampled cine-data. As shown before, each technique alone yielded a three-fold gain in speed, while CS followed by parallel imaging yielded an up to 9-fold theoretical acceleration of the experiment. Fig. (**11**) shows an end-diastolic frame of a mid-ventricular slice across a normal mouse heart comparing the fully sampled image to the corresponding frames with under-sampling factors 4, 8, 9 and 16, respectively. Preliminary quantitative analysis of LV functional parameters demonstrated a generally good agreement between values obtained from unaccelerated and with those from accelerated data [103].

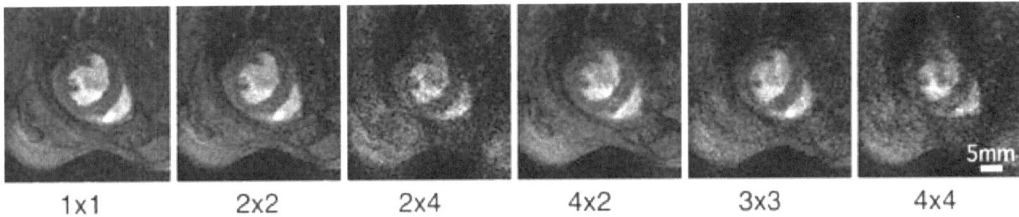

| 1x1 | 2x2 | 2x4 | 4x2 | 3x3 | 4x4 |

Figure 11: (Left to right) - fully sampled, and reconstructions of retrospectively undersampled end-diastolic frames through a mid-ventricular slice across a mouse heart in end-diastole. The scale bar indicates 5mm, and the acceleration factors are given as $R_{CS} \times R_{PI}$.

CONCLUSIONS

This chapter introduced and discussed various ways to speed up the MR imaging process. The heart is particularly suitable for the application of various acceleration techniques such as *k-t* BLAST or Compressed Sensing due its periodic motion patterns. The development of fast imaging techniques is predominantly driven by the clinical need to reduce costs of health care and to improve patient care. However, there is also an imperative need to develop techniques for speeding up the data acquisition process in preclinical MR for several reasons: (1) it is important to realize that MRI is an inherently expensive imaging modality, impacting on the clinical and the preclinical domain in a similar magnitude. While clinical routine scanning provides revenue to cover these costs, preclinical research has to rely on alternative funding streams, potentially adding significant costs, for example to a research proposal; (2) faster techniques will reduce the scan time per specimen, resulting in increased throughput, which in turn makes this technique more cost-efficient. Furthermore, there are major research programmes underway (such as for example the IMPC[3]) aiming to determine the function of every gene in the mouse genome, and relies on high-throughput phenotyping techniques to achieve this goal. In this context, CMR has to compete with other imaging modalities (such as micro computed

---

[3]http://www.mousephenotype.org

tomography - μCT) with respect to scientific value and cost efficiency; (3) reducing the scan time will decrease the anesthetic burden, which will particularly benefit very sick animals. Short scanning protocols may be therefore, vital for the survival of for example hemodynamically compromised rodent models of cardiovascular disease, as mentioned above; (4) faster methods will allow the employment of several different MR imaging/spectroscopy sequences during the same examination, as routinely used in the clinical CMR practice. Such an approach will facilitate multi-parametric information collection for each specimen and thus, provide not only a more powerful statistical analysis in an inhomogeneous population (each animal can serve as its own control) but potentially reduce the animal numbers used for research. While this has to be an ethical imperative for every scientist, it simultaneously reduces the costs of any preclinical research study.

CONFLICT OF INTEREST

This is to certify that the author does not have any conflict of interest.

ACKNOWLEDGEMENTS

Jürgen E. Schneider is a British Heart Foundation Senior Basic Science Research Fellow. He also acknowledges funding from the British Heart Foundation grant RG/10/002/28187 and the Wellcome Trust Core Award, Grant 090532/Z/09/Z. Furthermore, he would like to thank Dr. L. Diffley for proof-reading the manuscript, and Drs. B.J. van Nierop and G.J. Strijkers from the Department of Biomedical Engineering, University of Technology, Eindhoven, The Netherlands for kindly providing the images shown in Fig. (**6**).

REFERENCES

[1]   Poon M, Fuster V, Fayad Z. Cardiac magnetic resonance imaging: a "one-stop-shop" evaluation of myocardial dysfunction. Current opinion in cardiology. 2002 Nov;17(6):663-70.

[2]   Korosoglou G, Dengler TJ, Osman NF, Giannitsis E, Katus HA. Single coronary artery arising from the right sinus of valsalva: 'one-stop-shop' of coronary anatomy and functional significance by cardiovascular magnetic resonance. Clinical research in cardiology : official journal of the German Cardiac Society. 2009 Feb;98(2):133-6.

[3]   Ma H, Liu J, Wang B, Lin K, Wang Y, Yang J. "One-stop-shop" cardiac MRI at 3.0T for the detection of coronary artery disease. International journal of cardiology. 2012 Oct 4;160(2):e21-2.

[4]   Schneider JE, Lanz T, Barnes H, Stork LA, Bohl S, Lygate CA, *et al.* Accelerated cardiac magnetic resonance imaging in the mouse using an eight-channel array at 9.4 Tesla. Magn Reson Med. 2011 Jan;65(1):60-70.

[5]   Schneider JE, Wiesmann F, Lygate CA, Neubauer S. How to Perform an Accurate Assessment of Cardiac Function in Mice using High-Resolution Magnetic Resonance Imaging. J Cardiovasc Magn Reson. 2006;8(5):693-701.

[6]   Geelen T, Paulis LE, Coolen BF, Nicolay K, Strijkers GJ. Contrast-enhanced MRI of murine myocardial infarction - Part I. NMR in Biomedicine. 2012 Feb 6.

[7]   Coolen BF, Paulis LE, Geelen T, Nicolay K, Strijkers GJ. Contrast-enhanced MRI of murine myocardial infarction - Part II. NMR in Biomedicine. 2012 Feb 6.

[8]   Resonancia Magnetica. 2012. Available from: http://resonancia-magnetica.org/MagRes Chapters/21_02.htm.

[9]   Ruff J, Wiesmann F, Hiller KH, Voll S, von Kienlin M, Bauer WR, *et al.* Magnetic resonance microimaging for noninvasive quantification of myocardial function and mass in the mouse. Magn Reson Med. 1998;40:43-8.

[10]   Wiesmann F, Ruff J, Hiller KH, Rommel E, Haase A, Neubauer S. Developmental changes of cardiac function and mass assessed with MRI in neonatal, juvenile, and adult mice. Am J Physiol Heart Circ Physiol. 2000;278:H652-H7.

[11]   Schneider JE, Cassidy PJ, Lygate C, Tyler DJ, Wiesmann F, Grieve SM, *et al.* Fast, high-resolution *in vivo* cine magnetic resonance imaging in normal and failing mouse hearts on a vertical 11.7 T system. J Magn Reson Imaging. 2003 Dec;18(6):691-701.

[12]   Sosnovik DE, Dai G, Nahrendorf M, Rosen BR, Seethamraju R. Cardiac MRI in mice at 9.4 Tesla with a transmit-receive surface coil and a cardiac-tailored intensity-correction algorithm. J Magn Reson Imaging. 2007;26(2):279-87.

[13]   Fan X, Markiewicz EJ, Zamora M, Karczmar GS, Roman BB. Comparison and evaluation of mouse cardiac MRI acquired with open birdcage, single loop surface and volume birdcage coils. Phys Med Biol. 2006 Dec 21;51(24):N451-9.

[14]   Bucholz E, Ghaghada K, Qi Y, Mukundan S, Johnson GA. Four-dimensional MR microscopy of the mouse heart using radial acquisition and liposomal gadolinium contrast agent. Magn Reson Med. 2008 Jul;60(1):111-8.

[15]   Streif JU, Nahrendorf M, Hiller KH, Waller C, Wiesmann F, Rommel E, *et al. In vivo* assessment of absolute perfusion and intracapillary blood volume in the murine myocardium by spin labeling magnetic resonance imaging. Magn Reson Med. 2005 Mar;53(3):584-92.

[16]   Hiba B, Richard N, Thibault H, Janier M. Cardiac and respiratory self-gated cine MRI in the mouse: comparison between radial and rectilinear techniques at 7T. Magn Reson Med. 2007 Oct;58(4):745-53.

[17]   Roemer PB, Edelstein WA, Hayes CE, Souza SP, Mueller OM. The NMR phased array. Magn Reson Med. 1990 Nov;16(2):192-225.

[18]   Constantinides CD, Westgate CR, O'Dell WG, Zerhouni EA, McVeigh ER. A phased array coil for human cardiac imaging. Magn Reson Med. 1995 Jul;34(1):92-8.

[19]   Bottomley PA, Lugo Olivieri CH, Giaquinto R. What is the optimum phased array coil design for cardiac and torso magnetic resonance? Magn Reson Med. 1997 Apr;37(4):591-9.

[20]   Weiger M, Pruessmann KP, Leussler C, Roschmann P, Boesiger P. Specific coil design for SENSE: a six-element cardiac array. Magn Reson Med. 2001 Mar;45(3):495-504.

[21]   Wichmann T, Gareis D, Griswold M, Neuberger T, Wright S, Faber C, et al. A four channel transmit receive microstrip array for 17.6T. Proc Intl Soc Mag Reson Med. 2004:1578.

[22]   Armenean M, Hiba, B., Saint-Jalmes, H., Janier, M. and Beuf, O. Capacitive Decoupled two Element Phased Array Coil for Mouse Cardiac MRI at 7 T. Proc Intl Soc Mag Reson Med. 2005;13:927.

[23]   Ramirez MS, Bankson JA. Multiple-Mouse MRI with Multiple Arrays of Receive Coils (MARCs). Proc Intl Soc Mag Reson Med. 2008:1106.

[24]   Hardy CJ, Cline HE, Giaquinto RO, Niendorf T, Grant AK, Sodickson DK. 32-element receiver-coil array for cardiac imaging. Magn Reson Med. 2006 May;55(5):1142-9.

[25]   Zhu Y, Hardy CJ, Sodickson DK, Giaquinto RO, Dumoulin CL, Kenwood G, et al. Highly parallel volumetric imaging with a 32-element RF coil array. Magn Reson Med. 2004 Oct;52(4):869-77.

[26]   Schmitt M, Potthast A, Sosnovik DE, Polimeni JR, Wiggins GC, Triantafyllou C, et al. A 128-channel receive-only cardiac coil for highly accelerated cardiac MRI at 3 Tesla. Magn Reson Med. 2008 Jun;59(6):1431-9.

[27]   Hardy CJ, Giaquinto RO, Piel JE, Rohling KW, Marinelli L, Blezek DJ, et al. 128-channel body MRI with a flexible high-density receiver-coil array. J Magn Reson Imaging. 2008 Nov;28(5):1219-25.

[28]   Bock NA, Konyer NB, Henkelman RM. Multiple-mouse MRI. Magn Reson Med. 2003 Jan;49(1):158-67.

[29]   Dazai J, Bock NA, Nieman BJ, Davidson LM, Henkelman RM, Chen XJ. Multiple mouse biological loading and monitoring system for MRI. Magn Reson Med. 2004 Oct;52(4):709.

[30]   Bishop J, Feintuch A, Bock NA, Nieman B, Dazai J, Davidson L, et al. Retrospective gating for mouse cardiac MRI. Magn Reson Med. 2006 Mar;55(3):472-7.

[31]   Lanz T, Muller M, Barnes H, Neubauer S, Schneider JE. A high-throughput eight-channel probe head for murine MRI at 9.4 T. Magn Reson Med. 2010 Jul;64(1):80-7.

[32]   Constantinides C, Angeli S, Gkagkarellis S, Cofer G. Intercomparison of Performance of Rf Coil Geometries for High Field Mouse Cardiac Mri. Concepts in magnetic resonance Part A, Bridging education and research. 2011 Sep;38A(5):236-52.

[33]   Parallel Imaging in Clinical MR Applications. Baert AL, Knauth M, Sartor K, editors: Springer; 2007.

[34]   Handbook of MRI Pulse Sequences: Elsevier; 2004.

[35]   Larkman DJ, Nunes RG. Parallel magnetic resonance imaging. Phys Med Biol. 2007 Apr 7;52(7):R15-55.

[36]   Niendorf T, Sodickson D. [Acceleration of cardiovascular MRI using parallel imaging: basic principles, practical considerations, clinical applications and future directions]. Rofo. 2006 Jan;178(1):15-30.

[37]   Niendorf T, Sodickson DK. Parallel imaging in cardiovascular MRI: methods and applications. NMR Biomed. 2006 May;19(3):325-41.

[38]   Deshmane A, Gulani V, Griswold MA, Seiberlich N. Parallel MR imaging. J Magn Reson Imaging. 2012 Jul;36(1):55-72.

[39]   Pruessmann KP, Weiger M, Scheidegger MB, Boesiger P. SENSE: sensitivity encoding for fast MRI. Magn Reson Med. 1999 Nov;42(5):952-62.

[40] Griswold MA, Jakob PM, Heidemann RM, Nittka M, Jellus V, Wang J, *et al.* Generalized autocalibrating partially parallel acquisitions (GRAPPA). Magn Reson Med. 2002 Jun;47(6):1202-10.

[41] Blaimer M, Breuer F, Mueller M, Heidemann RM, Griswold MA, Jakob PM. SMASH, SENSE, PILS, GRAPPA: how to choose the optimal method. Top Magn Reson Imaging. 2004 Aug;15(4):223-36.

[42] Griswold MA, Kannengiesser S, Heidemann RM, Wang J, Jakob PM. Field-of-view limitations in parallel imaging. Magn Reson Med. 2004 Nov;52(5):1118-26.

[43] Goldfarb JW. The SENSE ghost: field-of-view restrictions for SENSE imaging. J Magn Reson Imaging. 2004 Dec;20(6):1046-51.

[44] Breuer FA, Kannengiesser SA, Blaimer M, Seiberlich N, Jakob PM, Griswold MA. General formulation for quantitative G-factor calculation in GRAPPA reconstructions. Magn Reson Med. 2009 Sep;62(3):739-46.

[45] Sodickson DK, Manning WJ. Simultaneous acquisition of spatial harmonics (SMASH): fast imaging with radiofrequency coil arrays. Magn Reson Med. 1997 Oct;38(4):591-603.

[46] Griswold MA, Jakob PM, Nittka M, Goldfarb JW, Haase A. Partially parallel imaging with localized sensitivities (PILS). Magn Reson Med. 2000;44:602-9.

[47] Seiberlich N, Ehses P, Duerk J, Gilkeson R, Griswold M. Improved radial GRAPPA calibration for real-time free-breathing cardiac imaging. Magnetic resonance in medicine : official journal of the Society of Magnetic Resonance in Medicine / Society of Magnetic Resonance in Medicine. 2011 Feb;65(2):492-505.

[48] Joseph AA, Merboldt KD, Voit D, Zhang S, Uecker M, Lotz J, *et al.* Real-time phase-contrast MRI of cardiovascular blood flow using undersampled radial fast low-angle shot and nonlinear inverse reconstruction. NMR Biomed. 2012 Jul;25(7):917-24.

[49] Zhang S, Uecker M, Voit D, Merboldt KD, Frahm J. Real-time cardiovascular magnetic resonance at high temporal resolution: radial FLASH with nonlinear inverse reconstruction. J Cardiovasc Magn Reson. 2010;12:39.

[50] Schneider JE, Lanz T, Barnes H, Medway D, Stork LA, Lygate CA, *et al.* Ultra-fast and accurate assessment of cardiac function in rats using accelerated MRI at 9.4 Tesla. Magn Reson Med. 2008 Mar;59(3):636-41.

[51] Breuer FA, Kellman P, Griswold MA, Jakob PM. Dynamic autocalibrated parallel imaging using temporal GRAPPA (TGRAPPA). Magn Reson Med. 2005 Apr;53(4):981-5.

[52] Ramirez MS, Esparza-Coss E, Bankson JA. Multiple-mouse MRI with multiple arrays of receive coils. Magn Reson Med. 2010 Mar;63(3):803-10.

[53] Piechnik SK, Ferreira VM, Dall'Armellina E, Cochlin LE, Greiser A, Neubauer S, *et al.* Shortened Modified Look-Locker Inversion recovery (ShMOLLI) for clinical myocardial T1-mapping at 1.5 and 3 T within a 9 heartbeat breathhold. Journal of cardiovascular magnetic resonance: official journal of the Society for Cardiovascular Magnetic Resonance. 2010;12:69.

[54] Dall'Armellina E, Piechnik SK, Ferreira VM, Si QL, Robson MD, Francis JM, *et al.* Cardiovascular magnetic resonance by non contrast T1-mapping allows assessment of severity of injury in acute myocardial infarction. J Cardiovasc Magn Reson. 2012;14:15.

[55] Ferreira VM, Piechnik SK, Dall'Armellina E, Karamitsos TD, Francis JM, Choudhury RP, *et al.* Non-contrast T1-mapping detects acute myocardial edema with high diagnostic accuracy: a comparison to T2-weighted cardiovascular magnetic resonance. J Cardiovasc Magn Reson. 2012;14:42.

[56] Look DC, Locker DR. Time saving in measurement of NMR and EPR relaxation times. Rev Sci Instr. 1969;41(2):250-51.

[57] Deichmann R, Haase A. Quantification of T1 values by SNAPSHOT-FLASH NMR imaging. J Magn Reson. 1992;96:608-12.

[58] Kober F, Iltis I, Izquierdo M, Desrois M, Ibarrola D, Cozzone PJ, *et al.* High-resolution myocardial perfusion mapping in small animals *in vivo* by spin-labeling gradient-echo imaging. Magn Reson Med. 2004 Jan;51(1):62-7.

[59] Kober F, Iltis I, Cozzone PJ, Bernard M. Myocardial blood flow mapping in mice using high-resolution spin labeling magnetic resonance imaging: influence of ketamine/xylazine and isoflurane anesthesia. Magn Reson Med. 2005 Mar;53(3):601-6.

[60] Bohl S, Lygate CA, Barnes H, Medway D, Stork LA, Schulz-Menger J, *et al.* Advanced methods for quantification of infarct size in mice using three-dimensional high-field late gadolinium enhancement MRI. Am J Physiol Heart Circ Physiol. 2009 Apr;296(4):H1200-8.

[61] Ratering D, Baltes C, Dorries C, Rudin M. Accelerated cardiovascular magnetic resonance of the mouse heart using self-gated parallel imaging strategies does not compromise accuracy of structural and functional measures. J Cardiovasc Magn Reson. 2010;12:43-55.

[62] Ratering D, Baltes C, Lohmann C, Matter CM, Rudin M. Accurate assessment of carotid artery stenosis in atherosclerotic mice using accelerated high-resolution 3D magnetic resonance angiography. MAGMA. 2011 Feb;24(1):9-18.

[63] Wiesmann F, Ruff J, Engelhardt S, Hein L, Dienesch C, Leupold A, *et al.* Dobutamine-stress magnetic resonance microimaging in mice: acute changes of cardiac geometry and function in normal and failing murine hearts. Circ Res. 2001;88:563-59.

[64] Lygate CA, Hunyor I, Medway D, de Bono JP, Dawson D, Wallis J, *et al.* Cardiac phenotype of mitochondrial creatine kinase knockout mice is modified on a pure C57BL/6 genetic background. Journal of Molecular and Cellular Cardiology. 2009;46(1):93-9.

[65] Coolen BF, Moonen RP, Paulis LE, Geelen T, Nicolay K, Strijkers GJ. Mouse myocardial first-pass perfusion MR imaging. Magn Reson Med. 2010 Dec;64(6):1658-63.

[66] van Nierop BJ, Coolen BF, Dijk WJ, Hendriks AD, de Graaf L, Nicolay K, *et al.* Quantitative first-pass perfusion MRI of the mouse myocardium. Magn Reson Med. 2012 Aug 20.

[67] Liang ZP, Boada FE, Constable RT, Haacke EM, Lauterbur PC, Smith MR. Constrained reconstruction methods in MR imaging,. Rev Magn Reson Med. 1992;4:67-185.

[68] McGibney G, Smith MR, Nichols ST, Crawley A. Quantitative evaluation of several partial Fourier reconstruction algorithms used in MRI. Magn Reson Med. 1993 Jul;30(1):51-9.

[69] Hu X, Parrish T. Reduction of field of view for dynamic imaging. Magn Reson Med. 1994 Jun;31(6):691-4.

[70] Madore B, Glover GH, Pelc NJ. Unaliasing by fourier-encoding the overlaps using the temporal dimension (UNFOLD), applied to cardiac imaging and fMRI. Magn Reson Med. 1999 Nov;42(5):813-28.

[71] Tsao J. On the UNFOLD method. Magn Reson Med. 2002 Jan;47(1):202-7.

[72] Jones RA, Haraldseth O, Muller TB, Rinck PA, Oksendal AN. K-space substitution: a novel dynamic imaging technique. Magn Reson Med. 1993 Jun;29(6):830-4.

[73] van Vaals JJ, Brummer ME, Dixon WT, Tuithof HH, Engels H, Nelson RC, *et al.* "Keyhole" method for accelerating imaging of contrast agent uptake. J Magn Reson Imaging. 1993 Jul-Aug;3(4):671-5.

[74]   Riederer SJ, Tasciyan T, Farzaneh F, Lee JN, Wright RC, Herfkens RJ. MR fluoroscopy: technical feasibility. Magn Reson Med. 1988 Sep;8(1):1-15.

[75]   Parrish T, Hu X. Continuous update with random encoding (CURE): a new strategy for dynamic imaging. Magn Reson Med. 1995 Mar;33(3):326-36.

[76]   Zaitsev M, Zilles K, Shah NJ. Shared k-space echo planar imaging with keyhole. Magn Reson Med. 2001 Jan;45(1):109-17.

[77]   Tsao J, Boesiger P, Pruessmann KP. k-t BLAST and k-t SENSE: dynamic MRI with high frame rate exploiting spatiotemporal correlations. Magn Reson Med. 2003 Nov;50(5):1031-42.

[78]   Tsao J, Behnia B, Webb AG. Unifying linear prior-information-driven methods for accelerated image acquisition. Magn Reson Med. 2001 Oct;46(4):652-60.

[79]   Kozerke S, Tsao J, Razavi R, Boesiger P. Accelerating cardiac cine 3D imaging using k-t BLAST. Magn Reson Med. 2004 Jul;52(1):19-26.

[80]   Marshall I, Jansen MA, Tao Y, Merrifield GD, Gray GA. Accelerated mouse cardiac imaging using threefold undersampling and kt-BLAST reconstruction. Proc Intl Soc Mag Reson Med. 2012;20:3847.

[81]   Pedersen H, Kozerke S, Ringgaard S, Nehrke K, Kim WY. k-t PCA: temporally constrained k-t BLAST reconstruction using principal component analysis. Magn Reson Med. 2009 Sep;62(3):706-16.

[82]   Makowski M, Jansen C, Webb I, Chiribiri A, Nagel E, Botnar R, *et al*. First-pass contrast-enhanced myocardial perfusion MRI in mice on a 3-T clinical MR scanner. Magn Reson Med. 2010 Dec;64(6):1592-8.

[83]   Lustig M, Donoho D, Pauly JM. Sparse MRI: The application of compressed sensing for rapid MR imaging. Magn Reson Med. 2007 Dec;58(6):1182-95.

[84]   Gamper U, Boesiger P, Kozerke S. Compressed sensing in dynamic MRI. Magn Reson Med. 2008 Jan 2008;59(2):365-73.

[85]   Jung H, Sung K, Nayak KS, Kim EY, Ye JC. k-t FOCUSS: a general compressed sensing framework for high resolution dynamic MRI. Magn Reson Med. 2009 Jan;61(1):103-16.

[86]   Candes EJ, Wakin MB. An Introduction To Compressive Sampling. Signal Processing Magazine, IEEE. 2008;25(2):21-30.

[87]   Lustig M, Donoho DL, Santos JM, Pauly JM. Compressed Sensing MRI. Signal Processing Magazine, IEEE. 2008;25(2):72-82.

[88]   Jung H, Ye JC, Kim EY. Improved k-t BLAST and k-t SENSE using FOCUSS. Phys Med Biol. 2007 Jun 7;52(11):3201-26.

[89]   Jung H, Park J, Yoo J, Ye JC. Radial k-t FOCUSS for high-resolution cardiac cine MRI. Magn Reson Med. 2010 Jan;63(1):68-78.

[90]   Wech T, Lemke A, Medway D, Stork LA, Lygate CA, Neubauer S, *et al*. Accelerating cine-MR imaging in mouse hearts using compressed sensing. Journal of magnetic resonance imaging : JMRI. 2011 Nov;34(5):1072-9.

[91]   Tropp JA, Gilbert AC. Signal recovery from random measurements *via* orthogonal matching pursuit. Ieee T Inform Theory. 2007 Dec;53(12):4655-66.

[92]   Ma S, Yin W, Zhang Y, Chakraborty A. An efficient algorithm for compressed MR imaging using total variation and wavelets. Proc IEEE Conference on Computer Vision and Pattern Recognition CVPR 2008. 2008:1-8.

[93]   Wech T, Medway D, Lygate CA, Neubauer S, Köstler H, Schneider JE. Accurate infarct-size measurements from accelerated, compressed sensing reconstructed cine-MRI images in mouse hearts. J Cardiovasc Magn Reson. 2012;14(Suppl 1):P57.

[94]   Takagawa J, Zhang Y, Wong ML, Sievers RE, Kapasi NK, Wang Y, *et al.* Myocardial infarct size measurement in the mouse chronic infarction model: comparison of area- and length-based approaches. J Appl Physiol. 2007 Jun;102(6):2104-11.

[95]   Motaal AG, Coolen BF, Abdurrachim D, Castro RM, Prompers JJ, Florack LM, *et al.* Accelerated high-frame-rate mouse heart cine-MRI using compressed sensing reconstruction. NMR Biomed. 2012 Oct 29.

[96]   Stuckey DJ, Carr CA, Tyler DJ, Aasum E, Clarke K. Novel MRI method to detect altered left ventricular ejection and filling patterns in rodent models of disease. Magn Reson Med. 2008 Sep;60(3):582-7.

[97]   Coolen BF, Abdurrachim D, Motaal AG, Nicolay K, Prompers JJ, Strijkers GJ. High frame rate retrospectively triggered Cine MRI for assessment of murine diastolic function. Magn Reson Med. 2013 Mar 1;69(3):648-56.

[98]   Waghorn B, Edwards T, Yang Y, Chuang KH, Yanasak N, Hu TC. Monitoring dynamic alterations in calcium homeostasis by T (1)-weighted and T (1)-mapping cardiac manganese-enhanced MRI in a murine myocardial infarction model. NMR Biomed. 2008 Nov;21(10):1102-11.

[99]   Li W, Griswold M, Yu X. Fast cardiac T1 mapping in mice using a model-based compressed sensing method. Magn Reson Med. 2012 Oct;68(4):1127-34.

[100]   Li W, Griswold M, Yu X. Rapid T(1) mapping of mouse myocardium with saturation recovery look-locker method. Magn Reson Med. 2010 Jul 14;64:1296-303.

[101]   Feng L, Srichai MB, Lim RP, Harrison A, King W, Adluru G, *et al.* Highly accelerated real-time cardiac cine MRI using k-t SPARSE-SENSE. Magn Reson Med. 2012 Aug 6.

[102]   Kim D, Dyvorne HA, Otazo R, Feng L, Sodickson DK, Lee VS. Accelerated phase-contrast cine MRI using k-t SPARSE-SENSE. Magn Reson Med. 2012 Apr;67(4):1054-64.

[103]   Wech T, Thornton V, Lygate CA, Neubauer S, Köstler H, Schneider JE. Highly Accelerated Cine-MRI in Mouse Hearts Using Compressed Sensing and Parallel Imaging at 9.4T. Proc Intl Soc Mag Reson Med. 2012;20:1130.

[104]   Lustig M, Santos JM, Donoho DL, Pauly JM. k-t SPARSE: High frame rate dynamic MRI exploiting spatio-temporal sparsity. Proc Intl Soc Mag Reson Med. 2006;14:2420.

Send Orders for Reprints to reprints@benthamscience.net

Latest Advances in Clinical and Pre-Clinical Cardiovascular MRI, 2014, Vol. 1, 163-198   **163**

CHAPTER 7

Regional Cardiac Function: Across Mammalian Species Comparison - the Paradigm of Murine MR Image-Based Phenotyping

Stelios Angeli [1] and Christakis Constantinides [2,*]

[1]*Prognosis Advanced Diagnostics Center and* [2]*Chi-Biomedical Ltd., Nicosia, Cyprus*

Abstract: This chapter summarizes regional cardiac functional studies using MRI that span the past 25 years. In addition to the comparison of the three major MRI techniques that achieve detailed studies of myocardial mechanics, an extensive reference to DENSE-MRI and its imaging and image-processing features is presented. The mouse paradigm, as a direct manifestation of international efforts for image-based phenotyping in health, disease and post-transgenetic modification, is also introduced. The appropriateness of extrapolations of inferences drawn from mouse studies to man are well-justified from presented evidence on isometric and allometric scaling of global and regional cardiac functional indices, however, noted mismatches of the fiber structure, force-frequency and energetic/metabolic reserves exist between the two species. While such arguments limit the range of possible pathological models that can associate human and murine disease, the mouse still remains a potentially attractive animal model for cardiovascular research today.

Keywords: Mouse paradigm, rat, heart, myocardium, cardiovascular disease, MRI, tagging, DENSE, HARP, Functional quantification, regional cardiac function, image-based phenotyping.

INTRODUCTION

The prominent role of cardiac MRI (CMR) in clinical practice and management arose/evolved from its unique ability to assess global and local morphology and function in a non-invasive manner [1-3], thereby becoming an invaluable tool to ascertain the etiology and disease prognosis, aiding the pharmacological and therapeutic regimes of treatment and progress monitoring.

---

*Address correspondence to Christakis Constantinides: Chi-Biomedical Ltd., Nicosia, Cyprus; Tel: (357) 22 345 839; E-mail: Christakis.Constantinides@gmail.com

With excellent tissue contrast, spatial resolution, signal-to-noise ratio characteristics, free of geometric constraints or assumptions, and with the synergistic help of developed image processing tools and techniques (registration, segmentation, filtering), CMR routinely allows quantification of global cardiac functional estimates, including (but not limited to) mass [5, 6], end-diastolic (EDV), end-systolic volumes (ESV), stroke volume (SV), ejection fraction (EF), cardiac output (CO), wall motion (WM), and wall thickening (WT) [6-12].

Despite the usefulness of global cardiac indices and their comparisons thereof, the value and importance of regional cardiac functional analyses in disease has been established as paramount over recent years. Not only are global measures of function insensitive to regional patterns of functional-structural changes in focal disease, they also often mask underlying regional dysfunction [13, 14], as it has been repetitively proven in disease states [15]. In most such cases, results either exemplify normal EF estimates [16] - despite significant ultra-structural changes and regional tissue dysfunction - or exhibit a highly heterogenous regional pattern of myocardial motion, and developed stress and strain.

This chapter provides a comprehensive overview and a detailed reference to the major MRI techniques that emerged over the past 25 years to assess regional cardiac function, with a detailed emphasis on displacement encoding with stimulated echoes (DENSE) [17]. The emergence of the mouse as one of the most attractive animal models of research and its potential role for the study of cardiac pathology in humans are then considered. Analogies with humans are drawn given recent evidence for isometric and allometric functional scaling in global and regional functional indices, including radial, longitudinal and circumferential strain, twist and torsion. Reference is also made to MR image-based phenotyping attempts and association of accumulated knowledge to human cardiac pathology.

QUANTIFICATION OF REGIONAL CARDIAC FUNCTION USING MRI

Regional functional CMR techniques emerged soon after the inception of the MRI phenomenon and its migration to clinical practice in the early-late 1980's. Currently, there is a number of major MRI techniques that allow quantitative evaluation of regional cardiac function, both in humans and animals: myocardial spin-tagging [18, 19], harmonic phase (HARP) imaging [20], displacement encoding with stimulated echoes (DENSE) [17], phase contrast (PC) velocity imaging [21, 22] and strain encoding (SENC) [23].

All such methods can be classified into magnitude-based (tagging), and phase-based (HARP, DENSE, PC, and SENC). Of these, tagging, HARP and DENSE have been widely used (both in humans and mice) for regional strain quantification. While PC imaging is associated with increased spatial resolution and is able to provide voxel-velocity estimates, it is nevertheless, subject to accumulating integration errors when the motion-displacement field is estimated [24]. SENC, a HARP-based variant, has only recently emerged, and its value and applicability to the assessment of cardiac functional performance remains to be determined.

The three established and widely used techniques and their most prominent features (imaging and post-processing) are summarized in Fig. (**1**). For example, tagging [18, 19] employs a generic spatial-modulation of magnetization (SPAMM) pulse sequence [19] that uses spatial pre-saturation pulses to modulate the intensity of the magnetization vector in the magnitude images at right-angled planes to the selected slice, resulting in patterns of low signal intensity (lines, grids, radial stripes *etc.*) within the image (tags). Tags then deform in accordance to the heart wall motion and fade based on the value of the myocardial T_1. To-date, two-dimensional (2D) tagging has been implemented along the short and long cardiac axes in standard or CINE modes [25]. It has undergone numerous improvements and modifications that include the delay alternating with mutations for tailored excitation (DANTE) implementation [26], CSPAMM [27], slice-following with CSPAMM [27], localized SPAMM [28], variable density SPAMM [30], single breath-hold with CSPAMM [31], and others.

HARP [20] is a tagging variant but operates in k-space, and is associated with increased processing efficiency for quantitative estimation of regional functional indices. It's based on the realization that tagging generates a spectral peak modulation pattern and that tagging information resides (and can be extracted through spectral filtering) in the signal peak of the first harmonic. The HARP image results from the multiplication of the reconstructed (using the Fourier

Transform) magnitude and phase images. Upon phase-unwrapping of the composite image, motion can then be estimated through phase tracking of voxels of interest. HARP has been extensively used over the years in both human [32-34] and animal applications [35, 36] and strain estimates have been successfully validated against tagging [32]. In a similar fashion to tagging, it has also undergone multiple improvements over the years, including the real-time HARP implementation [37], 3D-HARP [38], zHARP [39], and fastHARP [40].

Despite the common fundamental basis on which both HARP and DENSE are based upon (reconstruction of the displacement-deformation field based on phase images and their subsequent processing) [41], DENSE originated [42] and was developed independently from HARP at the National Institutes of Health (NIH). DENSE is based on the Stimulated Echo Acquisition Mode (STEAM) pulse sequence, originally developed and used for MR spectroscopic applications. Displacement encoding of moving spins is achieved using an encoding gradient before the first and an un-encoding gradient (after the third) successive radiofrequency (RF) excitation pulse. The time interval between the consecutive second and third RF excitations (commonly known as the mixing-time interval) provides DENSE with the inherent advantage of black-blood imaging. The reconstructed phase images (subsequently processed for phase-unwrapping) are utilized to map phase to displacement and allow strain estimation. In its most basic 2D form, DENSE encodes displacement independently along each of the two orthogonal directions, but invariably requires a phase reference map to null baseline phase offsets or correlated residual phase errors, or hardware imperfections. Overall, four image acquisitions are necessary for 2D displacement mapping. Despite its early implementation and applications in humans [42] and canine [17], DENSE has also evolved over the years to both clinical (DENSE, fast-DENSE, meta-DENSE, DENSE with CANSEL) [17, 42-45] and pre-clinical applications (2D-DENSE, balanced multipoint-DENSE, Cine-DENSE, navigator-gated spiral-DENSE, 3D-DENSE) [46-50].

All three techniques have been extensively reported in the scientific literature, a discussion that is outside the scope of this chapter. The reader is, however, referred to a recent, comprehensive and excellent review on the subject matter [3].

Characteristic	Tagging	HARP	DENSE
Technique	SPAMM	SPAMM	STEAM
Pulse Sequence	RO PE SS RF	RO PE SS RF	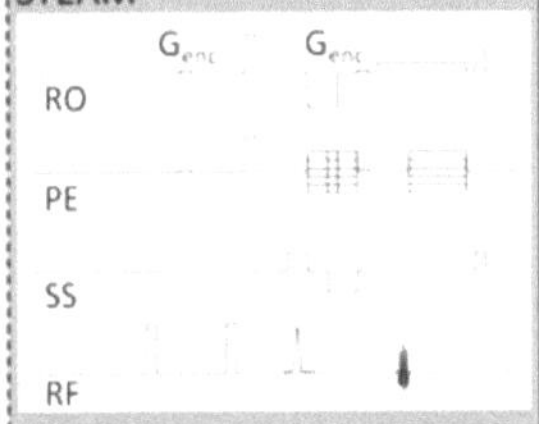 G_{enc} G_{enc} RO PE SS RF
Information Encoding	Magnitude Image	Magnitude & Phase Image	Phase Image
Dimensionality	2D (Short/Long Axis)	2D or 3D	2D or 3D
Contrast	Bright Blood	Bright Blood	Black Blood
Resolution	Limited tagging resolution	Limited tagging resolution on phase image	High spatial resolution
SNR	SNR T_1 dependence for tag intensity	Low SNR	SNR decreases over cardiac cycle
CINE Application	Yes	Yes	Yes
Postprocessing	Segment endo-,epicardial boarders, 3D active contour modeling	Isolation of 1st harmonic peak in k-space, tissue phase tracking	Segmentation, phase unwrap, tracking, strain calculation

Figure 1: Technical comparison of the major cardiac MRI functional quantification techniques developed over the last 25 years (myocardial spin-tagging, DENSE, and HARP). A common feature to all such techniques is their inherent ability to perform tissue tracking.

Inevitably, all three techniques are associated with shortcomings and limitations (as summarized in Fig. **1** above). Tagging is associated with low tag-resolution, T_1-dependence of tag-intensity over time (an issue prominent in humans, but not as critical in mice), inability to allow direct 3D-tagging, and complicated and time-consuming post-processing, with a concurrent demand for user-involvement. HARP on the other side, despite the improved efficiency in automated and faster data analysis, is also hampered by the inherently low spatial resolution of tags on the composite phase image. DENSE, despite its inherently low SNR performance (due to its association with stimulated echoes) and time-consuming acquisition scheme, is associated with increased (single-voxel) phase resolution, rapid image analysis, high displacement accuracy, the ability for Cine and 3D coverage, and exhibits an inherently increased myocardial-ventricular cavity contrast (black-blood imaging).

Given the attractive features and applicability and use of the DENSE technique over the past 15 years, both in the clinical and pre-clinical setting, the presented efforts on the study of myocardial mechanics that follow focus on such technique.

IMAGE-BASED PHENOTYPING - THE MOUSE PARADIGM

On the forefront of basic science, the mouse emerged as an attractive animal research model following the rapid advances in experimental molecular biology techniques that allowed targeted mutagenesis in single genes [51, 52]. Initial research efforts were supported by policies set forth at the US National level and implemented by initiatives, supported among others, by the human and mouse genome projects. Such projects, administered through NIH, aimed to the cloning and mapping of the entire human and mouse genomes [53, 54], and concluded successfully in 2003.

As the manipulation of the mammalian genome became routine, new avenues opened towards the generation of transgenic animal models for the study of cardiovascular function and dysfunction [55], marking the onset of the molecular physiology, proteomics, and (structural and functional) genomics era. Quantitative characterization of ventricular function had thus started to become critical for the phenotypic assessment of murine cardiac performance in health and in disease [56, 57].

Mouse cardiac MRI (Fig. **2**) emerged as a logical paradigm to human and mouse genome mapping initiatives, advances in human cardiac MRI, and image-based phenotyping attempts [58], focusing on highly efficient, high-throughput four-dimensional (4D) acquisition protocols *in vivo* [59].

Collectively, efforts over the past 15 years initially targeted the study of the global [4, 5, 10, 11, 60], and then the regional cardiac function [2, 36, 47-49, 61-64] in normal, wild-type control, and transgenic mice, as a basis for realizing the long-term goal of image-based phenotyping.

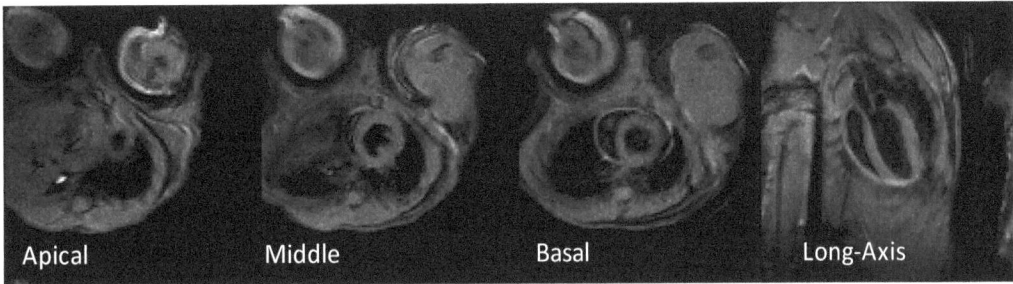

Figure 2: Typical short and long axis MR images of the murine heart at basal, middle, and apical myocardial locations of a C57BL/6 mouse, acquired using a conventional 2D FLASH pulse sequence under isoflurane anesthesia at 7T. All mouse studies were conducted in accordance to approved ACUC protocols.

The emergence and application of the various imaging attempts to characterize regional cardiac function in the mouse matched the evolution of the three major techniques (tagging, HARP and DENSE) in humans. The following sections summarize the technical development and flow of image processing steps associated with DENSE, before the applicability of all three techniques to mouse and human cardiac imaging are discussed and compared.

DENSE IMAGING

The pulse sequence is STEAM-based (Fig. **3**). A series of three consecutive α° RF pulses (typically with the first two being non-selective, and the third being a slice selective 90° pulse) precede the encoding and imaging scheme (which can be implemented as a spin-warp, echo-planar, fast-spin echo, spiral, or other). Encoding gradients (often referred to as G_{enc}) are placed after the first and third RF excitations to encode spin phase-displacement. Therefore, any moving spins will accumulate phase after the 'encoding gradient' is applied (immediately after the first RF excitation) which will not be reversed upon application of the 'unencoding' gradient, executed immediately after the third RF excitation. The accrued phase is directly proportional to the spin displacement during this interval. A simple phase-displacement mapping can reconstruct the displacement field.

Additionally, during the mixing time (the time interval between the second and third RF pulses) the magnetization is tipped to the negative z-direction and can thus be sensitized to T_1-weighting. Proper choice of the mixing time can achieve optimal contrast difference between the ventricular blood and the neighboring myocardium. Crushers and spoilers are also often employed (as seen in Fig. **3**) to null any residual magnetization during the mixing time, or post-completion of the unencoding module.

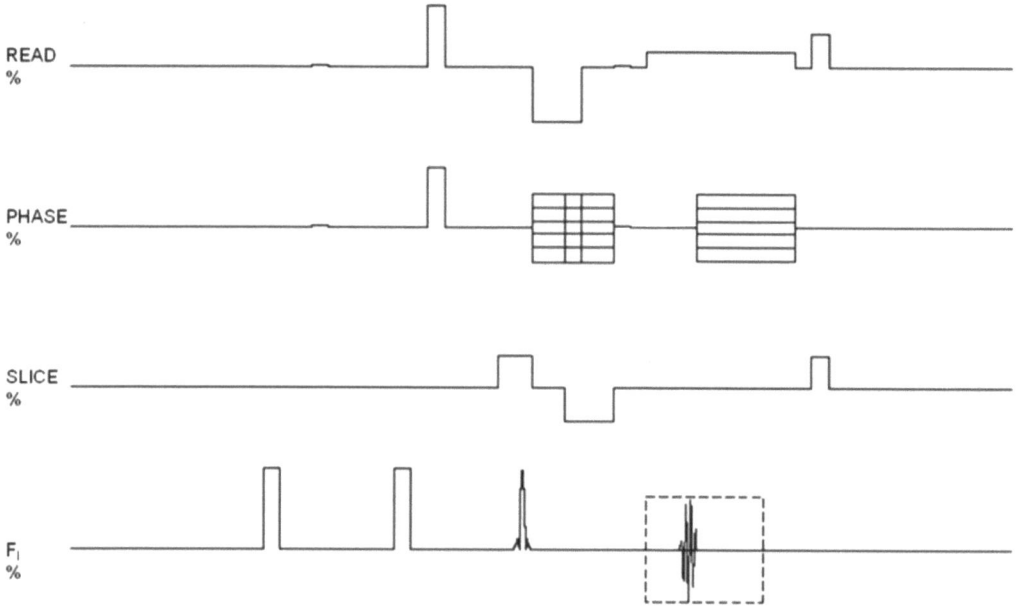

Figure 3: Schematic representation of the two-dimensional (2D) DENSE pulse sequence, based on a conventional stimulated echo (STEAM) pulse sequence. Evident are the motion encoding (and un-encoding) pulses immediately after the first non-selective 90° pulse and following the third slice selective 90° pulse, used to sensitize excited spins to motion (Figure compiled from the work of CC at the Mouse Image Facility at NIH during the period 2001-3-unpublished data).

STEAM-based sequences are associated with multiple echoes; a stimulated echo, a stimulated anti-echo, and a T_1 relaxation echo as previously reported [64]. Briefly, if the total magnetization M is expressed as a function of spin position r_i and time t, then immediately after the application of a displacement encoding gradient with value k_{enc}, the longitudinal magnetization vector M_z can be expressed as:

$$M_z(r_i,t) = M_0 \left[\cos(k_{enc}\, r_i) - 1 \right] e^{-\frac{t}{T_1}} + M_0 \qquad (1)$$

where M_0 denotes the equilibrium value of the total magnetization. Immediately after the application of the unencoding gradient (following the third α^o pulse), the total magnetization can be written as:

$$M_{xy}(r_i,t) = M_z(r_i,t)e^{-jk_{enc}(r_i+\Delta r_i)}\sin a \tag{2}$$

$$M_{xy}(r_i,t) = M_0\left[1-\left(1-\frac{e^{-jk_{enc}r_i}-e^{+jk_{enc}r_i}}{2}\right)e^{-\frac{t}{T_1}}\right]e^{-jk_{enc}(r_i+\Delta r_i)}\sin a \tag{3}$$

where Δr_i represents the spin-displacement during the mixing time. Expanding Equation (3) leads to:

$$M_{xy}(r_i,t) = \left(\frac{M_0}{2}e^{-jk_{enc}\Delta r_i}e^{-\frac{t}{T_1}}+\right.$$

$$+\frac{M_0}{2}e^{-jk_{enc}\Delta r_i}e^{-j2k_{enc}r_i}e^{-\frac{t}{T_1}} \tag{4}$$

$$\left.+M_0\left(1-e^{-\frac{t}{T_1}}\right)e^{-jk_{enc}\Delta r_i}e^{-jk_{enc}r_i}\right)\sin a$$

Each of the three terms of Equation 4, correspond sequentially to the stimulated echo, the anti-echo, and the T_1-relaxation echo. Practically, the presence and effects of such echoes can be visualized using phantom imaging as presented in the example of Fig. (**4**). Evident in the reconstructed DENSE magnitude image (due to the presence of all echoes) is a striation pattern in the magnitude image. The anti-echo can be removed upon application of a larger k_{enc}, eventually shifting it outside the field of view (as shown in the k-space images of Fig. **4**). While potentially a similar strategy can be endorsed to remove the T_1-relaxation echo, nevertheless, k_{enc} may become prohibitively large, thereby minimizing the sensitivity of displacement encoding (given a specific motional pattern for moving spins).

Alternative strategies to null the T_1-relaxation echo have been introduced, including an inversion recovery (IR) approach [43], a complementary data acquisition (at zero encoding strength) followed by subtraction of the two phase images [64], or a more recently proposed phase cycling scheme [44]. Unfortunately, the IR approach suffers due to the spatial heterogeneity of T_1, and the subtraction methodology requires additional time and is subject to heart-rate variability (an effect which may be more prominent to mice, studied under anesthesia [65]).

In practical applications, both the phase cycling and the subtraction approaches are used. An example of cardiac DENSE imaging using the latter methodology is shown in Fig. (**5**) for end-diastolic (ED) and end-systolic (ES) imaging in the anesthetized mouse. Evident in both the phase difference images is phase wrapping (more prominent at ES), associated with increased motion during the contractile part of the cardiac cycle, an issue that is ameliorated with phase-unwrapping algorithms, as explained below.

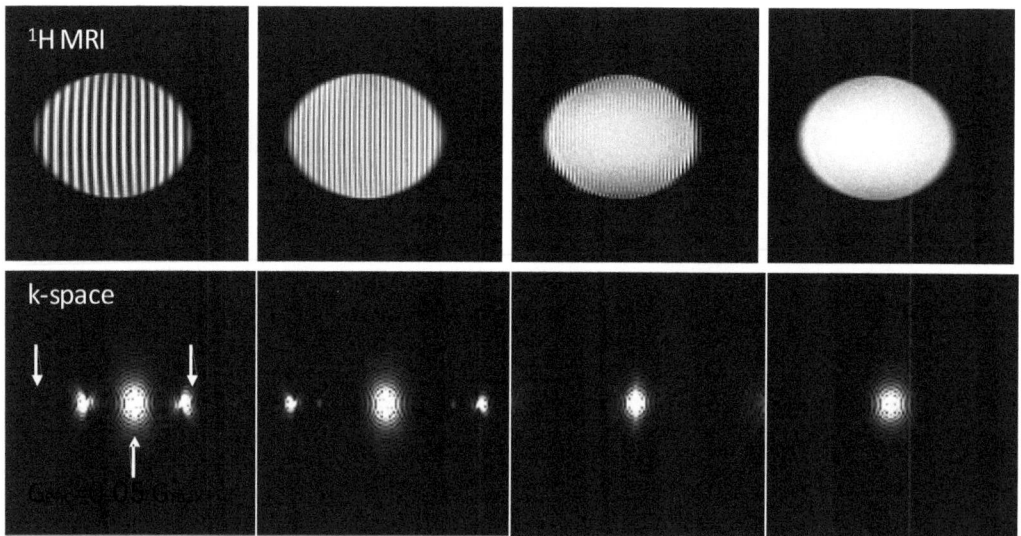

Figure 4: (Top row) Magnitude image, and (bottom row) corresponding k-space representation of oblique views of a gel phantom imaged using the 2D-DENSE pulse sequence. Indicative (in the k-space representations) are the echo, the anti-echo and the T_1-relaxation echo. Shown also is the anti-echo removal at increased encoding gradient strengths (leading to the elimination of the striation pattern on the magnitude image, as shown on top). Encoding values ranged between 0.1-0.5 cycles/mm and were in agreement with previously published reports (Figure compiled from the work of CC at the Mouse Image Facility at NIH during the period 2001-3-unpublished data).

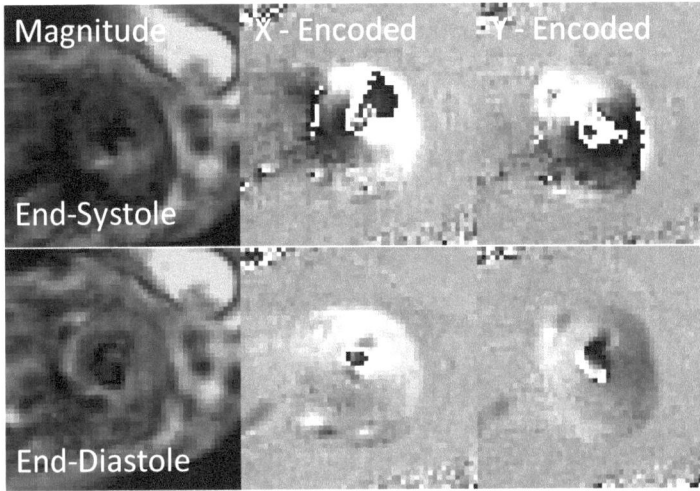

Figure 5: (Top row, left) End-systolic mid-ventricular magnitude ^{1}H cardiac MRI of a C57BL/6 mouse in a short axis view, (top row, right) end-systolic x-, and y-encoded 2D-DENSE phase difference images; (bottom row) corresponding end-diastolic magnitude and phase difference images.

DENSE Image Processing

A number of processing steps are associated with DENSE strain quantification. These are summarized in sequential order in Fig. (**6**) below, and discussed analytically in the sections that follow.

Segmentation

The first step in the post-processing flow of cardiac DENSE is the generation of binary masks of the myocardium (Fig. **6**). Such a task involves the definition of the myocardial epicardial and endocardial contours from the DENSE magnitude images by an expert user. Multiple manual [66, 67], semi-automatic [68-71] or template-matching techniques [72-75] can be utilized. Such techniques, often employ seed-point spline contours [75], active contours [68, 69], shape-template matching [71], or probabilistic- or anatomical atlas-based segmentation [76] for all the acquired slices throughout the cardiac cycle. Such a processing step can become tedious, time-consuming and computationally intensive. To overcome such difficulties, Spottiswoode *et al*. [70] recently proposed a methodology for the semi-automated motion-guided segmentation of cine DENSE datasets based on the encoded motion of a manually selected myocardial region through time.

| Set encoding strength k. Acquire DENSE magnitude and phase images at G_{enc}=0,+X, +Y | Use Magnitude image (Im) to segment myocardial mask (M). Generate Dense$_{masked}$=Im*M |
| | Phase unwrap (Quality Guided, Goldstein 2D) is optional and subject to specific conditions |

Magnitude   Masked
Wrapped   Unwrapped
X Encoded

| Calculate the distance vector **q** from the position vector **u**, assuming N_n closest neighboring points | Decode and calculate position vector u $$\nabla_r u = -\frac{1}{k}\nabla\phi_{unwrapped} \qquad \begin{pmatrix} 2k_{enc}\Delta x \\ 2\Delta\theta_b \end{pmatrix} = \begin{pmatrix} 1 & -1 \\ 1 & 1 \end{pmatrix}\begin{pmatrix} \phi_1 \\ \phi_2 \end{pmatrix}$$ |

| Track and compute the distance undeformed vectors in tensor **A** and deformed vectors in tensor **A'** | $A = [q_1,...,q_{N_n}]$ $A' = [q_{1'},...,q_{N_n'}]$ $A' = F.A$ |

d_{t9} d_{t11} d_{t13} d_{t15}
d_{t7} d_{t5} d_{t3} d_{t1}

| Estimate Deformation tensor F | Construction of the deformation tensor matrix **(3D)** $$F = A'.A(A.A^T)^{-1}$$ |

$\overline{F}$
$\chi(\overline{X},t)$
$\overline{X}$ $\overline{x}$
$\chi^{-1}(\overline{x},t)$
$\overline{X} = \overline{X}_{.J}.\overline{e}_J$ F^{-1} $\overline{x} = \overline{F}_{Ik}\overline{X}_{.k}.\overline{e}_I$
Initial Reference Configuration B_o (Langrangian)
Current Deformed Configuration B_t (Eulerian)

| Use Single-Value-Decomposition to avoid ill-conditioning problems | $A.A^T = U.S.V^T$ $F = A'.A.V.S_o.U^T$ $S_o = \begin{cases} S_{o,ik} = S_{t,k} & i \neq k \\ S_{o,ij} = 1/S_{t,j} & i = k \end{cases}$ |

| Compute Lagrangian/ Eulerian strain E | $E = \frac{1}{2}(F^TF - I)$ $E = \frac{1}{2}((FF^T)^{-1} - I)$ |

| Decompose Strain into longitudinal, second (circumferential) and first (radial) principle strain components | L=Longitudinal C=Circumferential R=Radial |

| Compute torsion and twist angles | $Torsion = \left(\frac{\theta_{apex} - \theta_{base}}{l_{LV}}\right)R_{LV}$ |

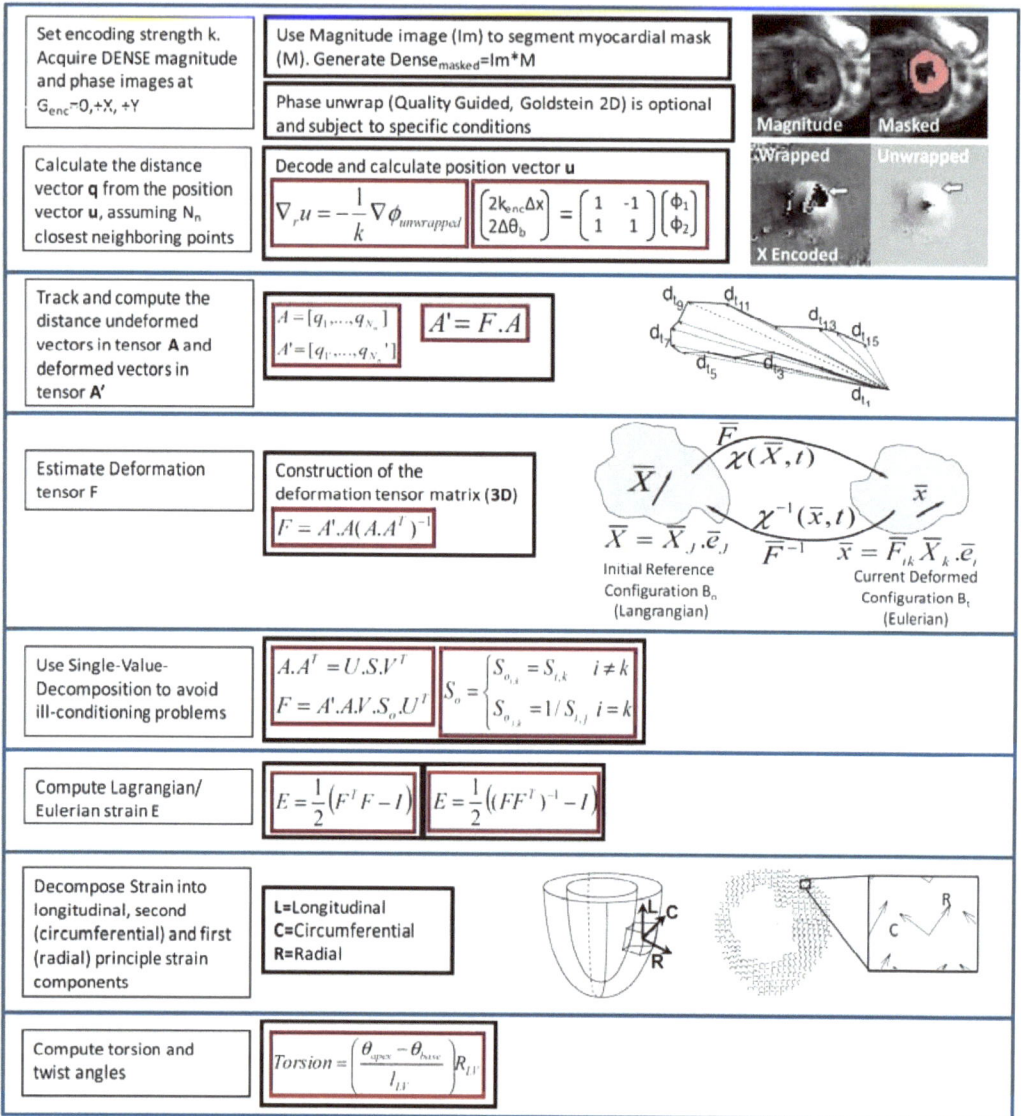

Figure 6: Flow diagram summarizing the post-processing steps for strain map calculation from DENSE image datasets. Characteristic figure examples of theoretical background and results of each processing step are shown in the right column of the chart.

Phase Unwrapping

The phase values in the DENSE images can only take values with the range of [-π, π], thereby often causing the phase to wrap during the cardiac contraction

(Fig. **6**) [77-80]. While it is possible to set the encoding frequency k_{enc} to be sufficiently small so that no phase wrapping occurs, this action will lead to an associated decrease in the displacement sensitivity [81]. Consequently, the practical choice of k_{enc} values, inevitably lead to phase wrapping, requiring the implementation of phase unwrapping algorithm (Fig. **6**) [17, 82]. Such algorithms attempt to restore the correct phase values of each myocardial voxel and allow the tissue tracking algorithms to reconstruct the motion pattern for subsequent strain estimation.

The relation of the measured/wrapped phase value $\varphi_{i,j}$ for each voxel, with the true phase value $\omega_{i,j}$ is given by the equation $\omega_{i,j} = \varphi_{i,j} + 2\pi n_{i,j}$ where $n_{i,j}$ specifies the correction required to restore the actual phase at each voxel (i, j) [79, 81, 83]. The phase unwrap problem is therefore reduced to the calculation of the $n_{i,j}$ for each imaged voxel. In CMR, the solution of such a problem can become complicated due to image noise and the relatively small transmural myocardial thickness (of only of a few voxels) [81], especially in the case of the mouse.

Phase unwrap algorithms typically fall into two major categories: a) the path-following algorithms, and b) the minimum L^p - norm algorithms. The first class unwrap the phase along a predetermined path in which phase consistency is met according to a quantitative measure [77, 78, 81, 84]. The second class of algorithms use a more global approach, aiming to minimize the integral of absolute and wrapped phase differences in an L^p - norm sense [81, 83, 85].

While the L^p - norm methods are typically more robust, computationally they are very demanding. Furthermore, the continuity of the myocardium provides a reliable path for the path-following algorithms, and are therefore favoured during the phase unwrap step of DENSE image processing. Specifically, widely used algorithms in this category are the Goldstein [84] and the Quality Guided algorithms [81].

Newer approaches to phase-unwrapping have led to an adaptive phase-unwrapping (APU) technique which incorporates the location of the myocardial wall into the quality map of the path-following algorithms, resulting in a reduced failure rate of the generic phase-unwrap algorithm, as reported recently [86].

Displacement Mapping and Material Point Tracking

During DENSE imaging, each voxel encodes the phase shift that spins accumulate from the initiation of the displacement encoding until the end of the acquisition for each cardiac frame (Figs. **3**, **5**). Therefore, in a DENSE displacement field for a cardiac frame, all vectors represent the encoded displacement of each myocardial voxel from the initial reference configuration to the deformed configuration, at the end of the frame. A two-dimensional (2D) plot of such displacement vectors often depicts vector arrows having their heads (targets) pointing to the center of the myocardial voxels at each imaged frame (Figs. **6**, **7**) [80, 81, 87]. Direct use of these displacement fields is limited because they only provide a net voxel displacement from the initial reference position (Eulerian displacement), instead of the frame-to-frame position change (Lagrangian displacement). The latter can be used to calculate Lagrangian strain [45, 87]. In order to reconstruct the frame-to-frame motion of myocardial voxels through the cardiac cycle, a material point tracking algorithm must be developed and used.

Initially, an arbitrary starting material point (x_0, y_0) is empirically chosen within the myocardium at end-diastole. For the subsequent frame, the three closest vector tails to the location of the material point of interest are identified within the displacement map. Identification is achieved by calculating the distances of all the vector tails within a sufficiently large circular region-of-interest chosen around the point of interest.

The identified vectors are then used to calculate their 2D-weighted average vector. The resulting interpolated vector is considered to be the displacement vector stemming from the original material point (x_0, y_0). Once all acquired frames have been analyzed, subtraction of interpolated vectors of consecutive (in time) cardiac frames, reconstruct the frame-to-frame motional pattern of the specific arbitrary material point [81, 87] (Figs. **6**, **7**).

In an effort to improve the accuracy of the resulting myocardial trajectory field, a number of spatial filters have been proposed for use [70] preventing the choice of erroneous closest vector tails. Upon application of such filters, nine closest vector tails are chosen instead of three, and a mean vector is calculated, as determined by their mean magnitude and spatial orientation. Subsequently, a magnitude and orientation deviation threshold is set in order to filter out erroneously selected vectors and the three closest tails fulfilling the set threshold requirements are chosen, before linear interpolation is applied [70, 80, 86]. Furthermore, in order to smooth and de-noise the resulting trajectories, temporal fitting can be performed using Fourier basis functions or higher order polynomials, shown to be able to better characterize the myocardial motion [70, 80, 81, 87, 88].

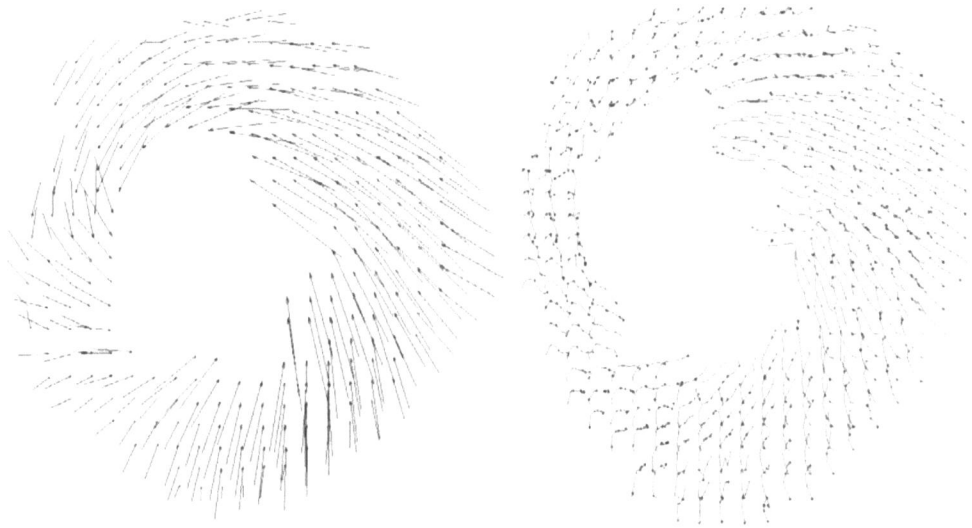

Figure 7: (Left) A typical murine left ventricular end-systolic displacement map. (Right) Filtered, unfitted tracked trajectories (from end-diastole to end-systole) of myocardial voxels at a mid-ventricular slice of the murine heart. The pattern shows the myocardial trajectories over the systolic contractile period.

Strain and Torsion Quantification

Following the application of the tracking algorithm - that allows the mapping of the trajectory of each myocardial voxel in time - an additional algorithm is employed to estimate its elicited strain. Initially, for a given point within the myocardium, its four neighboring voxels are selected. The vertical and lateral distances (q-entries) from the selected neighboring points are recorded in a constructed matrix A (Fig. **6**), whereas the accumulated deformed distances during a subsequent frame are recorded in a new matrix A'. Once all the distances are entered, the matrices A, A' have a rank of $n \times N_n$, where n is the number of directions (2 for 2D, 3 for 3D) and N_n is the number of the selected neighbouring points [48, 49, 81, 87] (Fig. **6**).

The calculation of the deformation tensor F requires inversion of the product AA^T. However, this may not always be possible because the inverse of AA^T may not exist (singular). To overcome the problem, one must ensure that the number of chosen neighbouring voxels is greater than the number of dimensions, and that the chosen neighbouring voxels span all possible directions. An alternative approach to avoid the ill-conditioned problem is to perform singular value decomposition of AA^T, followed by inversion of the diagonal entries of the constructed S matrix, as that is defined in Fig. (**6**) [48, 49, 87].

Lagrangian strain (E) is also calculated according to $E = 1/2(F^T F - I)$ and plotted for typical short axis MR images of a typical C57BL/6 mouse in Fig. (**8**). The process described above is repeated for all voxels within the myocardium and for all acquired temporal frames of the cardiac cycle (Fig. **9**) [36, 48, 49, 81, 87]. Once the strain values of all voxels are calculated, it can be easily appreciated that erroneous strain values arise at the endocardial and epicardial borders of the myocardium. Such errors result because the strain-matrix template partly resides outside the myocardium when strain is computed at the myocardial borders. To ameliorate the problem, the strain tensor is intentionally zeroed at the voxel locations of the two boundaries.

For torsion calculations, the radial vector (r) of a voxel of interest is defined in basal myocardium (as the vector originating from the image slice center of gravity to the voxel of interest), at end-diastole [ED] and at the end-systole [ES] (r′). Identification of the position of the voxel of interest in the end systolic frame is achieved with the use of the results of the tracking algorithm. The twist angle, θ_{base}, is then calculated using:

$$\theta_{base} = \cos^{-1}\left(\frac{r_x r_x' + r_y r_y' + r_z r_z'}{\sqrt{r_x^2 + r_y^2 + r_z^2}\sqrt{r_x'^2 + r_y'^2 + r_z'^2}} \right) \tag{5}$$

Similarly, the angle θ_{apex} is also calculated at the same radial ED position in an apical myocardial slice. Torsion is then computed according to:

$$Torsion = \left(\frac{\theta_{apex} - \theta_{base}}{l_{LV}}\right)R_{LV} \qquad\qquad (6)$$

where $\theta_{base}, \theta_{apex}$ are the calculated angles in the base and apex, respectively, l_{LV} is the length of the left ventricle (LV) and R_{LV} is the mean radius of the left ventricle [49].

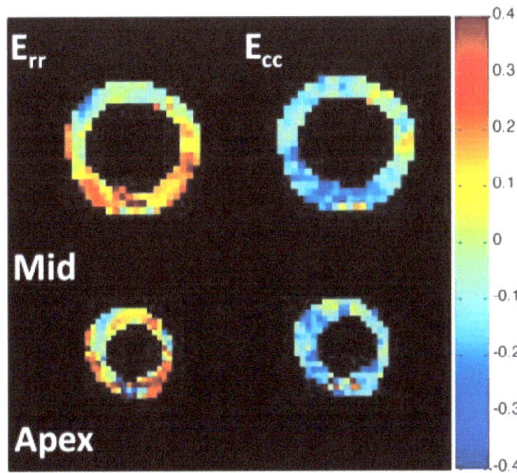

Figure 8: Lagrangian end-systolic (left) radial (Err) and (right) circumferential (Ecc) strain maps generated from (top) middle, and (bottom) apical ventricular short-axis slices of a murine heart. Mean strain values (within the various areas of the myocardium) vary between 8 - 11% for Err and -9 - -10% respectively, results which are in the range of previously reported values.

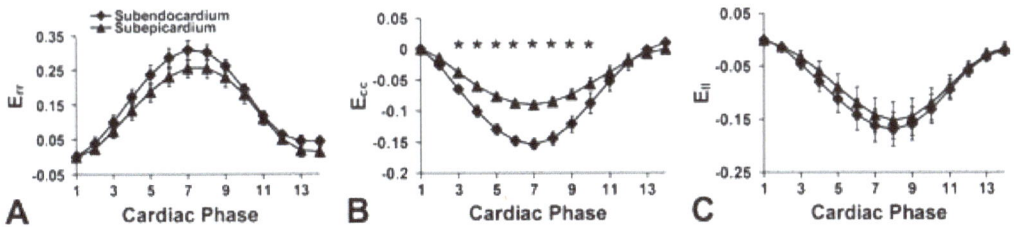

Figure 9: **(A)** Radial, **(B)** circumferential and **(C)** longitudinal strain as a function of cardiac phase measured using a 3D cine DENSE pulse sequence from seven C57BL/6 mice. Shown in the plots is an increase in the exhibited myocardial strain during systole followed by relaxation at diastole. In each plot two curves are presented corresponding to the sub-endocardial and the sub-epicardial regions of the LV observed to have statistically significant difference only at the circumferential component of strain (Reproduced from Zhong *et al.* Comprehensive Cardiovascular magnetic resonance of myocardial mechanics in mice using three-dimensional cine DENSE. Journal of Cardiovascular Magnetic Resonance 2011; 13:83, with permission (open access)).

Strain Tensor Decomposition - Cylindrical Coordinate Reference System

Once the strain tensors have been calculated, they are decomposed along the local RCL cylindrical coordinate system that best matches the prolate spheroidal anatomy of the heart [89]. Such a basis system consists of three principal unitary vectors along the radial (R) [pointing from the endo- to the epicardium], the longitudinal (L) (pointing from apex to base) and the circumferential (C) directions (often defined as the cross-product of the longitudinal and radial vectors) (Figs. **6-9**).

REGIONAL STRAIN QUANTIFICATION: ACROSS SPECIES COMPARISON

Regional LV systolic function is complex and entails a series of coordinated events characterized by respective strain components, including longitudinal contraction (Ell), circumferential shortening (Ecc) and radial thickening (Err). As cardiac muscle contracts, Ell and Ecc become increasingly negative in value, in comparison to Err that reflects chamber dilation, with an elicited positive strain. In accordance to the American Heart Association's (AHA) segmentation standards and nomenclature, such values are often reported in basal, middle, and apical myocardial regions, through a sectorial representation of the myocardium in a short axis representation [90].

Following the introduction of tagging [18, 19] and HARP [20], the assessment of LV systolic function focused initially on human and canine studies. It spanned a number of clinical and research efforts, including studies on normal LV and right-ventricular (RV) contractility and torsional patterns, but expanded to include coronary artery disease (CAD), ischemic heart disease (IHD), myocardial infarction (MI), dilated and hypertrophic cardiomyopathies (DCM, HCM), congenital disease, resynchronization therapy, valvular disease, and others [3]. Explicit reference to all the studies is impossible to include herein and it is beyond the scope of this chapter. The reader is, however, referred to excellent reviews that summarize all such efforts, including those by Petitjean *et al.* [91], Pai *et al.* [92] and Ibrahim [3].

In its independent development and evolution, DENSE [17], was employed for initial human [42, 93] and canine [17] validation studies, to find its way to the clinical setting for study of volunteers [45, 48, 86, 88, 94] and patients [86, 95], including but not limited to hypertension [86], coronary artery disease [86, 95], type II diabetes [86], non-ischemic cardiomyopathy, congestive heart failure, myocardial infarction [95-97], and others [98]. More recently, DENSE has been applied to the study of RV function [99] and in carotid artery wall strain imaging [100].

On the forefront of mouse cardiac MRI, the initial regional cardiac characterization efforts (that adapted from prior work in humans), included the tagging studies by Kolandaivelu on strain quantification [101], the study of Henson *et al.* [61] on torsional patterns of mouse and man, and subsequent works by Epstein *et al.* [13] on strain quantification in infacted mice, Zhou *et al.* [63] and Heijman *et al.* [2] on regional strain in normal [2, 63] and infarcted mice [2]. Such studies constituted the impetus for subsequent regional cardiac mouse publications, extending the initial 2D-tagging to a number of additional tagging [14, 102-104], HARP [35, 50, 105], and DENSE mouse studies [36, 46, 49].

While most studies report patterns of normal systolic strain indices, some extend to LGE-MI [102], dobutamine stimulation [36], heart failure following DCM [103] or compensated hypertrophy [106], and to gene-targeted mice including a vinculin (VclKO) knockout [104], a cardiac myosing binding protein C (cMyBPC) knockout [107], or to combined DENSE-Manganese Enhanced MRI eNOS and nNOS mice [108], before, and after β-adrenergic stimulation. For a recent, comprehensive review of MRI studies on murine models of pathology (that include metabolic, perfusion, transgenic, and other) the reader is referred to a review article by Epstein [62].

Comparison of Contractile Patterns of Motion and Strain in Human and Mouse

Moore *et al.* [89], Young *et al.* [109], and Petitjean *et al.* [76] summarize in an excellent fashion the motional contractile-relaxation patterns of myocardial motion through the cardiac cycle, from tagging data acquired from normal humans. Briefly, a homogeneous radial contractile pattern is observed over the LV with a mean inward displacement of 5 mm [76]. A mean clockwise basal twisting of -4.4° is counterbalanced by an anticlockwise mean apical twisting of 10°. At the onset of systole an initial anticlockwise basal rotation has also been noted [76, 89]. A mean Ecc value of -23±4.9% is observed, with a transmural variation from epicardium (lower strain) to the endocardium (larger strain). Ecc is also greater in value at the apex compared to base, and on the anterior and lateral walls. A graded pattern of longitudinal displacement is recorded with increased value at the base (mean value of 11.2 mm) compared to the middle-myocardium (mean value of 6.9 mm) and to the apex (mean value of 2.6 mm), exhibiting a larger value in the inferior wall.

For the RV, radial shortening is larger along the long-axis (mean value of 26.9%) compared to the short-axis plane (mean value of 17%), with higher values in the apical compared to the basal regions.

Importantly, disparities exist in radial displacements, longitudinal contraction, and radial strains reported by the two most prominent publications of Moore *et al.* [89] and Young *et al.* [109]. Such have been attributed to differences in the characteristics of the studied populations, slice level variations, motion estimation techniques and algorithms employed, and to other methodological differences (low tag-resolution, *etc.*).

For the mouse, a radial LV contractile pattern is reported with a mean inward displacement of 0.35 mm [64]. In contrast to the human, almost no apical longitudinal displacement (0.06 mm) is encountered in mice, whereas the corresponding basal displacement is reported to be approximately -0.5 mm [64]. The basal twisting (reported to range between +1.3 - -4.1°) is also counterbalanced by an anticlockwise mean apical twisting reported in the range of 3.3 - 8.7° [14, 36, 49, 64]. A mean Ecc value of -12.3±5.5 % (Ecc, peak=-18±2 %) is observed, with a transmural variation from epicardium (lower strain) to the endocardium (larger strain), in agreement with the human strain-development pattern. Ecc is also greater in value at the apex compared to base, and on the anterior and lateral walls [63, 64, 104]. A mean Err value of 21.8±8.8 % (Err=39.4±1.3 %) while the corresponding mean Ell values are -12.8±2.6% (Ell=-18±14 %).

Isometric and Allometric Scaling - Across Species Comparison - Strain Quantification

For proper comparisons between mouse and man in cardiac studies of pathology, it has become critical to ascertain the existence of isometric or allometric scaling for global and regional hemodynamics and indices of contractile function. Despite the fact that global hemodynamic parameters have been investigated long ago [110], and were recently summarized [111], data supportive of isometric/allometric scaling associations between mouse and man, regional systolic indices have only been diffusely compared through various publications over recent years, or occasional review articles [62]. Table **1** below (adopted from Dawson [57] and Weinberg *et al.* [111]) summarizes global hemodynamic parameter dependence from prior work [62, 57, 111], and lists our summary findings for regional systolic contractile parameters from an extensive (and exhaustive) literature search of human and murine publications, as tabulated in Table **2** below. Results are supportive of isometric and allometric scaling in accordance to the law: $Y = aBW^{b}$, where BW is the body weight, and a and b are constants.

Despite the isometric dependence of regional cardiac functional (wall-thickening, wall-motion and regional EF) as reported previously [58], and strain components (Ecc, Err, Ell) [results in Tables **1** and **2** and Figs. (**10**, **11**) of this work], paradoxical discrepancies between mammalian species still remain [49, 61]. For example, normalized torsion (between mouse and man) and myocardial fiber structure (for pair-wise comparisons between mouse, sheep, and rabbit) [112] exhibit distinct differences. Further studies are guaranteed to ascertain the exact physiological reasoning and on whether such findings can be explained by an increased cardiac mechanical efficiency in the mouse (as a result of a more efficient contractile machinery), or possibly due to differences in the metabolic/enzymatic activity, especially as it relates to differential phosphorylation patterns and kinetics.

MYOCARDIAL MECHANICS AND CARDIAC PATHOLOGY

Prior reference justifies the extensive applicability of regional CMR functional characterization techniques to mouse and human pathology including IHD, MI, HCM, DCM, and in various transgenetic models of hypertrophy, cardiomyopathy, and others.

Table 1: Summary of the most important morphological, functional, global and regional hemodynamic parameters and contractile indices of function between mammals, exhibiting isometric and allometric scaling. Adopted from Dawson [Dawson 1991] and Weinberg *et al.* [Weinberg 2007]. Mean BW values for each species was obtained from published results (mouse=25 g, canine=22 kg, porcine=30 kg, sheep=35 kg, human=80 kg).

Hemodynamic Parameter	Isometric/Allometric Scaling Law $Y=aBW^b$
Body mass	$a\,BW^1$
Heart weight	$a\,BW^1$
LV volume (EDV, ESV)	$a\,BW^1$
Stroke volume	$a\,BW^1$
Blood volume	$a\,BW^1$
Elastic modulus	$a\,BW^0$
Arterial pressure	$a\,BW^0$
PW velocity	$a\,BW^0$
Diameter pulsation	$a\,BW^0$
Coronary reserve	$a\,BW^0$
Blood viscosity	$a\,BW^0$
Blood velocity	$a\,BW^0$
Heart Rate	$a\,BW^{-1/4}$
Heart Period	$a\,BW^{1/4}$
Circulation time	$a\,BW^{1/4}$
Cardiac output	$a\,BW^{3/4}$
Acceleration, dP/dt	$a\,BW^{-1/4}$
Wall shear stress	$a\,BW^{-3/8}$
Temporal gradient of aortic wall shear stress	$a\,BW^{5/8}$
Artery length	$a\,BW^{1/4}$
Artery diameter	$a\,BW^{3/8}$
Total Peripheral Resistance	$a\,BW^{-3/4}$
Capillary diameter	$a\,BW^{1/12}$
Capillary length	$a\,BW^{5/24}$
Capillary number	$a\,BW^{5/8}$
Capillary velocity	$a\,BW^{-1/24}$
Cell number	$a\,BW^{5/8}$
Cell length	$a\,BW^{1/8}$
Cell volume	$a\,BW^{3/8}$
Aortic Reynolds number	$a\,BW^{3/8}$
Aortic Womersley number	$a\,BW^{1/4}$
Ecc	$-15.9\,BW^0$ (from results of this study)
Err	$24.2\,BW^0$ (from results of this study)
Ell	$-14.3\,BW^0$ (from results of this study)

Table 2: Quantitative comparison of regional strain and torsion estimates for the murine, sheep, porcine, canine and human hearts.

Species	ES Strain (%)			Torsion (°)	Twist (°)	Reference
	Base	**Mid**	**Apex**			
Mouse	*Radial*	*Radial*	*Radial*	5.6 ± 0.9^6	*Base*	[1]Gilson 2005 [46]
	$30\pm4*^1$	29 ± 17^6	$16\pm2*^1$	1.3 ± 0.23^1/mm	-0.2 ± 0.5^6	[2]Zhong J 2010 [36]
	21 ± 4^2	$30\pm4*^1$	27 ± 2^2	2.5 ± 0.5^2/mm	1.3 ± 0.6^1	[3]ZhongJ 2008 [50]
	12 ± 2^3	30 ± 7^3	12 ± 6^3	1.0 ± 0.25^{12}/mm	-1.7 ± 1.2^2	[4]Liu 2006 [14]
	10 ± 2^4	14 ± 3^4	13 ± 3^4	2.0 ± 1.5^{13}	-4.1 ± 1.8^4	[5]Chuang 2010 [104]
	$18\pm7.5*^5$	30 ± 7^5	$15.3\pm4.5*^5$	3.0 ± 0.7^{14}/mm	*Middle*	[6]Zhong 2011 [49]
	Circumferential	$25\pm13.5*^5$	*Circumferential*		3.3 ± 0.5^6	[7]Gilson 2004 [64]
	$-14\pm3*^1$	39.4 ± 1.3^7	$-13.3\pm1.5*^1$		2.9 ± 0.6^1	[8]Heijman 2004 [FVB] [2]
	-15 ± 1^2	*Circumferential*	-18 ± 1^2		*Apex*	[9]Epstein 2002 [13]
	-8 ± 1^3	-13 ± 3^6	-9 ± 2^3		7.1 ± 0.6^6	[10]Kolandaivelu 2000 [101]
	-13 ± 1^4	$-14.3\pm2.5*^1$	-18 ± 2^4		5.3 ± 0.5^1	[11]Young 2006 [102]
	$-8.3\pm4.1*^5$	-12 ± 2^3	$-12.7\pm4*^5$		3.3 ± 1.1^2	[12]Zhou 2003 [63]
	Longitudinal	-15 ± 2^4	*Longitudinal*		8.7 ± 3.2^4	[13]Henson 2000 [61]
	-11 ± 3^3	-9 ± 4^8	-10 ± 2^3			[14]Li 2010 [105]
	$-12.3\pm1.2*^5$	-12 ± 2^3	$-16\pm1*^5$			
		$-13\pm3.6*^5$				
		-14.5 ± 3.4^9				
		-16.4 ± 1.3^7				
		$-14 - -18\#^{10}$				
		-14 ± 1^{11}				
		Longitudinal				
		-18 ± 14^6				
		-11 ± 2^3				
		$-12.7\pm0.6*^5$				
		-13 ± 1^{11}				
Canine	*Radial*	*Radial*	*Radial*			[15]Rademakers 1994 [116]
	27.3 ± 16.5^{15}	20.8^{16}	40.3 ± 16.8^{15}			[16]Aletras 1999 [17]
	Fiber Direction:	35.8 ± 17.7^{15}	*Fiber Direction*			
	$-6.4\pm0.5*^{15}$	*Fiber Direction*	$-8.9\pm2.3*^{15}$			
	Cross-Fiber Dir	$-7.8\pm2.2*^{15}$	*Cross-Fiber Dir*			
	$-12\pm15*^{15}$	Cross-Fiber Dir:	$15.2\pm16*^{15}$			
		$-13.6\pm18.8*^{15}$				
Porcine		*Radial*				[17]Soleimanifard 2012 [117]
		16.4 ± 3.3^{17}				[18]Abd-Elmoniem2012 [118]
		Circumferential				
		-19.6 ± 3.7^{17}				
		-27 ± 1.6^{18}				
		Longitudinal				
		-21.7 ± 6.7^{17}				

(Table 2) contd.....

Species	ES Strain (%)			Torsion (°)	Twist (°)	Reference
	Base	Mid	Apex			
Sheep	*Circumferential* -12.5±2.5[#19] -10.1±2.6[#20] *Longitudinal* -13.0±2.6[#19] -10.5±2.8[# 20]	*Circumferential* -13.2±2.4[# 19] -9.5±2.1[#20] *Longitudinal* -16.2±0.3[#19] -10.2±3.4[#20]				[19]Guccione 2006 [119] [20]Zhang 2007 [120]
Human	*Radial* 21±3[#21] 45±4.9[#22] 35[23] 34[24] 21±2[4] *Circumferential* -19.5±1.3[#21] -18.5±2.4[#22] -19.4±2.7[#24] -27.2±5.5[#25] -17±5[10] -20±1[4] *Longitudinal* -16.7±2.6[#21] -14.7±0.5[#22] -17.7[23] -17[24]	*Radial* 33±10[26] 17.7±3.3[#21] 41.7±7.4[#22] 40.8[23] 29[24] 23±2[4] *Circumferential* -17±2[26] -20.5±1.3[#21] -19.2±3.8[#22] -32.3±2.7[#24] -29.6±3.8[#25] -18±4[10] -21±2[4] *Longitudinal* -16±2[26] -15.5±1.3[#21] -14.8±0.5[#22] -16.4[23] -16[24]	*Radial* 6.5±3.3[#21] 47.7±14[#22] 42[23] 28[24] 18±5[4] *Circumferential* -21.7±1.3[#21] -22.2±2.9[#22] -24.5±2.6[#24] -34±2.6[#25] -19±4[10] -22±3[4] *Longitudinal* -18.7±1[#21] -18.5±0.6[#22] -18.4[23] -18[24]	0.8±0.3[22]/mm 7.7±1.4[27] 7.9±0.5[26] 14.5±1.3[#21] 7.5±2.1[#21] 12±2*[22] 12.7±1.7[13] 12.1±1.9*[28]	*Base* -1±1.6[26] -1.8±1.5[#21] -4[29] -3.5±1[4] *Middle* 3.8±1.6[27] 6.4±1.4[26] 5.7±2.1[#21] 5*[29] *Apex* 15±1.2[26] 13±2[25] 10.5±2.1[29] 9.7±2.9[4]	[21]Young 1994 [109] [22]Moore 2000 [89] [23]Bogaert 2001 [124] [24]Kuijer 2002 [125] [25]Clark 1991 [122] [26]Zhong 2010 [48] [27]Russell 2008 [121] [28]Moore 2000 II [126] [29]Alouche 2001 [123]

#Values presented have been averaged over reported septal, posterior, anterior and lateral regions.
*Values presented have been averaged over reported transmural, epicardial, and endocardial regions.

While morphological and functional scaling from mouse to man has been proved (through consideration of global and regional cardiac function), for comparative interspecies studies of pathology, other integrative physiological responses also ought to be considered. Such include circulatory control, blood flow distribution and regulation, calcium storage and cycling, myosin light chain distribution, and force frequency reserve. Although evidence supports that bioenergetically and hemodynamically [57, 111] the mouse scales isometrically or allometrically with larger mammals and humans [113-115], exhibiting a similar maximal aerobic capacity with larger species [115], important considerations still remain. For example, metabolically the mouse still operates at the high end of its capacity and its reserve remains low. Given all considerations, extrapolations of inferences drawn from mouse studies to man are appropriate for proper models of cardiac disease, and therefore generalizations to all cardiac pathology may indeed be risky.

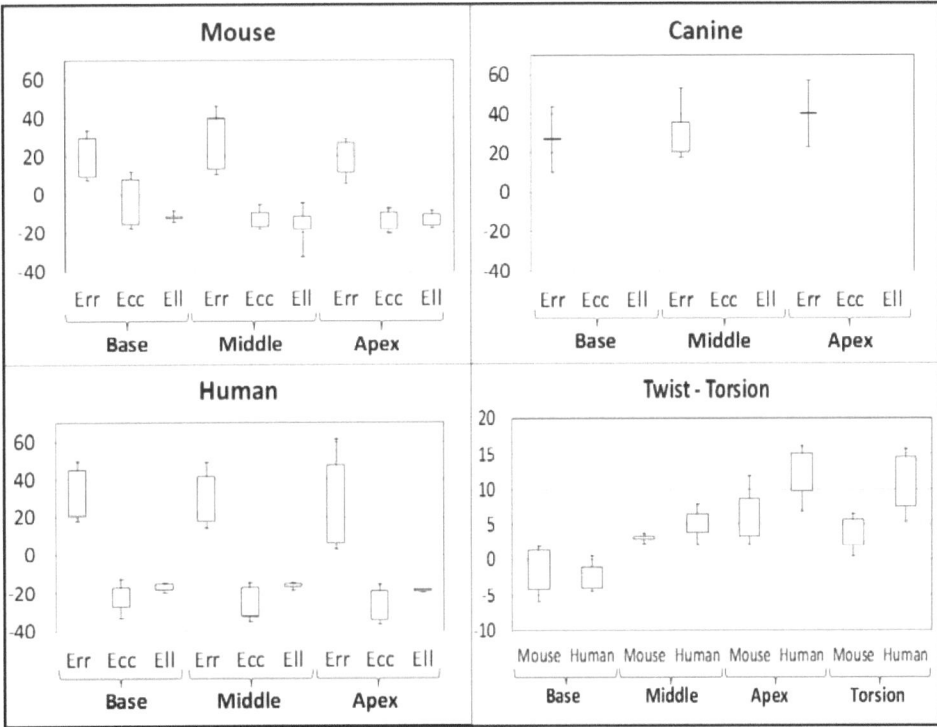

Figure 10: Regional strain distribution (Err, Ecc, Ell) in basal, middle, and apical areas of the murine, canine, and human myocardium, based on an extensive and exhaustive summary of studies and reports in the literature. Corresponding twist angle and torsion distribution (in degrees) in the murine and human myocardium, based on numerous studies and reports in the literature (see Table **2**). Data are plotted as minimum/maximum recorded value±SD (see Table **2**).

FUTURE DIRECTIONS

While image-based phenotyping has been a major long-term scientific goal, aiming to high-throughput cardiac studies of pathology, to-this-date, it still remains elusive. With the exemption of stem-cell strides (efforts that have evolved in an associative and translational manner within the scientific community), human and mouse cardiac pathological MRI studies have advanced mostly as parallel efforts, unsupported thus far by major National or International policies or consortia that would strategically coordinate multi-center studies, under carefully-controlled and normalized protocols. The latter, would certainly aid to establish the knowledge-platform to benefit cardiovascular disease, molecular genomics, or related/emerging technological advances, with an envisaged tremendous impact for translational research to man.

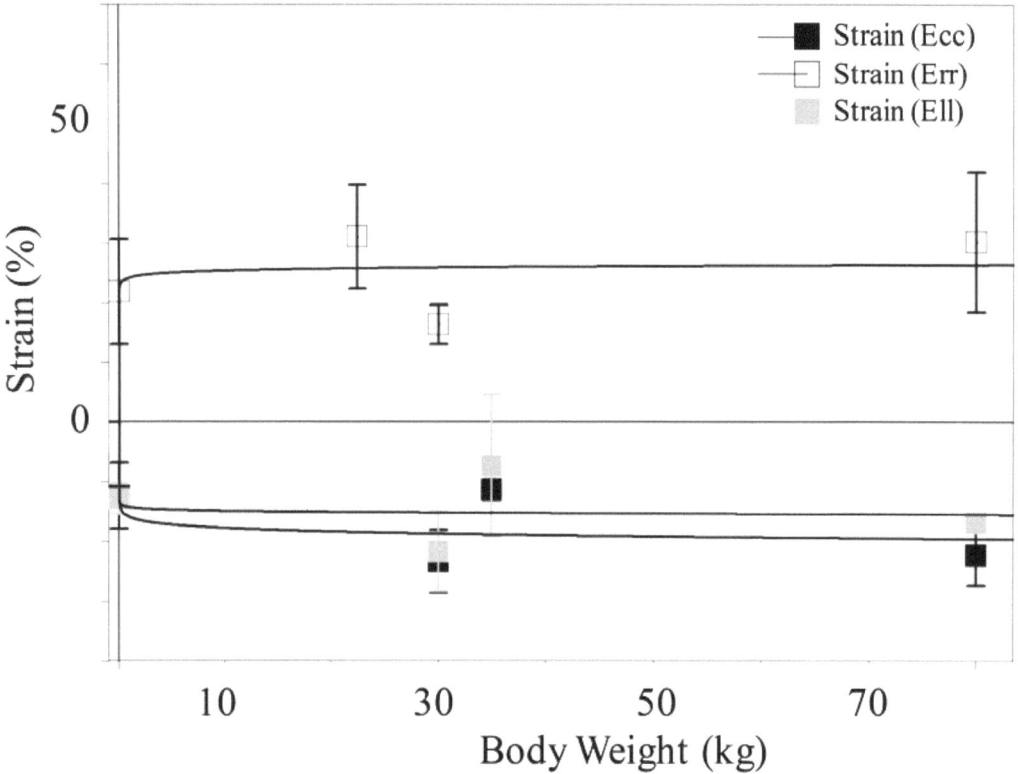

Figure 11: Isometric dependence of Ecc, Err and Ell across mammalian species, as supported by data in Table **2** and Fig. (**10**).

Recently funded European infrastructure roadmap efforts (Euro-Bioimaging, infrastructure for phenotyping and archiving of model mammalian genomes, European advanced translational research infrastructure in medicine), biobanks, and International mouse phenotyping consortia efforts (www.jax.org, www.mousephenotype.org, www.infrafrontier.eu, www.eatris.eu) target such critical areas in an associative and organized manner. While most of such attempts are still at infant stages, it is envisaged that they will develop to become the driving forces and repositories for the scientific community in upcoming years.

SUMMARY AND CONCLUSIONS

This chapter has summarized efforts of regional cardiac functional studies using MRI that span the past 25 years. In addition to the comparison of the three major MRI techniques that achieve detailed studies of myocardial mechanics, DENSE-MRI and its imaging and image-processing features has been emphasized. The mouse paradigm, as a direct manifestation of international efforts for image-based phenotyping in health, disease and post-transgenetic modification, has been introduced. The appropriateness of extrapolations of inferences drawn from mouse studies to man are well-justified from presented evidence on isometric and allometric scaling of global and regional cardiac functional indices. However, the reader's caution is drawn, given the mismatches of force-frequency and energetic/metabolic reserves between the two species. While such arguments limit the range of possible pathological models that can associate human and murine disease, the mouse is a potentially attractive animal model for cardiovascular research today.

CONFLICT OF INTEREST

Work for this project was partially pursued and completed at the Laboratory of Physiology and Biomedical Imaging, an ISO9001-certified lab, under the direction of CC, at the U. Cyprus. CC has been a consultant engineer for Chi-Biomedical Ltd. since 2004.

ACKNOWLEDGEMENTS

The authors acknowledge funding from the the Research Promotion Foundation under the grant RFP/TECHNOLOGY/MHXAN/0609(BE)/05. They [CC] would also like to thank Drs. R. Balaban, A. Koretsky, H. Wen, and Drs. A. Aletras, M. Lizak, and A. Silva at the National Heart Lung and Blood Institute (NHLBI) and the Mouse Imaging Facility at NINDS, at the National Institutes of Health for their instrumental support in the DENSE implementation effort in 2002-2003. They [CC] would also like to thank Professor E. McVeigh for the support and help with the gel phantom tagging studies in 1992-94, and [SA, CC] Professor. F.

Epstein at the University of Virginia Charlottsville and Dr. X. Zhong (currently at Siemens Inc.) for all their help and support during the past 3 years with the DENSE work. The University of Cyprus is also thanked for providing infrastructure support.

REFERENCES

[1] de Roos A, Kunz P, Lamb H, Kroft L, Langerak S, Doornbos J, van der We. Magnetic resonance imaging of ischemic heart disease: why cardiac magnetic resonance imaging will play a significant role in the management of patients with coronary artery disease. J Comp Assist Tomogr 1999; 23 (Suppl 1): S135-S141.

[2] Heijman E, Strijkers GJ, Habets J, Janssen B, Nicolay K. Magnetic resonance imaging of regional cardiac function in the mouse. MAGMA 2004; 17: 170-178.

[3] Ibrahim El-Sayed H. Myocardial tagging by cardiovascular magnetic resonance: evolution of techniques-pulse sequences, analysis algorithms, and applications. Journal of Cardiovascular Magnetic Resonance 2011; 13: 36.

[4] Manning WJ, Wei JY, Fossel ET, Burnstein D. Measurement of left ventricular mass in rats using electrocardiogram-gated magnetic resonance imaging. Am J Physiol 1990; 258: H1181-H1186.

[5] Shapiro EP. Evaluation of left ventricular hypertrophy by magnetic resonance imaging. Am J Card Imaging 1994; 8: 310-315.

[6] Florentine MS, Grosskreutz CL, Chang Q, Hartnett JA, Dunn VD, Ehrhardt JC, Fleagle SR, Collins SM, Marcus ML, Skorton DJ. Measurement of left ventricular mass *in vivo* using gated nuclear magnetic resonance imaging. J Am Coll Cardiol 1986; 8: 107-112.

[7] Semelka RC, Tomei E, Wagner S, Mayo J, Caputo G, O'Sullivan M, Parmley WW, Chatterjee K, Wolfe C, Higgins CB. Interstudy reproducibility of dimensional and functional measurements between cine magnetic resonance studies in the morphologically abnormal left ventricle. Am Heart J 1990; 119: 1367-1373.

[8] Semelka RC, Tomei E, Wagner S, Mayo J, Kondo C, Suzuki J, Caputo GR, Higgins CB. Normal left ventricular dimensions and function: interstudy reproducibility of measurements with cine MR imaging. Radiology 1990; 174: 763-768.

[9] Siri FM, Jelicks LA, Leinwand LA, Gardin JM. Gated magnetic resonance imaging of normal and hypertrophied murine hearts. Am J Physiology Am. J. Physiol. Heart Circ. Physiol. 1997; 272(41): H2394-H2402.

[10] Ruff J, Wiesmann F, Hiller KH, Voll S, von Kienlin M, Bauer WR, Rommel E, Neubauer S, Haase A. Magnetic resonance microimaging for noninvasive quantification of myocardial function and mass in the mouse. Magnetic Resonance in Medicine 1998; 40: 43-48.

[11] Slawson SE, Roman BB, Williams DS, Koretsky AP. Cardiac MRI of the normal and hypertrophied mouse heart. Magnetic Resonance in Medicine 1998; 39: 980-987.

[12] van der Geest RH, Reiber JH. Quantification in cardiac MRI. J Magn Reson Imaging 1999; 10: 602-608.

[13]   Epstein F, Yang z, Gilson WD, Berr SS, Cramer CM, French BA. MR Tagging early after myocardial infarction in mice demonstrates contractile dysfunction in adjacent and remote regions. Magn Reson Med 2002; 48: 399-403.

[14]   Liu W, Ashford MW, Chen J, Watkins MP, Williams TA, Wickline SA, Yu X. MR tagging demonstrates quantitative differences in regional ventricular wall motion in mice, rats, and men. Am J Physiol 2006; 291: H2515-H2521.

[15]   Young AA, Dokos S, Powell KA, Sturm B, McCulloch AD, Starling RC, McCarthy PM, White RD. Regional heterogeneity of function in nonischemic dilated cardiomyopathy. Cardiovascular Research 2001; 49: 308-318.

[16]   Chandra S, Skali H, Blankstein R. Novel techniques for assessment of left ventricular systolic function. Heart Fail Rev 2011; 16: 327-337.

[17]   Aletras AH, Ding S, Balaban RS, Wen H. DENSE: Displacement encoding with stimulated echoes in cardiac functional MRI. J Magn Reson 1999; 137: 247-252.

[18]   Zerhouni EA, Parish DM, Rogers WJ, Yang A, Shapiro EP. Human heart: tagging with MR imaging-a method for noninvasive assessment of myocardial motion. Radiology 1988; 169: 59-63.

[19]   Axel L, Dougherty L. MR imaging of motion with spatial modulation of magnetization. Radiology 1989; 171: 841-845.

[20]   Osman NF, Kerwin WS, McVeigh ER, Prince JL. Cardiac motion tracking using CINE harmonic phase (HARP) magnetic resonance imaging. Magnetic Resonance in Medicine 1999; 42: 1048-1060.

[21]   van Dijk, Noll DC, Pauly JM. Direct cardiac NMR imaging of heart wall and blood flow velocity. J Comp Assist Tomogr 1984; 8: 429-436.

[22]   Pelc NJ, Noll DC, Pauly JM. Method of noninvasive myocardial motion analysis using bidirectional motion integration in phase contrast MRI maps of myocardial velocity. US Patent 5257626, 1993.

[23]   Osman NF. Detecting stiff masses using strain-encoded (SENC) imaging. Magnetic Resonance in Medicine 2003; 49(3): 605-8.

[24]   Zhu Y, Drangova M, Pelc NJ. Estimation of deformation gradient and strain from cine-PC velocity data. IEEE Trans Med Imaging 16: 840-851, 1997.

[25]   McVeigh ER, Atalar E. Cardiac tagging with breath-hold CINE cardiac MRI. Magnetic Resonance in Medicine 1992; 28: 318-327.

[26]   Mosher TJ, Smith MB. A DANTE tagging sequence for the evaluation of translational sample motion. Magnetic Resonance in Medicine 1990; 15: 334-339.

[27]   Fischer SE, McKinnon GC, Maier SE, Boesinger P. Improved myocardial tagging contrast. Magnetic Resonance in Medicine 1993; 30: 191-200.

[28]   Fischer SE, McKinnon GC, Scheidegger MB, Prins W, Meier D, Boesiger P. True myocardial motion tracking. Magn Reson Med 1994; 31: 401-413.

[29]   Chandra SYY. Simulations and demonstrations of localized tagging experiments. J Magn Reson B 1996; 111: 285-288.

[30]   McVeigh ER, Bolster BD. Improved sampling of myocardial motion with variable separation tagging. Magnetic Resonance in Medicine 1998; 39: 657-661.

[31]   Stuber M, Spiegel MA, Fischer SE, Scheidegger MB, Danias PG, Pedersen EM, Boesiger P. Single breath-hold slice-following CSPAMM myocardial tagging. MAGMA 1999; 9: 85-91.

[32]   Castillo E, Lima JA, Bluemke DA. Regional myocardial function: advances in MR imaging and analysis. Radiographics 2003; 23: S127-S140.

[33]   Kraitchman DL, Sampath S, Castillo E, Derbyshire JA, Boston RC, Bluemke DA, Gerber BL, Prince JL, Osman NF. Quantitative ischemia detection during cardiac magnetic resonance stress testing by use of fastHARP. Circulation 2003; 107: 2025-2030.

[34]   Phatak NS, Maas SA, Veress AI, Pack NA, Di Bella EV, Weiss JA. Strain measurement in the left ventricle during systole with deformable image registration. Med Image Anal 2009; 13: 354-361.

[35]   Zhong J, Liu W, Yu X. Transmural myocardial strain in mouse: quantification of high-resolution MR tagging using HARP analysis. Magnetic Resonance in Medicine 2009; 61(6): 1368-1373.

[36]   Zhong J, Yu X. Strain and torsion quantification in mouse hearts under dobutamine stimulation using 2D multi-phase MR DENSE. Magnetic Resonance in Medicine 2010; 64(5): 1315-1322.

[37]   Sampath S, Derbyshire JA, Atalar E, Osman NF, Prince JL. Real-time monitoring of two-dimensional cardiac strain using a harmonic phase magnetic resonance imaging (HARP-MRI) pulse sequence. Magnetic Resonance in Medicine 2003; 50: 154-163.

[38]   Pan L, Prince JL, Lima JA, Osman NF. Fast tracking of cardiac motion using 3D-HARP. IEEE Trans Biomed Eng 2005; 52: 1425-1435.

[39]   Abd-Elmoniem KZ, Stuber M, Osman NF, Prince JL. ZHARP: three-dimensional motion tracking from a single image plane. Inf Process Med Imaging 2005; 19: 639-651.

[40]   Abd-Elmoniem KZ, Sampath S, Osman NF, Prince JL. Real-time monitoring of cardiac regional function using fastHARP MRI and region-of-interest reconstruction. IRRR Trans Biomed Eng 2007; 54: 1650-1656.

[41]   Kuijer JP, Hofman MB, Zwanenburg JJ, Marcus JT, van Rossum AC, Heethaar RM. DENSE and HARP: two views on the same technique of phase-based strain imaging. J Magn Reson Imaging 2006; 24: 1432-1438.

[42]   Aletras A, Balaban R, Wen H. High-resolution strain analysis of the human heart with fast-DENSE. Journal of Magnetic Resonance 1999; 140: 41-57.

[43]   Aletras AH, Wen H. Mixed echo train acquisition displacement encoding with stimulated echoes: an optimized DENSE method for *in vivo* function imaging of the human heart. Magnetic Resonance in Medicine 2001; 46: 523-534.

[44]   Epstein FH, Gilson WD. Displacement-encoded cardiac MRI using cosine and sine modulation to eliminate (CANSEL) artifact-generating echoes. Magnetic Resonance in Medicine 2004; 52: 774-781.

[45]   Kim D, Gilson WD, Kramer CM, Epstein FH. Myocardial tissue tracking with two-dimensional cine displacement-encoded MR imaging: development and initial evaluation. Radiology 2004; 230: 862-871.

[46]   Gilson WD, Yang Z, French BA, Epstein FH. Measurement of myocardial mechanics in mice before and after infarction using multislice displacement-encoded MRI with 3D motion encoding. Am J Physiol Heart Circ Physiol 2005; 288: H1491-H1497.

[47]   Zhong X, Helm PA, Epstein FH. Balanced multipoint displacement encoding for DENSE MRI. Magnetic Resonance in Medicine 2009; 61: 981-988.

[48]   Zhong X, Spottinswoode BS, Meyer CH, Kramer CM, Epstein FH. Imaging three-dimensional myocardial mechanics using navigator-gated volumetric spiral cine DENSE MRI. Magnetic Resonance in Medicine 2010; 64: 1089-1097.

[49]   Zhong X, Gibberman LB, Spottinswoode BS, Gilliam AD, Meyer CH, French BA, Epstein FH. Comprehensive cardiovascular magnetic resonance of myocardial mechanics in mice using three-dimensional cine DENSE. Journal of Cardiovascular Magnetic Resonance 2011; 13: 83.

[50]   Zhong J, Liu W, Yu X. Characterization of three-dimensional myocardial deformation in the mouse heart: An MR tagging study. Journal of Magnetic Resonance Imaging 2008; 27: 1263-1270.

[51]   Capecchi MR. The new mouse genetics: altering the genome by gene targeting. Trends Genet. 1989; 5(3): 70-6.

[52]   Capecchi MR. Altering the genome by homologous recombination. Science 1989; 244(4910): 1288-92.

[53]   Gregory SG, Sekhon M, Schein J, Zhao S, Osoegawak K, Scott CE, Evans RS, Burridge PW, Cox TV, Fox CA, Hutton RD, Mullenger IR, Phillips KJ, Smith J, Stalker J, Threadgold GJ, Birney E, Wylie K, Chinwalla A, Wallis J, Hillier L, Carter J, Gaige T, Jaeger S, Kremitzki C, Layman D, Maas J, McGrane R, Mead K, Walker R, Study of the Murine Cardiac Mechanical Function Using Magnetic Resonance Imaging: The Current Status, Challenges, and Future Perspectives 379 Jones S, Smith M, Asano J, Bosdet I, Chan S, Chittaranjan S, Chiu R, Fjell C, Fuhrmann D, Girn N, Gray C, Guin R, Hsiao L, Krzywinski M, Kutsche R, Sen Lee S, Mathewson C, McLeavy C, Messervier S, Ness S, Pandoh P, Prabhu A-L, Saeedi P, Smailus D, Spence L, Stott J, Taylor S, Terpstra W, Tsai M, Vardy J, Wye N, Yang G, Shatsman S, Ayodeji B, Geer K, Tsegaye G, Shvartsbeyn A, Gebregeorgis E, Krol M, Russell D, Overton L, Malek JA, Holmes M, Heaney M, Shetty J, Feldblyum T, Nierman WC, Catanesek JJ, Hubbard T, Waterston RH, Rogers J, de Jongk PJ, Fraser CM, Marra M, McPherson JD, Bentley DR. A Physical Map of the Mouse Genome. Nature 2002; 418: 743-750.

[54]   Collins FS, Green ED, Guttmacher AE, Guyer MS. A vision for the future of genomics research: A blueprint for the genomic era. Nature 2003; 422(6934): 835-847.

[55]   Ehmke H. Mouse gene targeting in cardiovascular physiology. Am J Physiol Regul Integr Comp Physiol 2003; 284: R28_R30.

[56]   Doevendans PA, Daemen MJ, de Muinck ED, Smits JR. Cardiovascular phenotyping in mice. Cardiovascular Research 1998; 39: 34-49.

[57]   Dawson TD. Engineering design of the cardiovascular system of mammals. Prentice Hall, 1991.

[58]   Constantinides C. Study of the murine cardiac mechanical function using magnetic resonance imaging: the current status, challenges, and future perspectives. Practical applications in Biomedical Engineering, Adriano O. Andrade, Adriano Alves Pereira, Eduardo L. M. Naves and Alcimar B. Soares (Ed.), ISBN: 978-953-51-0924-2, InTech, 2012.

[59]   Bucholz E, Ghaghada K, Qi Y, Mukundan S, Rockman H, Johnson GA. Cardiovascular phenotyping of the mouse heart using a 4D radial acquisition and liposomal Gd-DTPA-BMA. Magnetic Resonance in Medicine 2010; 63(4): 979-997.

[60]   Wiesmann F, Frydrychowicz A, Rautenberg J, Illinger R, Rommel E, Haase A, Neubauer S. Analysis of right ventricular function in healthy mice and a murine model of heart failure by *in vivo* MRI. Am J Physiol Heart Circ Physiol 2002; 283: H1065-H1071.

[61]   Henson RE, Song SK, Pastorek JS, Ackerman JJH, Lorenz CH. Left ventricular torsion is equal in mice and humans. Am J Physiol Circ Physiol 2000; 278: H1117-H1123.

[62] Epstein FH. MR in mouse models of cardiac disease. NMR in Biomedicine 2007; 20: 238-255.

[63] Zhou R, Pickup S, Glickson JD, Scott CH, Ferrari VA. Assessment of global and regional myocardial function in the mouse using cine and tagged MRI. Magnetic Resonance in Medicine 2003; 49(4): 760-764.

[64] Gilson WD, Yang Z, French BA, Epstein FH. Complementary displacement-encoded MRI for contrast enhanced infarct detection and quantification of myocardial function in mice. Magnetic Resonance in Medicine 2004; 51: 744-752.

[65] Constantinides C, Mean R, Janssen BJ. Effects of isoflurane anesthesia on the cardiovascular function of the C57BL/6 mouse. ILAR 2011; 52: e21-e31.

[66] Sato Y, Moriyama M, Hanayama M, Naito H, Tamura S. Acquiring 3D Models of Non-Rigid Moving Objects From Time and Viewpoint Varying Image Sequences: A Step Toward Left Ventricle Recovery. IEEE Transactions On Pattern Analysis And Machine Intelligence 1997; 19(3): 253-258.

[67] Frangi AF, Niessen WJ, Viergever MA. Three-dimensional modeling for functional analysis of cardiac images: a review. IEEE Trans Med Imaging 2001; 20: 2-25.

[68] Ranganath S. Contour extraction from cardiac MRI studies using snakes. IEEE Trans Med Imag 1995; 14(2): 328-338.

[69] Guttman MA, Zerhouni EA, McVeigh ER. Analysis of cardiac function from MR images. IEEE Comput Graph Appl 1997; 17: 30-38.

[70] Spottiswoode BS, Zhong X, Lorenz CH, Mayosi BM, Meintjes EM, Epstein FH. Motion-guided segmentation for cine DENSE MRI. Med Image Anal 2009; 13: 105-115.

[71] Papademetris X, Sinusas A, Dione D, Constable R, Duncan J. Estimating 3D left ventricular deformation from 3D medical image sequences using biomechanical models. IEEE Trans Med Imag 2002; 21 (7): 786-800.

[72] Lorenzo-Valdes M, Sanchez-Ortiz G, Elkington A, Mohiaddin R, Rueckert D. Segmentation of 4D cardiac MR images using a probabilistic atlas and the EM algorithm. Med Image Anal 2004; 8(3): 255-265.

[73] Lorenzo-Valdes M, Sanchez-Ortiz G, Mohiaddin R, Rueckert D. Atlas based segmentation and tracking of 3D cardiac MR images using non-rigid registration. In: Proceedings of Medical Image Computing and Computer- Assisted Intervention (MICCAI). LNCS 2002, Tokyo, Japan, pp. 642-650.

[74] Zhuang X, Hawkes D, Crum W, Boubertakh R, Uribe S, Atkinson D, Batchelor P, Schaeffter T, Razavi R, Hill D. Robust registration between cardiac MRI images and atlas for segmentation propagation. In: Society of Photo-Optical Instrumentation Engineers (SPIE) Conference, 2008, p. 691408.

[75] Perperidis D, Bucholz E, Johnson GA, Constantinides C. Morphological Studies of the Murine Heart Based on Probabilistic and Statistical Atlases. Computerized Graphics and Medical Imaging 2012; 36(2): 119-29.

[76] Petitjean C, Dacher JN. A review of segmentation methods in short axis cardiac MR images. Medical Image Analysis 2011; 15: 169-184.

[77] Huntley JM. Noise-immune phase unwrapping algorithm. Applied Optics 1989; 28(15): 3268-3270.

[78] Buckland JR, Huntley JM, Turner SRE. Unwrapping noisy phase maps by use of a minimum-cost-matching algorithm. Applied Optics 1995; 34(23): 5100-5108.

[79]   Chavez S, Xiang QS, An L. Understanding phase maps in MRI: A new cutline phase unwrapping method. IEEE Transactions on medical imaging 2002; 21(8): 966-977.

[80]   Gilliam AD, Epstein F, Acton ST. Cardiac motion recovery *via* active trajectory field models. IEEE Transactions Inf Technol Biomed 2009; 13(2): 226-235.

[81]   Spottiswoode BS, Zhong X, Hess AT, Kramer CM, Meintjes EM, Mayosi BM, Epstein FH. Tracking myocardial motion from cine DENSE images using spatiotemporal phase unwrapping and temporal fitting. IEEE Trans Med Imaging 2007; 26: 15-30.

[82]   Osman NF, McVeigh ER, Prince JL. Imaging heart motion using harmonic phase MRI. IEEE Trans Med Imaging 2000; 19: 186-202.

[83]   Bioucas-Dias JM, Valadao G. Phase unwrapping *via* graph cuts. LNCS 2005; 3522: 360-367.

[84]   Goldstein RM, Zebker HA, Werner CL. Satellite radar interferometry: Two-dimensional phase unwrapping. Radio Science 1988; 23(4): 713-720.

[85]   Kolmogorov V. What energy functions can be minimized *via* graph cuts? IEEE Transactions on Pattern Analysis and Machine Analysis 2004; 26(2): 147-159.

[86]   Wen H, Marsolo KA, Bennett EE, Lewis RP, Lipps DB, Epstein ND, Plehn JF, Croisille P. Adaptive postprocessing techniques for myocardial tissue tracking with displacement encoded MR Imaging. Radiology 2008; 246(1): 229-240.

[87]   Zhong X. Three-Dimensional Cine DENSE MRI. Ph.D. Thesis, University of Virginia, 2008.

[88]   Young A, Li B, Kirton RS, Cowan BR. Generalized spatiotemporal myocardial strain analysis for DENSE and SPAMM imaging. Magnetic Resonance in Medicine 2012; 67: 1590-1599.

[89]   Moore CC, Lugo-Olivieri CH, McVeigh ER, Zerhouni EA. Three-dimensional systolic strain patterns in the normal human left ventricle: characterization with tagged MR imaging. Radiology 2000; 214: 453-466.

[90]   Cerqueira MD, Weissman NJ, Dilsizian V, Jacobs AK, Kaul S, Laskey WK, Pennell DJ, Rumberger JA, Ryan T, Verani MS. Standardized myocardial segmentation and nomenclature for tomographic imaging of the heart: a statement for healthcare professionals from the cardiac imaging committee of the council on clinical cardiology of the American Heart Association. Circulation 2002; 105: 539-542.

[91]   Petitjean C, Rougon N, Cluzel P. Assessment of myocardial function: a review of quantification methods and results using tagged MRI. Journal of Cardiovascular Magnetic Resonance 2005; 7: 501-516.

[92]   Pai VM, Axel L. Advances in MRI tagging techniques for determining regional myocardial strain. Curr Cardiol Rep 2006; 8: 53-58.

[93]   Sigfridsson A, Haraldsson H, Ebbers T, Knutsson H, Sakuma H. Single breath-hold multi-slice DENSE MRI. Magnetic Resonance in Medicine 2010; 63: 1411-1411.

[94]   Hess AT, Zhong X, Spottinswoode BS, Epstein FH, Meintjes EM. Myocardial 3D strain calculation by combining Cine displacement encoding with Stimulated Echoes (DENSE) and Cine strain encoding (SENC) imaging. Magnetic Resonance in Medicine 2009; 62: 77-84.

[95]   Feng L, Donnino R, Babb J, Axel L, Kim D. Numerical and *in vivo* validation of fast cine displacement-encoded with stimulated echoes (DENSE) MRI for quantification of regional cardiac function. Magnetic Resonance in Medicine 2009; 62: 682-690.

[96]   Ashikaga H, Mickelsen SR, Ennis DB, Rodriguez I, Kellman P, Wen H, McVeigh ER. Electromechanical analysis of infarct border zone in chronic myocardial infarction. Am J Physiol Heart Circ Physiol 2005; 289: H1099-H1105.

[97]   Aletras AH, Tilak GS, Natanzon A, Hsu LY, Gonzalez FM, Hoyt RF, Arai AE. Retrospective determination of the area at risk for reperfused acute myocardial infarction with T2-weighted cardiac magnetic resonance imaging: histological and displacement encoding with stimulated echoes (DENSE) functional validations. Circulation 2006; 113: 1865-1870.

[98]   Spottinswoode BS, Russell JB, Moosa S, Meintjes EM, Epstein FH, Mayosi BM. Abnormal diastolic and systolic spetal motion following pericardietomy demonstrated by cine DENSE MRI. Cardiovasc J Afr 2008; 19: 208-209.

[99]   Auger DA, Zhong X, Epstein FH, Spottinswoode BS. Mapping right ventricular myocardial mechanics using 3D cine DENSE cardiovascular magnetic resonance. J Cardiovascular Magn Reson 2012; 14: 4. Doi: 10.1186/1532-429X-14-4.

[100]   Lin AP, Bennett E, Wisk LE, Gharib M, Fraser SE, Wen H. Circumferential strain in the wall of the common carotid artery: comparing displacement-encoded and cine MRI in volunteers. Magnetic Resonance in Medicine 2008; 60: 8-13.

[101]   Kolandaivelu A, Balaban RS. Quantitative evaluation of regional strain in mice using SPAMM tagging and DENSE. In: Proceedings of the 8th Annual Meeting of ISMRM, Denver 2000, p. 1610.

[102]   Young AA, French BA, Yang Z, Cowan BR, Gilson WD, Berr SS, Kramer CM, Epstein FH. Reperfused Myocardial Infraction in Mice: 3D Mapping of Late Gadolinium Enhancement and Strain. Journal of Cardiovascular Magnetic Resonance 2006; 8: 1-8.

[103]   Hankiewicz JH, Goldspink PH, Buttrick PM, Lewandowski ED. Principal strain changes precede ventricular wall thinning during transition to heart failure in a mouse model of dilated cardiomyopathy. American Journal of Physiology 2008; 294(1): H330-336.

[104]   Chuang JS, Zemljic-Harpf A, Ross RS, Frank LR, McCulloch AD, Omens JH. Determination of three-dimensional ventricular strain distributions in gene-targeted mice using tagged MRI. Magnetic Resonance in Medicine 2010; 64: 1281-1288.

[105]   Li W, Yu X. Quantification of myocardial strain at early systole in mouse heart: restoration of undeformed tagging grid with single-point HARP. J Magn Reson Imaging 2010; 32(3): 608-614.

[106]   van Nierop BJ, van Assen HC, van Deel ED, Niesen LB, Duncker DJ, Strijkers GJ, Nicolay K. Phenotyping of left and right ventricular function in mouse models of compensated hypertrophy and heart failure with cardiac MRI. PLoS One 2013; 8(2): e55424. Doi: 10.1371/journal.pone.0055424.Epub 2013.

[107]   Desjardins CL, Chen Y, Coulton AT, Hoit BD, Yu X, Stelzer JE. Cardiac myosin binding protein C insufficiency leads to early onset of mechanical dysfunction. Circ Cardiovasc Imaging 2012; 5: 127-136.

[108]   Vandsburger MH, French BA, Kramer CM, Zhong X, Epstein FH. Displacement-encoded and manganese-enhanced cardiac MRI reveal that nNOS, not eNOS, plays a dominant role in modulating contraction and calcium influx in the mammalian heart. American Journal of Physiology 2012; 302(2): H412-9. Soi: 10.1142/ajpheart.00705.2011.

[109]   Young A, Kramer C, Ferrari V, Axel L, Reichek N. Three-dimensional left ventricular deformation in hypertrophic cardiomyopathy. Circulation 1994; 90: 854-867.

[110] Holt JP, Rhode EA, Kines H. Ventricular volumes and body weight in mammals. Am J of Physiology 1968; 215(3): 704-715.

[111] Weinberg PD, Ethier CR. Twenty-fold difference in hemodynamic wall shear stress between murine and human aortas. J Biomech 2007; 40(7): 1594-1598.

[112] Healy L, Jiang Y, Hsu EW. Quantitative comparison of myocardial fiber structure between mice, rabbit, and sheep using diffusion tensor cardiovascular magnetic resonance. Journal of Cardiovascular Magnetic Resonance 2011; 13: 74.

[113] Dobson GP, Headrick JP. Bioenergetic scaling: Metabolic design and body-size constraints in mammals. Proc. Natl. Acad. Sci. USA 1995; 92: 7317-7321.

[114] Nielsen KS, Larimer JL. Oxygen Dissociation Curves of Mammalian Blood in Relation to Body Size. Am. J. Physiol. 1958; 195(2): 424-428.

[115] Phillips D, Covian R, Aponte A, Glancy B, Taylor JF, Chess D, Balaban RS. Regulation of oxidative phosphorylation complex activity: effects of tissue specific metabolic stress within an allometric series and acute changes in workload. Am J Physiol Regul Integr Comp Physiol. 2012; 302(9): R1034-48.

[116] Rademakers FE, Rogers WJ, Guier WH, Hutchins GM, Siu CO, Weisfeldt ML, Weiss JL, Shapiro EP. Relation of regional cross-fiber shortening to wall thickening in the intact heart. Three-dimensional strain analysis by NMR tagging. Circulation 1994; 89: 1174-1182.

[117] Soleimanifard S, Abd-Elmoniem KZ, Sasano T, Agarwal HK, Abraham MR, Abraham TP, Prince JL. Three-dimensional regional strain analysis in porcine myocardial infarction: a 3T magnetic resonance tagging study. Journal of Cardiovascular Magnetic Resonance 2012; 14: 85.

[118] Abd-Elmoniem KZ, Tomas MS, Sasano T, Soleimanifard S, Vonken E-JP, Youssef A, Agarwal H, Dimaano VL, Calkins H, Stuber M, Prince JL, Abraham TP, Abraham MR. Assessment of distribution and evolution of mechanical dyssynchrony in a porcine model of myocardial infarction by cardiovascular magnetic resonance. Journal of Cardiovascular Magnetic Resonance 2012; 14: 1.

[119] Guccione JM, Walker JC, Beitler JR, Moonly SM, Zhang P, Guttman MA, Ozturk C, McVeigh ER, Wallace AW, Saloner DA, Ratcliffe MB. The effect of anteroapical aneurysm plication on end-systolic three dimensional strain in the sheep: A magnetic resonance imaging tagging study. J Thorac Cardiovasc Surg 2006; 131(3): 579-586.e3.

[120] Zhang P, Guccione JM, Nicholas SI, Walker JC, Crawford PC, Shamal A, Acevedo-Bolton G, Guttman MA, Ozturk C, McVeigh ER, Saloner DA, Wallace AW, Ratcliffe MB. Endoventricular patch plasty for dyskinetic anteroapical left ventricular aneurysm increases systolic circumferential shortening in sheep. J Thorac Cardiovasc Surg 2007; 134(4): 1017-1024.

[121] Russell IK, Gotte MJ, Kuijer JP, Marcus JT. Regional assessment of left ventricular torsion by CMR tagging. Journal of Cardiovascular Magnetic Resonance 2008; 10: 26.

[122] Clark N, Reichek N, Bergey P, Hoffman E, Brownson D, Palmon L, Axel L. Circumferential myocardial shortening in the normal human left ventricle: assessment by magnetic resonance imaging using spatial modulation of magnetization. Circulation 1991; 84: 67-74.

[123] Allouche C, Makram-Ebeid S, Ayache N, Delingette H. A new kinetic modeling scheme for the human left ventricle wall motion analysis with MR-tagging imaging. In: Katila T, Magnin I, Clarysse P, Montagnat J, Nenonen J, eds. Functional Imaging and Modeling of

the Heart (FIMH'01). Lecture Notes in Computer Science, Helsinki, Finland, 2001; 2230: 61-68.

[124] Bogaert J, Rademakers F. Regional nonuniformity of normal adult human left ventricle. Am J Physiol, Heart Circ Physiol 2001; 280: 610-620.

[125] Kuijer J, Marcus J, Gtte M, van Rossum A, Heethaar R. Three dimensional myocardial strains at end-systole and during diastole in the left ventricle of normal humans. Journal of Cardiovascular Magnetic Resonance 2002; 4(3): 341-351.

[126] Moore CC, McVeigh ER, Zerhouni EA. Quantitative Magnetic Resonance Imaging of the Normal Human Left Ventricle. Topics in Magnetic Resonance Imaging 2000; 11(6): 359-371.

Send Orders for Reprints to reprints@benthamscience.net

CHAPTER 8

Mapping Myocardial Fiber Structure Using Diffusion Tensor Imaging

Osama Abdullah, Arnold David Gomez, Christopher L. Welsh and Edward Hsu[*]

Department of Bioengineering, University of Utah, Utah, USA

Abstract: Understanding of the structural-functional relationships of the heart, in both normal and diseased states, is not complete without incorporating precise knowledge of the underlying tissue microstructure, in terms of myocyte organization and orientation. By probing the effects on the diffusion of water molecules exerted by their microscopic environment, magnetic resonance diffusion tensor imaging (MR-DTI, or DTI for short) has emerged as a promising alternative to conventional histology for mapping fiber organization in ordered tissues such as the myocardium. In this chapter, the basic principles and recent advances in mapping myocardial structure using DTI are reviewed. Instances when DTI has advanced the understanding of the functional-structural relationship in the heart are also highlighted.

Keywords: Diffusion-weighted MRI, diffusion tensor imaging (DTI), helix angle, sheet angle, fractional anisotropy, mean diffusivity, tractography, myocardium, left ventricle, right handed fibers, left handed fibers, circumferential fibers, motion effects, ischemic disease, non-ischemic disease, hypertrophic cardiomyopathy, dyssynchronous heart failure.

INTRODUCTION

The intricate organization of the cardiac microstructure is a key determinant in the remarkably orchestrated atrial and ventricular activities. For example, each cardiac myocyte conducts an electrical impulse, contracts at the appropriate moment, at the right speed, and to the necessary extent [1]. The arrangement of the ventricular myocytes is involved in coordinating systolic contraction, in such ways that the efficiencies of blood ejection and fiber strain distribution are maximized [2]. Because electrical impulses propagate faster parallel to the main axis cardiomyocytes than perpendicular to them [3], mapping myofiber

*Address correspondence to Edward Hsu: Department of Bioengineering, University of Utah, Utah, USA; Tel: 801-585-7550; Fax: 801-587-8357; E-mail: edward.hsu@utah.edu

orientation is an essential element for understanding the structural-functional relationship not only in the normal heart, but also in disease conditions.

Over time, several conceptual and theoretical models have been proposed for different aspects of the heart incorporating progressively sophisticated interpretations of fiber structures made available by advancing technologies [4] (and references therein). Examples in cardiac biomechanics included constitutive modeling of tissue as an elastic material [5] and holistic understanding of the heart as a pump [1,6,7]. Experimental observations, like mechanical testing of myocardial tissue have shown that mechanical properties are dependent of tissue microstructure, in particular, fiber orientation, lamination (*i.e.*, sheet-like formation of fibers) and the associated arrangement of the extracellular matrix. To reach physiologically relevant results from the application of these models, both, information on tissue geometry and anisotropic tissue properties are necessary [8]. Similar requirements are related to modeling of cardiac tissue electrophysiology [9], including simulation of electrical propagation. It is well established that electrical conductivities of cardiac tissues are anisotropic [3,10] and that those are determined by tissue microstructure, in particular, the local orientation [11] and apparent laminar structure of cardiac fibers [12]. In general, anisotropic description of tissue properties is a crucial component for electro-mechanical modeling of the heart [13]. Electro-mechanical applications require the integrative modeling of electrical activation, force development, and mechanical deformation based on anisotropic tissue properties. Likewise, anisotropic cardiac tissue properties have been used to produce comprehensive models seeking to provide explanations for the basic mechanisms for ventricular contraction, expansion, and torsion [14], or to explain the nature of myocardial fiber arrangement [15,16].

By quantifying the effects on the translational motility of water molecules exerted by the microscopic environment, magnetic resonance diffusion tensor imaging (MR-DTI, or DTI for short) [17] has emerged as a unique, noninvasive and nondestructive alternative to histology for characterizing myocardial tissue microstructure. DTI yields information on the diffusion anisotropy, in terms of both its direction and magnitude, which can be used to elucidate the nature of the organization, geometry and content of the tissue. In this chapter, we will provide the basics of DTI theory, and summarize the latest progress that has been reported in relating the radiological findings provided by DTI to the known structural changes in cardiac disease, such ischemic or non-ischemic heart failure.

EARLIER OBSERVATIONS OF CARDIAC FIBER STRUCTURE

Structural observations have been associated with fundamental changes in our understanding of the heart as an organ from the early days of the study of anatomy and physiology. An early example came about in 1664, when Niels Stensen published comparative observations between dissections of cardiac and skeletal muscle tissues, both which resembled each other by their fibrous appearance, thus allowing the identification of the heart as a muscle [18]. As more detailed observations became documented, the fundamental tool used to identify transmural variations of myocardial tissue orientation *i.e.*, gross dissection of excised hearts (Lower *et al.* [19]), became insufficient for microstructural analysis and was aided by microscopes [20,21]. Ever since, analysis of cardiac microstructure in terms of fiber organization is often linked to the available technology.

Histological sections provided quantifiable investigations that allowed modeling of the heart, so that fiber orientation could be modeled and predicted by a mathematical formula, and to explain quantifiable differences between man and other species [11,22-24]. Specifically, Streeter and others observed that the sub-epicardial layer contains myofibers pointing "downward" toward the apex. The sub-endocardial layer contains myofibers pointing "upwards" toward the base of the heart. And the mid-wall fibers run circumferentially parallel to the heart equator. This unique fiber orientation patterns provided the basis to coin the term "double helical fiber structure" of the heart [22]. The sub-endocardial layer was assigned a positive helix angle, which is referred to as the right handed fibers (RHF). The sub-epicardial layer was assigned a negative helix angle, and referred to as the left handed fibers (LHF). And the mid-wall layer was referred to as the circumferential fibers (CF), because the fibers in this layer mostly run parallel to the cardiac short axis.

Cardiac modeling and the development of structure-function theories continues to be an active area of research today [4], and the adoption of a comprehensive heart model is still controversial [1,6,7,16]. The introduction of digital image processing permitted more comprehensive analysis of histology, which sometimes included the use of volumetric statistics [25-28]. Likewise, more sophisticated optical methods like electron microscopy were later used to observe intermediate structures like myocardial sheets [12], and more recently, subcellular organization with the use of confocal microscopy [29].

The advent of radiological imaging has allowed noninvasive and nondestructive quantification of the myocardial fiber structure, which is highly desirable for preserving valuable samples or for evaluating the tissue *in vivo*. Specific techniques include X-ray diffraction [30,31], contrast-enhanced computer tomography [32] and MRI. The latter, stands alone in terms of soft tissue sensitivity and safety considerations, and can provide fiber orientation information *via* either susceptibility mapping [33] or diffusion tensor imaging (DTI) [34-38]. Recent technological advances like *in vivo* DTI [39-42] hold the potential to not only improve the general understanding of cardiac structure and function, but also to provide subject-specific modeling of normal and diseased hearts.

BASICS OF DIFFUSION MRI

Diffusion refers to the random displacement of water molecules due to their thermal energy, also referred to as Brownian motion. It is important to distinguish diffusion from other transport mechanisms such as coherent blood flow in vessels. In statistical sense, the average displacement along a given axis in space, $\langle r \rangle$, of diffusing water molecules is related to the diffusion coefficient, D (in mm^2/s), *via* the Einstein's equation:

$$\langle r \rangle = \sqrt{2D\Delta} \quad \ldots \tag{1}$$

where Δ is the diffusion time. The diffusion coefficient D is typically slower in biological tissues compared to free water due to the obstructions imposed by tissue microstructure (*e.g.,* cell membranes, fibers, *etc.*).

The effect of diffusion on the magnetic resonance signal has been observed and quantified well before the invention of the MRI scanner [43,44]. Stejskal and Tanner proposed the pulsed-field-gradient (PFG) preparation to measure diffusion [45]. In the PFG preparation shown in Fig. (**1**), suppose a unit MRI signal (called "spin") at an initial position r_1 experiences a short diffusion-weighting gradient pulse, and the same spin randomly moves to location r_2 at some duration Δ (referred to as diffusion time) later when it experiences a second gradient pulse of equal amplitude but opposite polarity to the first. The net phase ϕ_{net} imparted on the spin will be proportional to its relative displacement $(r_2 - r_1)$ given by:

$$\phi_{net} = -\gamma G \cdot (r_2 - r_1) \, \delta \ \ldots \tag{2}$$

where γ is the gyromagnetic ratio for the spin (hydrogen for most DTI applications), G and δ are the amplitude and widths of the diffusion encoding gradient pulses, respectively. Note that the direction of G dictates the axis in which diffusion motion is measured - for example, G_x will encode water displacements in the x direction only.

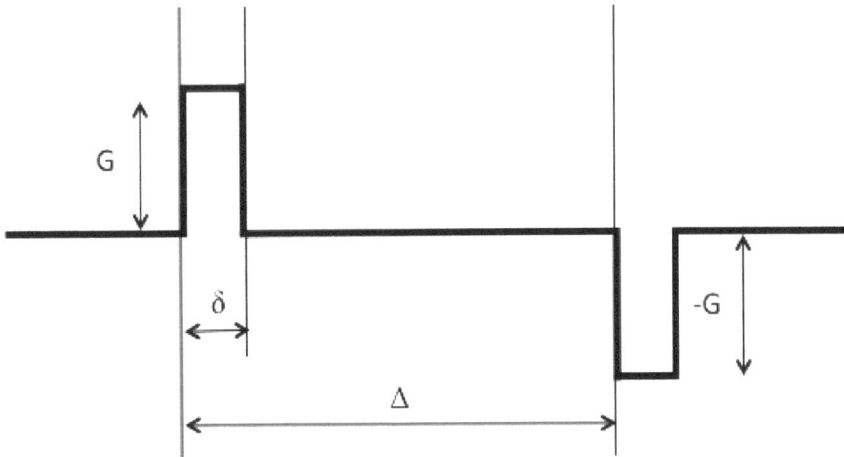

Figure 1: Pulsed field gradient preparation as proposed by Stejskal and Tanner [45].

The Brownian translational motion of spins due to diffusion is a random process that is subject to the conditional probability density function P specified by a normal distribution with a standard deviation indicated by equation (1). The detected MRI signal after PFG preparation can be obtained by calculating the expected value of the phase dispersion for an ensemble of spins over the probability density function according to:

$$I = I_0 \int exp(i\phi_{net}) P(r_2 | r_1) d\phi \quad \dots \tag{3}$$

where I_0 is the diffusion-independent image intensity. The solution of the above equation for isotropic case can be expressed as [45]:

$$I = exp\left(-\gamma^2 G^2 \delta^2 \left(\Delta - \frac{\delta}{3}\right) D\right) \quad \dots \tag{4}$$

Equation (4) is often rewritten as

$$I = I_0 exp(-bD) \tag{5}$$

$$\text{with } b = \gamma^2 G^2 \delta^2 \left(\Delta - \frac{\delta}{3}\right) \quad \dots$$

Equation (5) conveniently separates the exponent into an intrinsic tissue property term, D, and a single parameter, the so-called diffusion-weighting b factor (typically expressed in units of s/mm^2), that combines all the MRI prescription variables. Equation (5) states that the effect of diffusion manifests as attenuation of the image intensity, which behaves inverse-exponentially with respect to both the diffusivity and the applied diffusion encoding gradient parameters.

MRI of Anisotropic Diffusion

Diffusion in an anisotropic medium will manifest in directionally dependent Brownian motion. Axons, ligaments, and muscle fibers are all example of anisotropic tissues, which impose a preferential direction for diffusing water molecules, where, one would intuitively expect that water diffusion will be more free and faster along the direction of the fibers but is more hindered and slower across the fibers. The orientation-dependent behavior gives rise to the anisotropic diffusion property probed in DTI. In a PFG preparation, when the diffusion encoding gradient is applied parallel to the fibers, the image intensity I in Equation (5) will contain higher diffusion contribution than in the case when the encoding gradient is applied perpendicular to the fibers. Higher diffusion contribution in certain direction translates to higher attenuation in signal intensity. Fig. (**2**) illustrates the anisotropic diffusion behavior in a perfused guinea pig heart. Fig. (**2a**) is an anatomical image without diffusion weighting, while Fig. (**2b, c**) are diffusion-weighted images showing different contrasts due to the different diffusion encoding direction in each case.

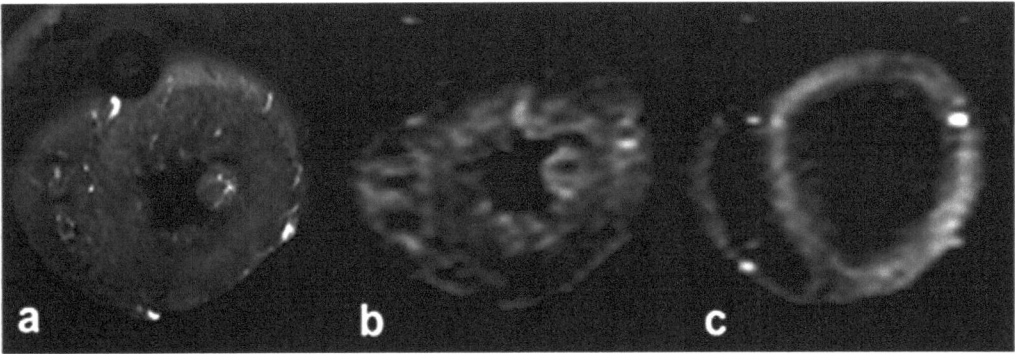

Figure 2: Anisotropic diffusion contrast in a perfused guinea pig heart. (**a**) anatomical gradient-echo image without diffusion weighting. Diffusion-weighted image (b = 500 s/mm^2) with diffusion encoding gradient applied in left-right direction (**b**), and in-out of page (**c**). Animal procedures were conducted with protocols approved by the Institutional Animal Care and Use Committee at the University of Utah.

Anisotropic diffusion in 3D space cannot be fully characterized by a single diffusion coefficient. Instead, a tensor, appropriately called diffusion tensor, is required [17]. The MRI signal of spins diffusing in an anisotropic medium can be explained by considering the special case where the principal axes of diffusion of certain anisotropic tissue have diffusivities D_1, D_2, and D_3 along the three orthogonal principal directions (in descending order), and that diffusion is encoded along the same direction as the principal diffusivities *via* the diffusion encoding gradients $G(t)$. If the encoding gradients have identical timings and only differ in their directions, then $G(t)$ can be written as:

$$G(t) = \begin{bmatrix} G_1(t) \\ G_2(t) \\ G_3(t) \end{bmatrix} = \boldsymbol{u} \cdot \|\boldsymbol{G}(t)\| = \begin{bmatrix} u_1 \\ u_2 \\ u_3 \end{bmatrix} \cdot \|\boldsymbol{G}(t)\| \qquad \ldots \qquad (6)$$

where u is a unit vector defining the direction of the encoding gradients (which coincides with principal diffusion axis). Following the notation of Equation (4), the signal intensity satisfies:

$$I = I_0 \exp\left(-bu^T \cdot \begin{bmatrix} D_1 & 0 & 0 \\ 0 & D_2 & 0 \\ 0 & 0 & D_3 \end{bmatrix} \cdot u\right) = I_0 \exp(-bu^T \cdot D_\Lambda \cdot u) \quad \ldots \tag{7}$$

where the effective diffusivity can be defined as: $D_{eff} = u^T \cdot D_\Lambda \cdot u$.

Now let's generalize the special case introduced in Equation (6) and (7) when the diffusion encoding gradients direction g does not coincide with the principal diffusion axis, the former can be translated to the principal diffusion axis *via* a rotation matrix R, such that: $u = Rg$. Then, Equation (7) becomes:

$$I = I_0 \exp(-b\, g^T R^T \cdot D_\Lambda \cdot R\, g) = I_0 \exp(-b\, g^T \cdot D \cdot g) \quad \ldots \tag{8}$$

where $D = R^T \cdot D_\Lambda \cdot R$ corresponds to the diffusion tensor. The diffusion tensor is a symmetric, 2nd rank tensor, containing 6 independent elements, 3 describing the magnitude and another 3 describing the principal direction of diffusion.

Although Equation (8) provides a convenient and intuitive link between the MRI signal and the principal diffusion directions, it does not take into account the effect of the co-called gradient cross terms [17]. A more general expression for the diffusion tensor formalism can be written as:

$$I = I_0 \exp\left(-\sum_{i=x,y,z} \sum_{j=x,y,z} b_{ij} D_{ij}\right) \quad \ldots \tag{9}$$

where x,y,z represent the laboratory frame of reference. In Equation (9), the diffusion tensor can be written in a matrix form as:

$$D = \begin{pmatrix} D_{xx} & D_{xy} & D_{xz} \\ D_{xy} & D_{yy} & D_{yz} \\ D_{xz} & D_{yz} & D_{zz} \end{pmatrix} \quad \ldots. \tag{10}$$

And b_{ij} is the b-matrix [17] which can be calculated according to:

$$b = \gamma^2 \int_0^{TE} \left[\left(\int_0^t G(t')dt' \right)^T \left(\int_0^t G(t')dt' \right) \right] dt \quad \ldots \tag{11}$$

and G is an arbitrary time-varying diffusion-weighting vector of any orientation:

$$G(t) = [G_x(t), G_y(t), G_z(t)] \quad \ldots \tag{12}$$

Regardless on whether Equation (8) or (9) is used, the typical DTI experiment consists of acquiring series of diffusion-weighted MRI scans with diffusion encoding gradients encoded along at least six non-collinear directions. Estimation of the diffusion tensor is usually performed on a voxel-by-voxel basis, *via* appropriate curve fitting of the observed signals to the signal attenuation equation. The estimated diffusion tensor in Equation (10) bears little use for inferring the tissue microstructure, since the relevant information is embedded in the tensor elements. Hence, the concept of "diffusion ellipsoid" has been proposed [17] to simplify the interpretation of the diffusion tensor. The diffusion ellipsoid is a 3-dimensional representation of the displacement profile covered in space by diffusing molecules during the diffusion time Δ [46]. The principal axes of the diffusion ellipsoid can be calculated by performing eigenvalue decomposition of Equation (10) where the diffusion tensor gets converted into a product between a diagonal matrix of its eigenvalues (D_1, D_2, and D_3) and transformation (or rotation) matrix consisting of its eigenvectors (e_1, e_2, and e_3). The eigenvalues and the eigenvectors of the diffusion tensor correspond to the diffusivities as observed along the principal axes of diffusion ellipsoid and the orientations of its axes, respectively. The central premise of DTI is that the direction in which water diffusion is the fastest, which is the eigenvector of the largest diffusion tensor eigenvalue, coincides with the local tissue fiber orientation.

To make the derived eigenvalues from the diffusion tensor more intuitive, the diffusion tensor eigenvalues are commonly used to compute the mean diffusivity (MD) and fractional anisotropy (FA) index, given by:

$$MD = (D_1 + D_2 + D_3) / 3 \quad \ldots \tag{13}$$

$$FA = \sqrt{\frac{3}{2}} \sqrt{\frac{(D_1 - MD)^2 + (D_2 - MD)^2 + (D_3 - MD)^2}{D_1^2 + D_2^2 + D_3^2}} \qquad \ldots \qquad (14)$$

where D_1, D_2, D_3 represent the eigenvalues of the DT matrix (in descending order).

Mathematically, the MD is proportional to the average diffusion in the 3 principal axes. FA measures the fraction of the diffusion tensor that can be ascribed to anisotropic diffusion [46]. FA varies between 0 (isotropic diffusion) and 1 (infinite anisotropy). Lower FA values can be found in isotropic media (*e.g.,* free water in a beaker), whereas progressively higher FA reflects higher diffusion anisotropy (*e.g.,* brain white matter). In practice, MD and FA have the feature of being rotationally invariant, *i.e.,* do not depend on the orientations of the diffusion principal axes. This renders FA and MD as a convenient quantitative metrics that capture the overall magnitude of diffusion and the degree of diffusion anisotropy, respectively. Fig. (**3**) shows MD and FA pixel maps of a healthy human heart specimen.

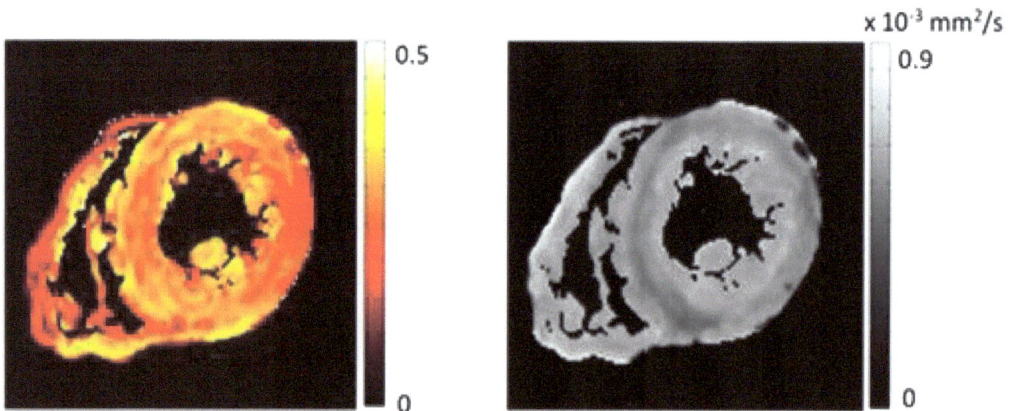

Figure 3: Pixel maps of Fractional Anisotropy (left) and Mean Diffusivity (right) obtained from a healthy human heart specimen. This study was approved by the Institutional Review Board at the University of Utah. Informed consent was obtained from all participating subjects.

DTI ASSESSMENT OF MYOCARDIAL STRUCTURE

The anisotropy and orientation of cardiomyocytes make the heart an excellent candidate for diffusion MRI techniques. Indeed, the first report documenting cardiac fiber mapping using DTI was published soon after DTI was introduced by Basser *et al.* [17]. In 1994, Garrido *et al.* [34] reported the detection of the known myocardial helical pattern in perfused rat heart by DTI, demonstrating the potential for utilizing DTI as a nondestructive technique to characterize the 3-dimensional myocardial fiber architecture.

Validation of DTI for Myocardial Fiber Orientation Mapping

As stated above, the main premise in DTI mapping of myocardial fiber structure is that the direction of fastest observed water diffusion (*i.e.*, the primary eigenvector of the diffusion tensor) coincides with local fiber orientation. Histological correlation studies performed in freshly excised [36], perfused [37], and formalin fixed [38] myocardium provided strong support for the premise.

Hsu *et al.* [36] correlated local fiber angle measurements obtained from DTI and histology, on a pixel-by-pixel basis, in a freshly excised specimen from the right ventricle of dog heart. Expanding on Hsu's study, Scollan *et al.* [37] used a perfused rabbit heart model to quantify and correlate DTI fiber orientation mapping with histology. Not only Scollan's study reaffirmed the findings by Hsu - that primary eigenvector obtained from DTI correlates closely with histological measures in the left ventricle, but they also demonstrated this correlation when the heart was perfused at physiologic conditions. Holmes *et al.* subsequently correlated the principal eigenvector obtained from DTI to histology in fixed rabbit hearts and reported less than 4° difference between fiber angles measured from DTI and histology. The latter two studies suggest that neither physiologic perfusion nor tissue fixation adversely impacted the accuracy of fiber orientation mapping using DTI.

Sheet Structure Mapping *via* DTI

In 1995, LeGrice *et al.* [12] proposed that the ventricular myocardium is further organized into laminar substructures, referred to as sheets, or "sheetlets" as they do not form continuous structure traversing the whole heart [47]. The sheetlet planes are approximately 4-5 cardiomyocyte thick, with the myocytes in each sheet tightly coupled with a collagen network, while the adjacent sheets loosely connected to allow for slippage [12, 48]. However, because the initial study was performed on fixed myocardium which was susceptible to artifacts (*e.g.,* shrinkage) related to the preparation, the existence of laminar structure (or sheets) has been debated by some researchers [1]. Nevertheless, several cardiac DTI reports have linked the tertiary (smallest) eigenvector of the DTI matrix to the normal of the sheet plane [37,47-49]. Scollan *et al.* [37] suggested that the secondary and tertiary eigenvector of the diffusion tensor form a systematic pattern similar to the sheet structure proposed by Le Grice [12]. Scollan suggested that the sheet planes lay horizontally in the LV mid-wall and become more vertically oriented at the epicardium and endocardium.

Tseng *et al.* [48] utilized optical images of inked prints obtained directly from the cut face of bovine heart specimens. The authors claimed that their inking method allows for DTI fiber mapping and the cleavage orientations in fresh specimens to be acquired under identical conditions, which minimizes the possibility of alterations of the tissue integrity between modalities (optical *vs* DTI). Together, although the supporting evidence is not as direct and unequivocal as the case of fiber orientation, results of cardiac DTI studies to date are consistent with the notion that the secondary and tertiary diffusion tensor eigenvectors respectively correspond to the orientation and the normal to the myocardial sheets.

DTI as Function of the Cardiac Cycle

It is accepted that blood is ejected by the heart mainly *via* the contraction of its cardiomyocytes. However, the increase in cardiomyocyte diameter during contraction accounts for only 20% of the observed systolic wall thickening [12], which suggests that the dynamically changing hierarchical organization of the myocardium also plays an important role. DTI can provide unique insights on the states of the fiber and sheet rearrangement during contraction. Although different groups attempted to conduct DTI at different points in the cardiac cycle [40, 50, 51], probably the most comprehensive investigation of myofiber rearrangement dynamics using DTI so far was the report by Hales *et al.* [47]. The authors imaged the same perfused heart (of a normal rat) at relaxed and contracted states. As shown in Fig. (**4**), the authors reported higher right-handed fibers percentage (in the endocardial wall) and lower left-handed fibers percentage (in the epicardial wall) in contracture state. They also suggested that the sheet angles follow a similar pattern of that demonstrated by Scollan [37] - in which the sheet planes at relaxed state lay parallel to the equatorial axis in the mid-wall, and become vertically orientated at the epi- and endocardial walls. Further, they also showed that the sheet angles rearrangement follows an accordion-like behavior in contracture state, in which the sheet planes become more vertically orientated (especially in the mid-wall) at contracture as shown in Fig. (**4b**). This study elegantly proposed a mechanism in which an accordion-like rearrangement of sheets combined with inter-sheet slippage can contribute to ventricular deformation, including centripetal wall-thickening (*i.e.*, toward the center of the LV cavity) and baso-apical shortening.

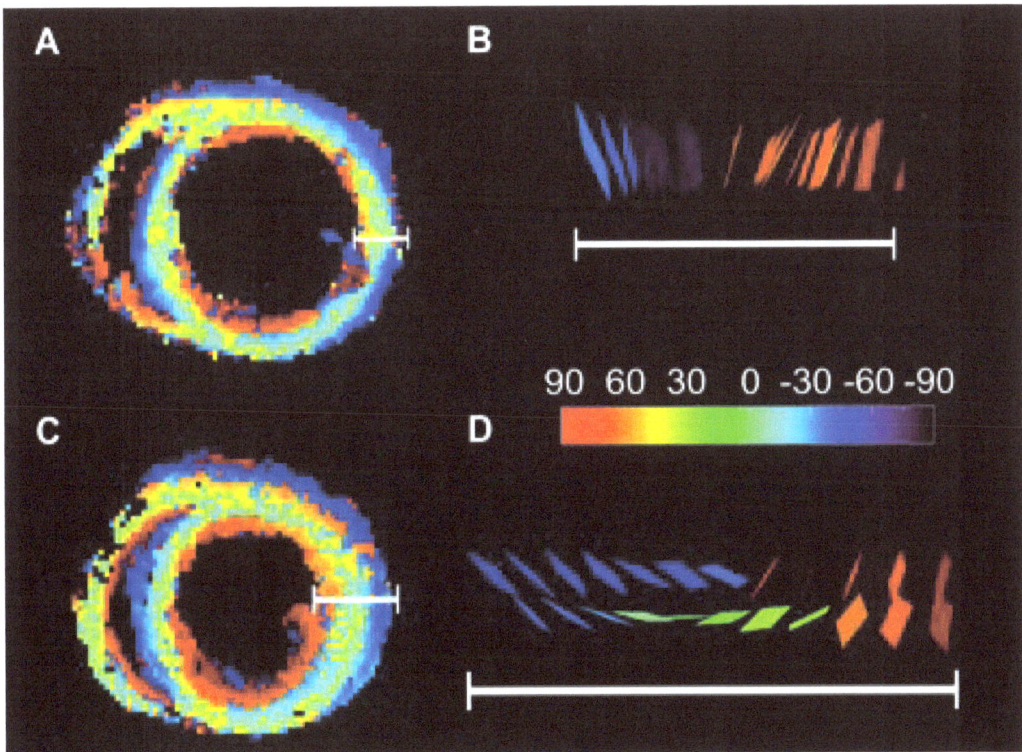

Figure 4: Helix angle maps of relaxed (**A**) and contracted states (**C**). Helix angles are represented by the color bar. Color-coded rectangles on the right represent profiles of sheet arrangement in the transmural direction (taken from the white-bars) in relaxed (**B**) and contracted states (**D**). The sheet angles in B and D were calculated as the planes perpendicular to the smallest eigenvector obtained from the diffusion tensor. Reprinted from Hales *et al.* [47]; with permission from Elsevier.

Cardiac DTI in Mammalian Species

To date, DTI has been used to characterize the fiber structure of normal hearts in several small and large animal species, including mouse, rat, rabbit, sheep, dog, in addition to human [34,51-54]. Despite differences in mammalian hearts, the general myocardial fiber architecture detected by DTI displays high degree of general similarity among different species, albeit there also exist important differences. Healy *et al.* [55] compared the helix angle between mouse, rabbit and sheep. As shown in Fig. (**5**), although all three species showed the well-known counterclockwise rotation of the fiber helix angle in the LV, the range of endocardial to epicardial helix angle was significantly different among the species. The structural differences exist among hearts at least from animals of different sizes, suggesting caution is needed when extrapolating myocardial structures from one species to another in, for example, myocardial functional modeling studies.

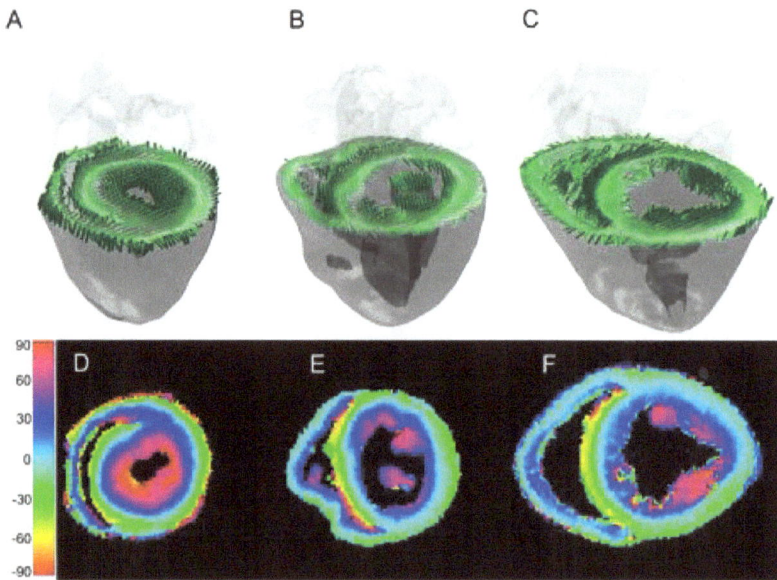

Figure 5: Myocardial fiber orientation in mouse (**A**, **D**), rabbit (**B**, **E**), and sheep (**C**, **F**). Top row shows cylindrical rods rendering of the fiber structure, while the bottom row show the color-coded helix angle map on pixel-by-pixel basis in short axis configuration. The color bar on the left reports angles in degrees. Despite similarities of helix angle across species, significant differences exist in the range of fiber rotation from endocardium to epicardium. Figure obtained from Healy *et al.* [55] with permission.

Applications in Cardiac Pathology

DTI has also been utilized to study cardiac pathologies in humans and animals for ischemic and non-ischemic cardiac disease, both *in vivo* and *ex vivo* [56-63]. The main parameters that have been reported are the scalar DTI parameters (especially FA and MD), and myocardial fiber orientation (helix and sheet angles).

For ischemic disease in animal models and humans, nearly all studies reported a decrease in FA and increase in MD in the infarcted myocardium compared to remote, unaffected normal regions of the same heart or to healthy control group [57, 59-62]. One infarcted mouse heart study reported the opposite trend in the infarct zone (*i.e.*, lower MD and higher FA in infarct zone depending on heart extraction time post myocardial infarction) [64].

The known helical pattern in the infarct and remote zones retains its general behavior (*i.e.*, endocardium has positive right-handed helix fiber angles, denoted as RHF, and the epicardium has negative left-handed helix fiber angles, denoted as LHF). Most studies reported higher fiber angular deviation in the infarct compared to remote zone or in normal subjects. The fiber angular deviation was defined as the standard deviation of the helix angles in selected ROIs and used as a metric for the local fiber disarray. For example, a rat infarct model by Chen *et al.* [56] reported higher angular deviation in the infarcted myocardium and correlated the measurements from DTI with histology. Chen's finding was supported by Wu *et al.* [59] who reported in an infarcted porcine model higher angular deviation and lower helix angle range (defined as sub-endocardial minus sub-epicardial helix angle) in the infarct zone. Another study by Wu *et al.* [61] of infarcted porcine model reported lower RHF and higher LHF in the infarct and remote zones, which the authors referred to as "left-handed shift of fibers around the infarct zone".

In vivo DTI in human patients with acute myocardial infarction [58] and a follow up study on chronic infarct [60] was performed on the same subjects. In these human studies, the RHF percentage was decreased while the LHF increased in the infarct zone. Interestingly, these studies also reported that the opposite trend occur in the remote zone (*i.e.*, increase in RHF and reduction in LHF in remote zone)

[58], which is contrary to the porcine heart infarct study (in the remote zone) [61]. The authors hypothesized that compensatory responses affected the RHF and LHF in the remote and infarct zones such that the overall (LHF+RHF)/CF (where CF refers to mid-wall circumferential fibers percentage) would remain constant [58]. Collectively, a major finding [58, 60, 61] is that the sub-endocardial RHF is implicated in the remodeling and healing process in the infarcted heart, and this notion was supported by non-DTI studies (*e.g.,* [65]).

Recently, Mekkaoui *et al.* [62] expanded on the conventional region-of-interest-based analyses by utilizing statistical approach to characterize the 3D helical fiber architecture in the full left ventricle. Mekkaoui utilized tractography-based helix angle classification and introduced the tractography coherence index, and applied this approach to study normal human, normal rat, and normal and infarcted sheep hearts [62]. Since this approach eliminated the subjectivity of selecting ROIs in heart, and treated the heart fiber structure as a continuum, to date this study seems to be the most robust study for fiber angle analysis in the heart. In the infarcted sheep myocardium, Mekkaoui [62] confirmed some of the finding reported in the previous ischemic human studies [59, 61], in which the LHF decreased in the remote zone, and he also showed that remodeling in the remote zone implicate all layers (endocardium, epicardium, and mid-wall).

DTI has also been applied to study cardiac remodeling in the non-ischemic heart disease, such as the dyssynchronous heart failure [57], and in hypertrophic cardiomyopathy [63]. Helm *et al.* [57] used a canine heart model of dyssynchronous heart failure and performed 3D DTI acquisition on the excised specimens. In diseased hearts, they reported regional reduction in wall thickness (septal, anterior, and posterior), but not in the lateral wall. They showed that the regional differences in the wall thickness were associated with rearrangement of sheet angles, whereas the septal wall became more vertically oriented compared to the lateral wall. The authors hypothesized that vertically oriented sheet angles could explain the reduction of wall thickness in the septal wall. Because electrical propagation in myocytes favors the direction along the main fiber axis [3], the authors speculated that vertically-oriented sheet angles may be responsible for hindering the transmural electrical propagation, which may explain the observed dyssynchrony in certain segments of the diseased hearts.

In a study of hypertrophic cardiomyopathy by Tseng *et al.* [63], the authors performed *in vivo* DTI and strain imaging on human patients. They reported reduced fractional anisotropy and increased fiber disarray, which interestingly correlated with reduction in functional parameters (*e.g.,* fiber and cross fiber strains). The authors then concluded that myofiber disarray in hypertrophic cardiomyopathy is correlated with abnormalities of both passive and active myocardial function [63].

Applications in Small Animals

Mapping the 3D myocardial fiber architecture can be performed routinely and in a relatively short time, at least compared to reconstructing a 3D volume from 2D histological dissection. However, compared to many other MRI techniques, DTI is inherently challenging due to the prolonged scan time and its low SNR (from diffusion encoding *via* signal attenuation). In the small animals (*e.g.,* mouse), the challenges are exacerbated by the small imaging voxel size necessary to provide the anatomical details and, in the case of *in vivo* imaging, constraints imposed by the specific physiology (*e.g.,* high heart rate) of the animals. Nonetheless, state-of-the-art dedicated small animal MRI scanners equipped with high performance gradient sets are capable of producing high-quality DTI fiber maps in several hours. Fig. (**6**) shows 3D heart reconstruction from a mouse (left) and a rat (right), with the two images demonstrating one of the many possibilities to visualize the fiber structure in the heart. The simplest way to visualize the fiber orientation is by using the definition of the helix angle proposed by Streeter [11]. The helix angle can be obtained from each imaging voxel by projecting the principal eigenvector of the diffusion tensor onto the tangential plane and then taking the angle between this projection and the horizontal (or equatorial) axis. Each angle can be assigned a different false color depending on its value as shown in the color bar in Fig. (**6**). An alternative way to visualize fiber structure is by generating "tractography" [66] streamlines connecting principal eigenvectors of neighboring voxels as shown in the right panel of Fig. (**6**).

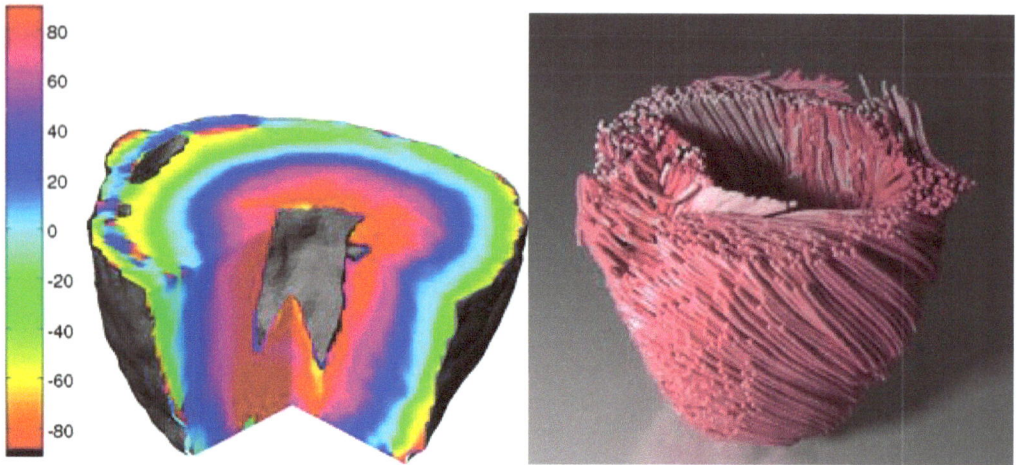

Figure 6: Left: color-coded helix angle map in *mouse* heart (resolution 100 *μm* isotropic, 12 diffusion gradient directions, scan time 9 hours). The color bar on the left represent the helix angle value for each imaging voxel (in degrees). Right: Myocardial fiber mapping using DTI-tractography in a *rat* heart (resolution 150 *μm* isotropic, 12 diffusion gradient directions, scan time 16 hours). Image on right is courtesy of Dr. Grant Gullberg from Berkeley National Lab.

Technical Consideration for *In Vivo* DTI in Small Animals

Despite challenges arising from the beating motion of the heart and the sensitivity of diffusion-encoding to strain-memory effect [36, 68], *in vivo* cardiac DTI has been shown feasible, at least in humans [36, 40-42, 61, 68]. Moreover, although additional challenges exist, the feasibility of *in vivo* cardiac DTI in the mouse has been demonstrated by recent reports, where diffusivity and fiber orientation information is used to characterize cardiac remodeling associated with ischemia and hypertrophy [69, 70].

Besides constraints imposed by scan time, resolution and SNR common to all DTI experiments, *in vivo* cardiac DTI in general face few additional challenges stem from the unique physiology of the heart. First, compared to other organs, the heart undergoes large and relatively periodic beating motion, which can cause pronounced ghosting and streaking artifacts along the phase encoding axis of an MR image. Although these motion artifacts can be greatly reduced by employing gated acquisitions (*e.g.,* dual cardiac and ventilation-gated MRI), the heightened sensitivity of diffusion MRI to motion leaves very little room for uncorrected instrument imperfections, such as errors in gradients calibration or uncompensated eddy current effects.

Second, to reduce the effects of bulk motion while providing sufficient degree of diffusion encoding, *in vivo* cardiac DTI is often performed using diffusion encoding pulses across not one but two cardiac cycles using stimulated echo-based pulse sequences [35]. The contraction and expansion of the myocardium between the diffusion encoding gradient pulses can lead to erroneous estimates of diffusion induced by strain-memory effects [36, 68, 71], since tissue strain alters the relative displacements and phases of spins from which diffusion is encoded. Depending on the nature of the strain, if uncorrected, the effect can be either over- or under-estimation of the diffusion measurements. Because cardiac strain can be separately quantified *via*, for example, phase-contrast methods, one solution is to subtract its effects and produce corrected fiber orientation measurements from *in vivo* cardiac DTI data [67]. A second solution, based on the fact that the strain effects are dependent on the average strain across the cardiac cycle, is to obtain strain-free *in vivo* cardiac DTI measurements by selecting the right timing delay in the cardiac-gated acquisition where the average strain is already zero [70].

Instead of working with myocardial strain, an alternative approach is to employ bipolar diffusion encoding gradient pulses, where spin phases are not left un-refocused across the cardiac cycle, which has been shown effective in minimizing the contribution of strain in *in vivo* cardiac DTI measurements [40, 41]. The main drawback of the approach is the reduced diffusion-weighting b-value that can be achieved using shortened diffusion times. Obviously the practical utility of bipolar gradient pulses depends on whether the required hardware, specifically whether high-performance gradients (in terms of both amplitude and slew rate), exists. Recently, advanced gradient hardware, capable of up to 300 mT/m for human brain imaging and 1500 mT/m in mouse systems as of the current writing, has been introduced. The latter has been credited for the feasibility of *in vivo* cardiac DTI in mice, where the fast heart rate of the animal (300—600 bpm) makes it all but impossible to conduct DTI without extremely large and narrow diffusion encoding pulses. Because the feasibility hinges on the availability of high-performance gradient systems relative to the animal heart rate, and that the performance of a gradient system in turn depends greatly on its size, the feasibility of *in vivo* cardiac DTI in other-size small animals (*e.g.,* rats) remains to be demonstrated.

Besides strain, another physiologic source that can complicate *in vivo* cardiac DTI is perfusion. Perfusion (in this case blood flow in the capillary bed) has long been known for causing additional spin phase dispersion and leading to overestimated diffusion coefficients *via* the so called intravoxel incoherent motion effect [71] in highly vascularized organs such as the liver [72]. Because the capillary flow is faster than the diffusion of water, the flow-mediated perfusion effects can be eliminated from diffusion measurements by employing sufficiently high (b > 200 s/mm^2) diffusion weighting. The perfusion dependence of diffusion MRI has been theorized [73,74] and recently empirically demonstrated *in vivo* [75] and for the perfused heart [76].

Combined, it is clear that the specific physiologies of the beating heart add technical challenges that need to be addressed for performing *in vivo* cardiac DTI. Technological advances have made most the known issues tractable, but there remains room for improvement. Until then, caution is warranted in interpreting *in vivo* cardiac DTI results.

CONCLUSION

Cardiac DTI has gained momentum in recent years. Advances in gradient hardware and motion compensation strategies allowed the acquisition of high quality DTI data in fixed and live, beating hearts. Not only cardiac DTI yields important information about the state of the cardiac microstructure, for example, *via* the fractional anisotropy or mean diffusivity indexes, but also reveals the dynamically changing hierarchical organization of the myocardium as manifested in the fiber and sheet angles. Cardiac DTI can potentially complement other well-established MRI techniques to monitor cardiac disease, such as late-gadolinium enhancement [77] to detect heart infarct, or T$_1$ mapping to detect diffuse fibrosis [78] in the non-ischemic heart failure.

CONFLICT OF INTEREST

This is to certify that the author does not have any conflict of interest.

ACKNOWLEDGEMENT

Edward Hsu is a Principle Investigator. He also acknowledges funding from NIH R01 HL102298.

REFERENCES

[1]   Anderson RH, Ho SY, Sanchez-Quintana D, Redmann K, Lunkenheimer PP. Heuristic problems in defining the three-dimensional arrangement of the ventricular myocytes. The Anatomical Record. 2006 Jun;288A(6):579-86.

[2]   Rijcken J, Bovendeerd PH, Schoofs a J, Van Campen DH, Arts T. Optimization of cardiac fiber orientation for homogeneous fiber strain during ejection. Annals of Biomedical Engineering. 1999;27(3):289-97.

[3]   Roberts DE, Hersh LT, Scher a. M. Influence of cardiac fiber orientation on wavefront voltage, conduction velocity, and tissue resistivity in the dog. Circ. Res. 1979 May 1;44(5):701-12.

[4]   Gilbert SH, Benson AP, Li P, Holden A V. Regional localisation of left ventricular sheet structure: integration with current models of cardiac fibre, sheet and band structure. European Journal of Cardio-Thoracic Surgery. 2007 Aug;32(2):231-49.

[5]   Guccione JM, Costat KD, Mccullocht AD. Finite ventricular element stress analysis of left mechanics in the beating dog heart. J Biomechanics. 1995;28(10).

[6]   Lunkenheimer PP, Redmann K, Kling N, Jiang X, Rothaus K, Cryer CW, *et al*. Three-dimensional architecture of the left ventricular myocardium. Anat. Rec. A. Discov. Mol. Cell Evol. Biol. 2006 Jun;288(6):565-78.

[7]   Torrent-Guasp F, Ballester M, Buckberg GD, Carreras F, Flotats A, Carrió I, *et al*. Spatial orientation of the ventricular muscle band: physiologic contribution and surgical implications. J. Thorac. Cardiovasc. Surg. 2001 Aug;122(2):389-92.

[8]   McCulloch AD. Cardiac biomechanics. In: Bronzino J, editor. The Biomedical Engineering Handbook. 2nd Editio. Boca Raton: CRC Press; 2000. p. 28-46.

[9]   Clayton RH, Bernus O, Cherry EM, Dierckx H, Fenton FH, Mirabella L, *et al*. Models of cardiac tissue electrophysiology: progress, challenges and open questions. Progress in Biophysics and Molecular Biology. Elsevier Ltd; 2011;104(1-3):22-48.

[10]   Clerc L. Directional differences of impulse spread in trabecular muscle from mammalian heart. J Physiol. 1976;255:335-46.

[11]   Streeter DD, Spotnitz HM, Patel DP, Ross J, Sonnenblick EH. Fiber orientation in the canine left ventricle during diastole and systole. Circ. Res. 1969 Mar;24(3):339-47.

[12]   LeGrice IJ, Smaill BH, Chai LZ, Edgar SG, Gavin JB, Hunter PJ. Laminar structure of the heart: ventricular myocyte arrangement and connective tissue architecture in the dog. Am. J. Physiol. 1995 Aug;269(2 Pt 2):H571-82.

[13]   Sachse FB. Computational cardiology: modeling of anatomy, electrophysiology, and mechanics. 1st ed. Goos G, Hartmanis J, van Leeuwen J, editors. New York, US: Springer; 2004. p. 322.

[14]   Hunter PJ, McCulloch AD, Ter Keurs HE. Modelling the mechanical properties of cardiac muscle. Prog. Biophys. Mol. Biol. 1998 Jan;69:289-331.

[15] Schmitt B, Fedarava K, Falkenberg J, Rothaus K, Bodhey NK, Reischauer C, *et al*. Three-dimensional alignment of the aggregated myocytes in the normal and hypertrophic murine heart. J Appl Physiol. 2009;921-7.

[16] Buckberg GD. Architecture must document functional evidence to explain the living rhythm. Eur. J. Cardiothorac. Surg. 2005 Feb;27(2):202-9.

[17] Basser PJ, Mattiello J, LeBihan D. MR diffusion tensor spectroscopy and imaging. Biophys. J. 1994 Jan;66(1):259-67.

[18] Tubbs RS, Gianaris N, Shoja MM, Loukas M, Cohen Gadol AA. "The heart is simply a muscle" and first description of the tetralogy of "fallot". early contributions to cardiac anatomy and pathology by bishop and anatomist niels stensen (1638-1686). Int. J. Cardiol. 2012 Feb 9;154(3):312-5.

[19] Lower R. Tractus de corde. London: Translation by K. Franklin, Oxford University Press, 1932.

[20] Gibson A. Report cix. on the primitive muscle tissue of the human heart. Br. Med. J. 1909 Jan 16;1(2507):148.4-150.

[21] Schäfer EA. A method of recording changes of volume by means of photography and its application to the plethysmographic record of the normal frog heart. J Physiol. 1884 Sep;5(3):[127]-129, 194-1.

[22] Streeter DD, Hanna WT. Engineering mechanics for successive states in canine left ventricular myocardium. Circ. Res. 1973 Dec;33(6):656-64.

[23] Armour JA, Randall WC. Structural basis for cardiac function. Am. J. Physiol. 1970 Jun;218(6):1517-23.

[24] Freeman GL, LeWinter MM, Engler RL, Covell JW. Relationship between myocardial fiber direction and segment shortening in the midwall of the canine left ventricle. Circ. Res. 1985 Jan;56(1):31-9.

[25] Tezuka F, Hart W, Lange PE, Nürnberg JH. Muscle fiber orientation in the development and regression of right ventricular hypertrophy in pigs. Pathology International. Wiley Online Library; 1990;40(6):402-7.

[26] McLean M, Prothero J. Myofiber orientation in the weanling mouse heart. Am. J. Anat. 1991 Dec;192(4):425-41.

[27] Pearlman ES, Weber KT, Janicki JS. Quantitative histology of the hypertrophied human heart. Fed. Proc. 1981 May 15;40(7):2042-7.

[28] Pearlman ES, Weber KT, Janicki JS, Pietra GG, Fishman AP. Muscle fiber orientation and connective tissue content in the hypertrophied human heart. Lab. Invest. 1982 Feb;46(2):158-64.

[29] Lasher R a, Hitchcock RW, Sachse FB. Towards modeling of cardiac micro-structure with catheter-based confocal microscopy : a novel approach for dye delivery and tissue characterization. IEEE. Trans. Med. Imaging. 2009 Aug;28(8):1156-64.

[30] Sowerby AJ, Harries J, Diakun GP, Towns-Andrews E, Bordas J, Stier A. X-ray diffraction studies of whole rat heart during anoxic perfusion. Biochem. Biophys. Res. Commun. 1994 Aug 15;202(3):1244-51.

[31] Yagi N, Shimizu J, Mohri S, Araki J, Nakamura K, Okuyama H, *et al*. X-ray diffraction from a left ventricular wall of rat heart. Biophys. J. 2004 Apr;86(4):2286-94.

[32] Aslanidi O V, Nikolaidou T, Zhao J, Smaill BH, Gilbert SH, Holden A V, *et al*. Application of micro-computed tomography with iodine staining to cardiac imaging,

segmentation, and computational model development. IEEE. Trans. Med. Imaging. 2013 Jan;32(1):8-17.

[33] Vignaud A, Rodriguez I, Ennis DB, DeSilva R, Kellman P, Taylor J, *et al*. Detection of myocardial capillary orientation with intravascular iron-oxide nanoparticles in spin-echo MRI. Magn Reson Med. 2006 Apr;55(4):725-30.

[34] Garrido L, Wedeen VJ, Kwong KK, Spencer UM, Kantor HL. Anisotropy of water diffusion in the myocardium of the rat. Circ. Res. 1994 May 1;74(5):789-93.

[35] Reese TG, Weisskoff RM, Smith RN, Rosen BR, Dinsmore RE, Wedeen VJ. Imaging myocardial fiber architecture *in vivo* with magnetic resonance. Magn Reson Med. 1995 Dec;34(6):786-91.

[36] Hsu EW, Muzikant AL, Matulevicius SA, Penland RC, Henriquez CS. Magnetic resonance myocardial fiber-orientation mapping with direct histological correlation. Am J Physiol Heart Circ Physiol. 1998 May;274(5 Pt 2):H1627-34.

[37] Scollan DF, Holmes A, Winslow R, Forder J, Gilbert SH, Benoist D, *et al*. Histological validation of myocardial microstructure obtained from diffusion tensor magnetic resonance imaging. Am J Physiol Heart Circ Physiol. 1998 Dec;275(6 Pt 2):H2308-H2318.

[38] Holmes A, Scollan DF, Winslow RL. Direct histological validation of diffusion tensor MRI in formaldehyde-fixed myocardium. Magn Reson Med. 2000 Jul;44(1):157-61.

[39] Dou J, Reese TG, Tseng W-YI, Wedeen VJ. Cardiac diffusion MRI without motion effects. Magn Reson Med. 2002 Jul;48(1):105-14.

[40] Gamper U, Boesiger P, Kozerke S. Diffusion imaging of the *in vivo* heart using spin echoes-considerations on bulk motion sensitivity. Magn Reson Med. 2007 Feb;57(2):331-7.

[41] Nielles-Vallespin S, Mekkaoui C, Gatehouse P, Reese TG, Keegan J, Ferreira PF, *et al*. *In vivo* diffusion tensor MRI of the human heart: reproducibility of breath-hold and navigator-based approaches. Magn Reson Med. in press. 2012; DIO 10.1002/mrm.24488.

[42] McGill L-A, Ismail TF, Nielles-Vallespin S, Ferreira P, Scott AD, Roughton M, *et al*. Reproducibility of *in vivo* diffusion tensor cardiovascular magnetic resonance in hypertrophic cardiomyopathy. J Cardiovasc Magn Reson. 2012 Dec 24;14(1):86.

[43] Hahn E. Spin echoes. Physical Review. 1950;80(4):580-94.

[44] Carr H, Purcell E. Effects of diffusion on free precession in nuclear magnetic resonance experiments. Physical Review. 1954;94(3):630-8.

[45] Stejskal EO, Tanner JE. Spin diffusion measurements: spin echoes in the presence of a time-dependent field gradient. J Chemical Physics. 1965;42(1):288.

[46] Le Bihan D, Mangin JF, Poupon C, Clark C a, Pappata S, Molko N, *et al*. Diffusion tensor imaging: concepts and applications. J Magn Reson Imaging. 2001 Apr;13(4):534-46.

[47] Hales PW, Schneider JE, Burton R a B, Wright BJ, Bollensdorff C, Kohl P. Histo-anatomical structure of the living isolated rat heart in two contraction states assessed by diffusion tensor MRI. Progress in Biophysics and Molecular Biology. 2012;110(2-3):319-30.

[48] Tseng W-YI, Wedeen VJ, Reese TG, Smith RN, Halpern EF. Diffusion tensor MRI of myocardial fibers and sheets: correspondence with visible cut-face texture. J Magn Reson Imaging. 2003 Jan;17(1):31-42.

[49] Chen J, Liu W, Zhang H, Lacy L, Yang X, Song S-K, *et al*. Regional ventricular wall thickening reflects changes in cardiac fiber and sheet structure during contraction: quantification with diffusion tensor MRI. Am J Physiol Heart Circ Physiol. 2005 Nov;289(5):H1898-907.

[50] Mekkaoui C, Nielles-vallespin S, Gatehouse PD, Jackowski MP, Firmin DN, Sosnovik DE. Diffusion MRI tractography of the human heart *in vivo* at end-diastole and end-systole. In Proceedings of the 15th Annual SCMR Scientific Sessions, Orlando, FL, USA. 2012;14(Suppl 1):O49.

[51] Jiang Y, Pandya K, Smithies O, Hsu EW. Three-dimensional diffusion tensor microscopy of fixed mouse hearts. Magn Reson Med. 2004 Sep;52(3):453-60.

[52] Dou J, Xia L, Zhang Y, Shou G, Wei Q, Liu F, *et al.* Mechanical analysis of congestive heart failure caused by bundle branch block based on an electromechanical canine heart model. Phys Med Biol. 2009 Jan 21;54(2):353-71.

[53] Jiang Y, Guccione JM, Ratcliffe MB, Hsu EW. Transmural heterogeneity of diffusion anisotropy in the sheep myocardium characterized by MR diffusion tensor imaging. Am J Physiol Heart Circ Physiol. 2007 Oct;293(4):H2377-84.

[54] Rohmer D, Sitek A, Gullberg GT. Reconstruction and visualization of fiber and laminar structure in the normal human heart from *ex vivo* diffusion tensor magnetic resonance imaging. Investigative Radiology. 2007;42(11):777-89.

[55] Healy LJ, Jiang Y, Hsu EW. Quantitative comparison of myocardial fiber structure between mice, rabbit, and sheep using diffusion tensor cardiovascular magnetic resonance. J Cardiovasc Magn Reson. 2011 Jan;13:74.

[56] Chen J, Song S-K, Liu W, McLean M, Allen JS, Tan J, *et al.* Remodeling of cardiac fiber structure after infarction in rats quantified with diffusion tensor MRI. Am J Physiol Heart Circ Physiol. 2003 Sep;285(3):H946-54.

[57] Helm PA, Younes L, Beg MF, Ennis DB, Leclercq C, Faris OP, *et al.* Evidence of structural remodeling in the dyssynchronous failing heart. Circ. Res. 2006 Jan 6;98(1):125-32.

[58] Wu M, Tseng W-YI, Su MM, Liu C, Chiou K-R, Wedeen VJ, *et al.* Diffusion tensor magnetic resonance imaging mapping the fiber architecture remodeling in human myocardium after infarction: correlation with viability and wall motion. Circulation. 2006 Sep 5;114(10):1036-45.

[59] Wu Y, Tse H-F, Wu EX. Diffusion tensor MRI study of myocardium structural remodeling after infarction in porcine model. IEEE Engineering in Medicine and Biology Society. 2006. p. 1069-72.

[60] Wu M-T, Su M-YM, Huang Y-L, Chiou K-R, Yang P, Pan H-B, *et al.* Sequential changes of myocardial microstructure in patients postmyocardial infarction by diffusion-tensor cardiac MR: correlation with left ventricular structure and function. Circ Cardiovasc Imaging. 2009 Jan;2(1):32-40.

[61] Wu EX, Wu Y, Nicholls JM, Wang J, Liao S, Zhu S, *et al.* MR diffusion tensor imaging study of postinfarct myocardium structural remodeling in a porcine model. Magn Reson Med. 2007 Oct;58(4):687-95.

[62] Mekkaoui C, Huang S, Chen HH, Dai G, Reese TG, Kostis WJ, *et al.* Fiber architecture in remodeled myocardium revealed with a quantitative diffusion CMR tractography framework and histological validation. J Cardiovasc Magn Reson. 2012 Jan;14(1):70.

[63] Tseng W-YI, Dou J, Reese TG, Wedeen VJ. Imaging myocardial fiber disarray and intramural strain hypokinesis in hypertrophic cardiomyopathy with MRI. J Magn Reson Imaging. 2006 Jan;23(1):1-8.

[64]   Strijkers GJ, Bouts A, Blankesteijn WM, Peeters THJM, Vilanova A, Van Prooijen MC, *et al*. Diffusion tensor imaging of left ventricular remodeling in response to myocardial infarction in the mouse. NMR in Biomedicine. 2009 Feb;22(2):182-90.

[65]   Natali AJ, Wilson LA, Peckham M, Turner DL, Harrison SM, White E. Different regional effects of voluntary exercise on the mechanical and electrical properties of rat ventricular myocytes. The Journal of Physiology. 2002 May 3;541(3):863-75.

[66]   Sosnovik DE, Wang R, Dai G, Reese TG, Wedeen VJ. Diffusion MR tractography of the heart. J Cardiovasc Magn Reson. 2009 Jan;11:47.

[67]   Reese T, Wedeen V, Weisskoff R. Measuring diffusion in the presence of material strain. J. Magn. Reson. 1996 Sep;112(3):253-8.

[68]   Huang S, Mekkaoui C, Chen HH, Wang R, Ngoy S, Liao R, *et al*. Serial diffusion tensor MRI and tractography of the mouse heart *in vivo*: impact of ischemia on myocardial microstructure. From 2011 SCMR/Euro CMR Joint Scientific Sessions Nice, France. 2011. p. O28.

[69]   Huang S, Polasek M, Chen H, Wang R, Ngoy S, Liao R, *et al*. Molecular and microstructural changes accompanying left ventricular hypertrophy revealed with *in vivo* diffusion tensor MRI (dti) and molecular imaging of the mouse heart. In Proceedings of the 19th Annual Meeting of ISMRM. 2011.

[70]   Tseng WI, Reese TG, Weisskoff RM, Wedeen VJ. Cardiac diffusion tensor MRI *in vivo* without strain correction. Magn Reson Med. 1999;403(May):393-403.

[71]   Le Bihan D, Breton E, Lallemand D, Aubin M-L, Vignaud J, Laval-Jeantet M. Separation of diffusion and perfusion in intravoxel incoherent motion MR imaging. Radiology. 1988;168(2):497-505.

[72]   Luciani A, Vignaud A, Cavet M, Van Nhieu JT, Mallat A, Ruel L, *et al*. Liver cirrhosis : intravoxel incoherent motion MR imaging — pilot study. Radiology. 2008;249(3):891-9.

[73]   Le Bihan D, Breton E, Lallemand D, Aubin M-L, Vignaud J, Laval-Jeantet M. Separation of diffusion and perfusion in intra voxel incoherent motion MR imaging. Radiology. 1988;168:497-505.

[74]   Le Bihan D, Turner R. The capillary network: a link between ivim and classical perfusion. Magn Reson Med. 1992 Sep;27(1):171-8.

[75]   Callot V, Bennett E, Decking UKM, Balaban RS, Wen H. *In vivo* study of microcirculation in canine myocardium using the IVIM method. Magn Reson Med. 2003 Sep;50(3):531-40.

[76]   Abdullah O, Gomez AD, Merchant S, Stedham O, Heidinger M, Poelzing S, *et al*. Effects of perfusion on cardiac MR diffusion measurements. Proceedings of the 21st Annual Meeting of ISMRM. Salt Lake City; 2012.

[77]   Kim RJJ, Fieno DSS, Parrish TBB, Harris K, Chen E, Simonetti O, *et al*. Relationship of MRI delayed contrast enhancement to irreversible injury, infarct age, and contractile function. Circulation. 1999;1992-2002.

[78]   Messroghli D, Nordmeyer S, Dietrich T, Dirsch O, Kaschina E, Savvatis K, *et al*. Assessment of diffuse myocardial fibrosis in rats using small animal look-locker inversion recovery (SALLI) T_1 mapping. Circulation Cardiovascular Imaging. 2011 Sep 14;4(6):636-40.

List of Abbreviations

AHA	=	American Heart Association
ACCF	=	The American College of Cardiology Foundation
ACR	=	American College of Radiology
AF	=	Atrial Fibrillation
AIF	=	Arterial input function
AMI	=	Acute myocardial infarction
APU	=	Adaptive phase-unwrapping
ARVC	=	Arrhythmogenic Right Ventricular Cardiomyopathy
AS-CMR	=	Adenosine stress cardiovascular magnetic resonance (AS-CMR) imaging
ASNC	=	American Society of Nuclear Radiology
ATP	=	Adenosine Triphosphate
BSA	=	Body Surface Area
BLAST	=	Broad-use Linear Acquisition Speed-up Technique
CABG	=	Coronary Artery Bypass Graft Surgery
CAD	=	Coronary artery disease
CE-MRA	=	Contrast enhanced magnetic resonance angiography
CF	=	Circumferential Fibers
CMR	=	Cardiovascular Magnetic Resonance

CMRA   = Coronary magnetic resonance angiography

CRT   = Cardiac Resynchronisation Therapy

CS   = Compressed Sensing

CSI   = Chemical Shift Imaging

CTCA   = Computer Tomography Coronary Angiography

CT-PET   = Computer Tomography Positron Emission Tomography

DCM   = Dilated Cardiomyopathy

DCE-MRI   = Dynamic Contrast Enhanced MRI

DENSE   = Displacement Encoding with Stimulated Echoes

DHE   = Delayed hyper-enhanced

DM   = Diabetes Mellitus

DSCMR   = Dobutamine stress CMR

DSE   = Dobutamine stress echocardiography

DT-MRI   = Diffusion Tensor MRI

Dy   = Dysprosium

ECV   = Extra Cellular Volume

ECG   = Electrocardiogram

EDV   = End Diastolic Volume

EF   = Ejection Fraction

ESV   = End Systolic Volume

FA   = Fractional Anisotropy

FDG   = Fluoro-Deoxy-Glucose

FLASH   = Fast Low Angle Shot

GFR   = Glomerulus Filtration Rate

GK   = Guanylate kinase

GRAPPA   = Generalized Auto-calibrating Partially Parallel Acquisitions

HARP   = Harmonic Phase Imaging

HCM   = Hypertrophic Cardiomyopathy

HE   = Hepatic Encephalopathy

HF   = Heart Failure

HFA   = Heart Failure Association

ICD   = Implantable cardioverter defibrillators

IHD   = Ischemic Heart Disease

IVC   = Inferior Vena Cava

LCA   = Left Coronary Artery

LDD   = Low Dose Dobutamine

LGE   = Late Gadolinium Enhancement

LPA   = Left Pulmonary Artery

LVH   = Left Ventricular Hypertrophy

LV   = Left Ventricle

LW	=	Left ventricular free wall
MD	=	Mean Diffusivity
MDCT	=	Multi detector computed tomography
MEMRI	=	Manganese Enhanced MRI
MI	=	Myocardial Infarction
MnDPDP	=	Manganese dipyridoxyl diphosphate
MPA	=	Main Pulmonary Artery
MRA	=	Magnetic Resonance Angiography
MRI	=	Magnetic Resonance Imaging
MRS	=	Magnetic Resonance Spectroscopy
MVO	=	Microvascular Obstruction
NASCI	=	North American Society for Cardiac Imaging
NCX	=	Sodium-Calcium Exchanger
NMR	=	Nuclear Magnetic Resonance
NSF	=	Nephrogenic Systemic Fibrosis
PAVR	=	Partial Anomalous Venous Return
PC	=	Phase Contrast
PCA	=	Principle Component Analysis
PCr	=	Phosphocreatine
PDE	=	Phosphomonoester

PET   = Positron Emission Tomography

PFC   = Perfluorocarbon

PMCA   = Plasma membrane calcium pump ATPase

PPCM   = Peripartum cardiomyopathy

PSF   = Point Spread Function

PV   = Pulmonary Valve

RA   = Right Atrium

RF   = Radio Frequency

RHF   = Right Handed Fibers

PFG   = Pulsed-Field Gradient

RMS   = Root Mean Square

ROC   = Receiver-Operating Curve

RPA   = Right Pulmonary Artery

RV   = Right Ventricle

RyR   = Ryanoid receptors

SCAI   = Society for Cardiovascular Angiography and Interventions

SCCT   = Society of Cardiovascular Computed Tomography

SCMR   = Society for Cardiovascular Magnetic Resonance

SENC   = Strain Encoded

SENSE   = SENSitivity Encoding

SIR   =   Society of Interventional Radiology

SLOOP   =   Spectral localisation with optimum point spread function

SNR   =   Signal-to-Noise Ration

SPECT   =   Single photon emission computed tomography

SPIO   =   Superparamagnetic Iron Oxide

SR   =   Sarcoplasmatic reticulum

SSFP   =   Steady State at Free Precession

STIR   =   Short Inversion Recovery Time

SVC   =   Superior Vena Cava

TAC   =   Transverse Aortic Contraction

TE   =   Echo Time

TL   =   True Lumen

Tm   =   Thulium

ToF   =   3D Time-of-Flight

TPSF   =   Transform Point Spread Function

TR   =   Repetition Time

VENC   =   Velocity Encoding Sensitivity

VNR   =   Velocity-to-Noise-Ratio

VSD   =   Ventricular Septal Defect

μCT   =   Micro-CT

1D   = One Dimensional

2D   = Two Dimensional

3D   = Three Dimensional

4D   = Four Dimensional

5F-BAPTA   = 1,2-bis(2-amino-5-fluorophenoxy)ethane-N,N,N',N'-tetraacetic acid

2,3-DPG   = 2,3-diphosphoglycerate

INDEX

A

H

I

www.ingramcontent.com/pod-product-compliance
Lightning Source LLC
Chambersburg PA
CBHW050823220326
41598CB00006B/302